Molecular Mechanisms of Neurotransmitter Release

For other titles published in this series, go to
www.springer.com
click on the series discipline: Biomedical Sciences
click on the heading "Series" or search for series name
click on the name of the series: Contemporary Neuroscience

Molecular Mechanisms of Neurotransmitter Release

Zhao-Wen Wang

Department of Neuroscience, University of Connecticut Health Center,
Farmington, CT, USA

Editor

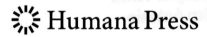 Humana Press

Editor:
Zhao-Wen Wang, Ph.D.
Department of Neuroscience
University of Connecticut Health Center
263 Farmington Avenue
Farmington, CT
USA
zwwang@uchc.edu

ISBN: 978-1-934115-38-1   e-ISBN: 978-1-59745-481-0
DOI:10.1007/978-1-59745-481-0

Library of Congress Control Number: 2008925596

Cover caption: Diagram illustrating two modes of synaptic vesicle exocytosis: full-collapse fusion and kiss-and-run. In full-collapse fusion, neurotransmitters are released from synaptic vesicles through the sequential steps of docking, priming, and fusion. Protein and lipid components of synaptic vesicles are then retrieved through clathrin-mediated endocytosis. The endocytosed vesicle may become part of an endosome, from which new synaptic vesicles are generated. In kiss-and-run, neurotransmitters are released through a transient fusion pore formed between the vesicle membrane and the plasma membrane. Drawing by Kaijie J. Wang.

Printed on acid-free paper

9 8 7 6 5 4 3 2 1

springer.com

Preface

Neurons in the nervous system organize into complex networks and their functions are precisely controlled. The most important means for neurons to communicate with each other is transmission through chemical synapses, where the release of neurotransmitters by the presynaptic nerve terminal of one neuron influences the function of a second neuron. Since the discovery of chemical neurotransmission by Otto Loewi in the 1920s, great progress has been made in our understanding of molecular mechanisms of neurotransmitter release. The last decade has seen an explosion of knowledge in this field. The aim of *Molecular Mechanisms of Neurotransmitter Release* is to provide up-to-date, in-depth coverage of essentially all major molecular mechanisms of neurotransmitter release. The contributors have made great efforts to write concisely but with sufficient background information, and to use figures/diagrams to present clearly key concepts or experiments. It is hoped that this book may serve as a learning tool for neuroscience students, a solid reference for neuroscientists, and a source of knowledge for people who have a general interest in neuroscience.

I was fortunate to be able to gather contributions from a group of outstanding scientists. I thank them for their efforts. In particular, I want to thank Dr. Erik Jorgensen who offered valuable suggestions about the book in addition to contributing an excellent chapter. I thank US National Science Foundation and National Institute of Health for their supports. I also thank my son Kaijie Wang for the drawing used on the book cover. Finally, I thank Humana Press for the opportunity of editing this book. Patrick Marton, a managing editor of the publisher, was especially helpful.

Zhao-Wen Wang

Contents

Contributors

Allen W. Chan
Genetics and Development Division, Toronto Western Research Institute,
Toronto, Ontario, Canada

Bojun Chen
Department of Neuroscience, University of Connecticut Health Center,
Farmington, CT, USA

Matthew Frerking
Neurological Sciences Institute, Oregon Health and Science University,
Beaverton, OR, USA

Kensuke Futai
RIKEN-MIT Neuroscience Research Center, Picower Institute
for Learning and Memory, Department of Brain and Cognitive Sciences,
Massachusetts Institute of Technology, Cambridge, MA, USA

Qian Ge
Department of Neuroscience, University of Connecticut Health Center,
Farmington, CT, USA

Yasunori Hayashi
RIKEN-MIT Neuroscience Research Center, Picower Institute for Learning
and Memory, Department of Brain and Cognitive Sciences, Massachusetts
Institute of Technology, Cambridge, MA, USA

Liming He
National Institute of Neurological Disorders and Stroke, National Institutes
of Health, Bethesda, MD, USA

Erik M. Jorgensen
Department of Biology and Howard Hughes Medical Institute, University
of Utah, Salt Lake City, UT, USA

Carin Loewen
Department of Biomedical Sciences, Program in Molecular, Cellular
and Integrative Neuroscience, Colorado State University, Fort Collins,
CO, USA

Benjamin D. McNeil
National Institute of Neurological Disorders and Stroke, National Institutes
of Health, Bethesda, Maryland, USA

Frederic A. Meunier
Queensland Brain Institute and School of Biomedical Sciences,
University of Queensland, St. Lucia, Queensland, Australia

Toshihisa Ohtsuka
Department of Clinical and Molecular Pathology, Graduate School
of Medicine/Faculty of Medicine, University of Toyama, Sugitani,
Toyama, Japan

Shona L. Osborne
Queensland Brain Institute and School of Biomedical Sciences,
University of Queensland, St. Lucia, Queensland, Australia

Mark T. Palfreyman
Department of Biology and Howard Hughes Medical Institute,
University of Utah, Salt Lake City, UT, USA

Richard J. Reimer
Department of Neurology and Neurological Sciences and Graduate Program
in Neuroscience, Stanford University School of Medicine, Stanford,
CA, USA

Noreen Reist
Department of Biomedical Sciences, Program in Molecular, Cellular
and Integrative Neuroscience, Colorado State University, Fort Collins,
CO, USA

Janet E. Richmond
Biological Sciences Department, University of Illinois at Chicago,
Chicago, IL, USA

Michael T. Roberts
Oregon Hearing Research Center/Vollum Institute, Oregon Health
and Science University, Portland, OR, USA

Zu-Hang Sheng
Synaptic Function Section, National Institute of Neurological Disorders
and Stroke, National Institutes of Health, Bethesda, Maryland, USA

Liesbet Smitz
VIB Department of Developmental Genetics, K.U. Leuven
Center for Human Genetics, Leuven, Belgium

Elise F. Stanley
Genetics and Development Division, Toronto Western Research Institute,
Toronto, Ontario, Canada

Yoshimi Takai
Division of Molecular and Cellular Biology, Department of Biochemistry and
Molecular Biology, Kobe University Graduate School of Medicine/Faculty of
Medicine, Kusunoki-cho, Chuo-ku, Kobe, Japan

Hiroaki Tani
Department of Neurology and Neurological Sciences and Graduate Program
in Neuroscience, Stanford University School of Medicine, Stanford,
CA, USA

Laurence O. Trussell
Oregon Hearing Research Center/Vollum Institute, Oregon Health
and Science University, Portland, OR, USA

Patrik Verstreken
VIB Department of Developmental Genetics, K.U. Leuven Center
for Human Genetics, Leuven, Belgium

Zhao-Wen Wang
Department of Neuroscience, University of Connecticut Health Center,
Farmington, CT, USA

Robby M. Weimer
Genentech, South San Francisco, CA, USA

Joyce Wondolowski
Neurological Sciences Institute, Oregon Health and Science University,
Beaverton, OR, USA

Ling-Gang Wu
National Institute of Neurological Disorders and Stroke, National Institutes
of Health, Bethesda, Maryland, USA

Pingyong Xu
National Laboratory of Biomacromolecules, Institute of Biophysics,
Chinese Academy of Sciences Beijing 100101, China; and College of Life
Science and Technology, Huazhong University of Science and Technology,
Wuhan, China

Tao Xu
National Laboratory of Biomacromolecules, Institute of Biophysics, Chinese
Academy of Sciences Beijing 100101, China; and College of Life Science
and Technology, Huazhong University of Science and Technology, Wuhan, China

Kimberly A. Zaia
Department of Neurology and Neurological Sciences and Graduate Program
in Neuroscience, Stanford University School of Medicine, Stanford,
CA, USA

R. Grace Zhai
Department of Molecular and Cellular Pharmacology, Leonard M. Miller
School of Medicine, University of Miami, Miami, FL, USA

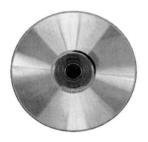

COMPANION CD

Illustrations listed here may be found on the Companion CD attached to the inside back cover. Figures available in color on the CD are indicated by boldface. See the README file on the CD for further details. The CD is compatible with both Mac and PC operating systems.

Chapter 1
The Architecture of the Presynaptic Release Site

R. Grace Zhai

Contents

Abstract The architecture of the presynaptic release site is exquisitely designed to facilitate the regulated tethering, docking, and fusing of synaptic vesicles with the plasma membrane. With the identification of some of the building blocks, we are beginning to understand the morphologic and functional properties of the synapse. Presynaptic release sites consist of a plasma membrane, a cytomatrix, and dense projections. These three components are morphologically distinct, yet they are intimately connected with each other and the postsynaptic nerve terminal, ensuring the fidelity of synaptic vesicle tethering, docking and fusion, as well as signal detection. Although the morphology of active zones and the molecular composition vary among species, tissues and cells, the architectural design of the release sites is likely conserved.

Keywords Ribbon synapses, T-bar, dense projections, cytomatrix, neuromuscular junction.

R. Grace Zhai
Department of Molecular and Cellular Pharmacology, Leonard M. Miller School of Medicine,
University of Miami, Miami, FL 33136
e-mail: gzhai@med.miami.edu

Z.-W. Wang (ed.) *Molecular Mechanisms of Neurotransmitter Release,*
© Humana Press 2008 a part of Springer Science+Business Media, LLC

In 1897 Sir Charles Sherrington (1) introduced the term *synapse* to explain the delay he observed in the spinal reflex at the junction between neurons, as he "felt the need of some name to call the junction between nerve-cell and nerve-cell, because the place of junction now entered physiology as carrying functional importance" (2). The notion of synapse contributed to the birth of the concept of chemical transmission, at first with adrenalin (3) and secondly with acetylcholine (ACh) (4,5). At the time, the concept of a synapse was purely physiologic, as no morphologic data were available to determine whether the connection was continuous or not. It was not until the mid-1940s that René Couteaux, a great French histologist, first morphologically identified synapses (6). By means of Janus Green B dye, Couteaux (7,8) revealed the membranous subneural apparatus related to the synaptic gutter. This discovery gave a morphologic basis to the physiologic term and defined synapses as specialized cell-cell contacts where signals are transduced from a neuron to its target cell.

In chemical synapses, signal transduction is achieved by converting an electrical signal into a chemical signal that diffuses between cells. This signal conversion occurs primarily at active zones—highly specialized sites on the presynaptic nerve terminal. The term *active zone* was coined in 1970 by Couteaux and Pecot-Dechavassine (9) during their ultrastructural studies of partially contracted frog muscles, where they observed that profiles of open synaptic vesicles occurred immediately adjacent to the presynaptic dense bands, and consequently they designated these dense bands "*les zones actives.*" Subsequently, similar observations were made in other types of synapses.

Ultrastructural studies of synapses in different organisms have revealed the following conserved morphologic features among active zones, regardless of their size, location, or types of neurons and their targets. First, the plasma membrane of the active zone appears to be electron-dense, suggesting its proteinaceous nature. Second, synaptic vesicles cluster, tether, and fuse at the active zone (9,10). Third, the active zone is closely and precisely aligned with a postsynaptic density (PSD) area, such that the active zone spans the same width as the PSD, and the extracellular space between the two membranes (synaptic cleft) is as narrow as 30 nm (11). The latter two morphologic characteristics suggest that active zones function as sites of synaptic vesicle exocytosis and neurotransmitter release. Over the last three decades these hypotheses have been supported by many neuroscientists through studies of synaptic vesicle exocytosis and postsynaptic neurotransmitter receptor function. It is important to note that more recent studies have suggested that neuronal exocytosis can occur at sites that are distant from active zones—the so-called ectopic release sites (12), indicating that cellular communication in the nervous system may be more versatile and dynamic than we have already known.

This chapter discusses the structural organization of active zones as the primary release sites in different types of synapses found in a variety of organisms, summarizes recent advances in the molecular characterization of the assembly of active zones, proposes that all active zones are organized according to the same pattern, and concludes by discussing the possible structural bases of ectopic release.

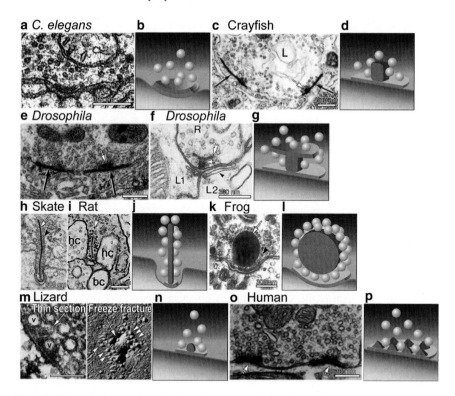

Fig. 1.1 Electron micrographs and schematic representations of the active zone structures found in different synapses of various organisms. Electron micrographs of synapses and schematic diagrams of the corresponding active zones are shown. (**a,b**) A *C. elegans* neuromuscular junction (NMJ) terminal (84) with a plaque-like active zone projection (white arrow). (**c,d**) A crayfish NMJ terminal (97) with a dense projection (white arrow). Active zones are indicated by black arrows. L: large diameter axon terminal. (**e**) A *Drosophila* NMJ terminal (115) with a dense projection called a T-bar (white arrow). Active zones are indicated by black arrows. (**f**) A *Drosophila* tetrad synapse between photoreceptor (R) and lamina monopolar cells (L1 and L2) (85). Dense projections (T-bar) consist of a platform (double arrowhead) and a pedestal (white arrow). Arrowhead indicates the postsynaptic cisternae. (**g**) Schematic diagram of a T-bar. (**h**) An electroreceptor in skate (82) with a long ribbon-like dense projection (arrow) and a halo of synaptic vesicles (arrowhead). (**i**) A triadic photoreceptor ribbon synapse between rod photoreceptor and horizontal cell (hc) and a rod bipolar cell (bc) in a rat (92). (**j**) Schematic diagram of a ribbon synapse. (**k,l**) A saccular hair cell in frog (82) with a spherical dense projection (arrow) and attached vesicles (arrowhead). (**m**) A thin section and a freeze fracture image of a lizard NMJ terminal (22). The dense projection is marked by arrows in both images, and the intramembraneous particles are marked by arrowheads. Vesicles docked at the active zone are marked by 'v'. (**n**) Schematic diagram of a NMJ. (**o**) An excitatory synaptic terminal in human hippocampus (78) with two active zones (arrows). (**p**) Schematic diagram of a human central nervous system (CNS) active zone

The Structure of Active Zones

Morphologically, active zones are defined as sites of synaptic vesicle docking and fusion, and physiologically they are defined as sites of neurotransmitter release. Based on these definitions, the active zone can be dissected into three morphologically and functionally distinct components: (1) the plasma membrane juxtaposed to the PSD where synaptic vesicle fusion occurs, (2) the cytomatrix immediately internal to the plasma membrane where synaptic vesicles dock, and (3) the electron-dense projections extending from the cytomatrix into the cytoplasm on which synaptic vesicles are tethered. All active zones have these three components although they vary in appearance, especially in the size and shape of dense projections. Figure 1.1 illustrates the ultrastructure of active zones found in nine different types of synapse, as well as the schematic representation of the three components in each type of active zone. Below, I discuss the molecular and functional properties of each component of the active zone.

The Plasma Membrane of the Active Zone

Besides separating the cytosol from the extracellular environment, the plasma membrane of the active zone has two "gates" essential for neurotransmission, one for Ca^{2+} entry, which is the voltage-gated Ca^{2+} channel, and the other for neurotransmitter exit, which is the synaptic vesicle fusion site. These two gates are thought to be in close proximity with each other based on several observations. First, the time delay between Ca^{2+} entry and synaptic vesicle fusion is only 0.2 ms (13,14). Second, theoretical analyses of calcium diffusion dynamics and quantal secretion have shown that the probability of secretion of a synaptic vesicle decreases threefold with the doubling of the distance between the calcium channel and the synaptic vesicle from 25 to 50 nm (15). It is thus likely that in most synapses the space between calcium channels and docked synaptic vesicles at the active zone is less than 50 nm (14,16). Numerous immunohistochemical studies have demonstrated the localization of calcium channels near the active zone (17–19); however, the organization and arrangement of calcium channels at active zones are best suggested by freeze-fracture studies on frog, lizard, and mammalian neuromuscular junctions (NMJs) (20–22). On freeze-fracture replicas of NMJ boutons, double rows of prominent intramembranous particles of 10 to 12 nm in diameter can be seen with occasional synaptic vesicles clustered closely beside them (Figs. 1.1M and 1.2C). These rows of particles are in exact register with postsynaptic folds in the underlying muscle (21) and are postulated to be voltage-gated calcium channels (18,23,24). The most direct evidence supporting this view comes from atomic force microscopy on the large calyciform synapse of the chick ciliary ganglion, showing a row-like arrangement of the immunolabeled calcium channels (25).

If the calcium channels are organized in orderly arrays at active zones, one would expect the other gates—the synaptic vesicle fusion sites—to be organized in a corresponding manner. The vesicle fusion sites are specialized to allow the lipid bilayers of synaptic vesicles and active zone plasma membrane to come together and form a hydrophilic fusion pore. The SNARE (soluble *N*-ethylmaleimide–sensitive factor attachment receptor) complex has been thought to be the driving force for bringing the membranes together, facilitating lipid bilayer mixing and subsequent

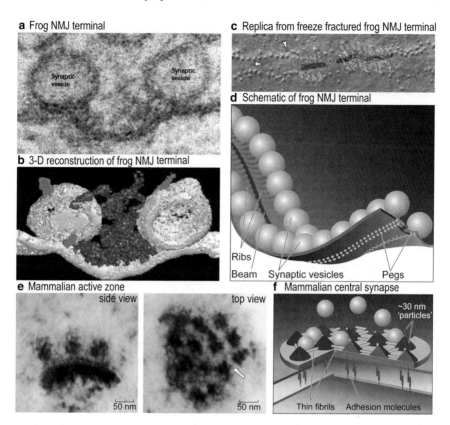

Fig. 1.2 Models of the active zone structure in frog NMJ and mammalian CNS synapses. (A–D) The active zone structure in frog NMJs (58). (E,F): The active zone structure in mammalian CNS synapses (59). (**a**) Transmission electron microscopy (TEM) micrograph of frog NMJ, where synaptic vesicles are docked to the plasma membrane through dense projections. (**b**) A three-dimensional reconstructed and surface-rendered view of the active zone material and docked vesicles. (**c**) A replica from a freeze-fractured frog NMJ showing a series of particles/macromolecules along each ridge with surface-rendered rib and beam assemblies. Sites of vesicle fusion can be seen as dimples next to the particles (arrowheads). (**d**) Schematic diagram of the arrangement of ribs, beams, and synaptic vesicles at frog NMJs. (**e**) TEM micrographs of purified active zones from mammalian CNS in side view and top view. Thin fibrils can be seen (arrow in top view). (**f**) Schematic diagram of the active zone structure of mammalian central synapses

membrane fusion (26,27). The t-SNAREs (target-SNAREs) syntaxin and SNAP-25 (synaptosome-associated protein of 25 kDa) have been localized to the presynaptic plasma membrane, although their distribution is not restricted to the active zone and the precise positioning and organization of t-SNAREs at the active zone are not clear (28–30). Biochemical analyses have demonstrated direct interactions between the t-SNAREs and calcium channels (31–34). This might be the mechanism for the close positioning of the fusion machinery and calcium channels required for Ca^{2+}-dependent exocytosis. Interestingly, a study in PC12 cells, a neurosecretory cell line, has shown that syntaxin and SNAP-25 form cholesterol-dependent clusters in the plasma membrane, and these clusters seem to define sites at which secretory vesicles dock and fuse with high preference. Cholesterol removal causes dispersion of the clusters and subsequent inhibition of exocytosis (35). This study provides a clue for the potential role of lipids in active zone plasma membrane specification.

Other important components of the plasma membrane are the adhesion molecules, which most likely mediate the precise alignment of the active zone with the PSD. Several classes of adhesion molecules have been shown to be present at the active zone: cadherins (36,37), protocadherins (38), nectins (39,40), neural cell adhesion molecule (NCAM) (41), fasciclin II (42), Aplysia cell adhesion molecule (apCAM) (43), Down Syndrome cell adhesion molecule (DsCAM) (44), syndecans (45), L1/neuroglian (46), integrins (47), neurexins (48), and sidekicks (49,50). All adhesion molecules share common protein motifs: an extracellular domain that mediates binding with the post- or presynaptic counterparts or extracellular matrix, a single-pass transmembrane domain or membrane anchor, and often an intracellular domain that binds to the cytoskeleton or intracellular scaffolding proteins (51,52). All of these adhesion molecules except neurexin, which is expressed presynaptically and binds its postsynaptic receptor neuroligin (49), are expressed in both pre- and postsynaptic terminals, and mediate adhesion through homophilic interactions. Adhesion molecules at the active zone are more than just "glue." They also mediate signaling within and between nerve terminals and modulate neurotransmission. Numerous reviews have commented on the detailed mechanisms of these molecules in synapse adhesion and regulation (40,53–55).

In summary, the primary function of the plasma membrane at the active zone during neurotransmitter release is to mediate the fusion of synaptic vesicles upon calcium entry. This is achieved by an array-like organization of calcium channels and localization of the fusion machinery at the membrane.

The Cytomatrix Underlying the Plasma Membrane of the Active Zone

When viewed by electron microscopy, the cytomatrix of the active zone is electron-dense and displays a "web"-like pattern, which was first noticed by Bloom and Aghajanian (56) and subsequently by Pfenninger and colleagues (57). Recently, elegant studies have provided the first three-dimensional views of the cytomatrix at the active zone of the frog NMJ and the mammalian central nervous system (CNS) synapse. By means of electron microscope tomography, Harlow and colleagues (58) revealed a striking array-like structure at the frog NMJ consisting of "beams" and "ribs" that connect docked synaptic vesicles with putative calcium channels (Fig. 1.2A-D). The beams run along the midline of the presynaptic ridge, and the ribs extend laterally from the beams and connect the synaptic vesicles near the vesicle-plasma membrane interface. In addition, the ribs are connected to the intramembrane macromolecules (pegs in Fig. 1.2D) resembling the putative calcium channels seen in freeze-fracture studies (Figs. 1.1M and 1.2C). With this organization, each docked vesicle is perfectly aligned with at least one calcium channel, which would allow high fidelity of coupling between them.

A picture of the mammalian CNS synapse was revealed by Phillips and colleagues (59). In this study, the authors purified a presynaptic particle web consisting of pyramidally shaped particles (~30 nm in dimension) interconnected by fibrils (Fig. 1.2E). The particles are evenly spaced by the fibrils at approximately 50- to 100-nm intervals, forming a web of 50- to 100-nm slots for synaptic vesicles to dock and fuse (Fig. 1.2F).

The electron-dense nature of the cytomatrix underlying the plasma membrane suggests that many proteins are localized there and that the cytomatrix at the active zone is important in regulating vesicle docking and fusion. In searching for the building blocks of this specialized cytomatrix, a number of protein components have been identified. Based on their function or putative function, proteins identified in the active zone cytomatrix can be classified into three categories. First are the classical cytoskeletal proteins corresponding to actin, tubulin, myosin, spectrin α chain and β chain, and β-catenin (59–61). They are the fundamental elements of the framework of active zone cytomatrix. Second are the scaffold proteins, including SAP90/PSD95/Dlg, SAP97, and CASK/LIN-2 (62–65). These proteins are not restricted to active zones. They also participate in clustering of postsynaptic receptors and are involved in the organization of a variety of cell junctions (66–68). If the cytoskeleton proteins form a grid-like structure at the active zone, these scaffolding proteins probably link the ion channels and the fusion machinery onto the grid to ensure proper active zone function. For example, CASK interacts with β-neurexin, syndecan 2, calcium channels, the cytosolic protein Veli/LIN-7, and the Munc18/n-Sec1–interacting protein Mint1 (64,69–71). Third are the active zone-specific proteins including RIM1, Munc13/UNC-13, Bassoon, Piccolo/Aczonin, and CAST/ERCs (72–77). Their active zone-specific localization and multidomain structure allow them to form large protein complexes, and participate in modulating synaptic vesicle docking, priming, and fusion as well as in initiating assembly of the active zone structure. Physiologic studies indicate that some of these proteins are involved in vesicle priming as well as synaptic transmission regulation (78–80).

In summary, the primary function of the cytomatrix at the active zone is to mediate docking of synaptic vesicles. The cytoskeletal and scaffolding proteins form a web-like structure consisting of slots for synaptic vesicle docking, and components of the cytomatrix regulate vesicle priming and fusion.

Synaptic Ribbons: The Electron-Dense Projections Extending from the Cytomatrix of the Active Zone

Some active zones have very prominent electron-dense projections extending from the cytomatrix into the cytoplasm. They were first described and characterized in vertebrate sensory synapses involved in vision, hearing, and balance (81–83). These dense projections, or synaptic ribbons, are ribbon-like or spherical, extend 0.5 to 1 μm into the cytoplasm, and always have a "halo" of synaptic vesicles tethered to their surface (Fig. 1.1H–L) (82). Due to their remarkable appearance, it has been thought that ribbon synapses are different from all other synapses, and the synaptic ribbons are exclusive to ribbon synapses in order to mediate the graded and sustained neurotransmitter release of these synapses (82,83). However, through careful examination and comparison of different types of synapses, a hypothesis emerges that electron-dense projections are not unique to ribbon synapses but rather are an integral part of the active zone, have an evolutionarily conserved structure, and function to tether synaptic vesicles at active zones.

Morphologically, dense projections have been observed in different types of synapses of different species. In *Caenorhabditis elegans*, dense projections at the NMJ appear as plaques (Fig. 1.1A) (84). In *Drosophila*, T-shaped dense projections can be seen at NMJs, tetrad synapses of the visual system (Fig. 1.1E–G), and CNS synapses (85,86). In crayfish, dense projections at the NMJ appear cylindrical (Fig. 1.1C,D) (87). In vertebrates, dense projections at the NMJ have been described for frog, lizard, and mammals (Fig. 1.1M,N) (10,20,22). Dense projections in mammalian CNS synapses were noted in electron microscopy (EM) studies as early as the 1960s, and recently have been purified and visualized in great detail (Fig. 1.2E) (56,59). Based on the size of dense projections, we can classify active zones into two types: those with prominent dense projections, including invertebrate synapses with T-bars and vertebrate ribbon synapses, and those with less prominent dense projections, including vertebrate NMJs and CNS synapses. Dense projections in the latter type of active zones are not very prominent and project less than 100 nm into the cytoplasm. As such, they are often considered to be part of the cytomatrix at the active zone (11,78,88).

Physiologically, numerous studies have demonstrated the tethering function of dense projections. At vertebrate sensory synapses, the motor protein KIF3A, which is a component of ribbons, likely mediates the tethering of synaptic vesicles (89). At frog NMJs, synaptic vesicles are tethered through ribs to the beams corresponding to the dense projections, as revealed by tomographic analyses (58). In crayfish and *Drosophila*, synaptic vesicles cluster around dense body (Fig. 1.1C,D) or T-bars (Fig. 1.1E–G), although the mechanism of tethering is not known. Recently, dense projections of mammalian CNS active zones have been biochemically purified and molecularly characterized (59). These dense projections are ~30 nm in size and pyramid-like in appearance (Figs. 1.1P and 1.2E), and contain synaptic vesicle binding proteins such as synapsin and RIM (59,76,90). These pyramid-like dense projections are thought to tether and cluster synaptic vesicles to the active zone.

Despite the proposed function of tethering synaptic vesicles, dense projections do not seem to be essential for neurotransmitter release, as suggested by a series of knockout studies. For example, Bassoon is a key component of the photoreceptor ribbon synapse in mammals (91). In the retina of homozygous *bassoon* mutant mouse, the number of ribbons is greatly decreased, and the remaining ones are freely floating in the cytoplasm with synaptic vesicles attached to them. Electroretinograms from the photoreceptors show that neurotransmission is maintained at low-intensity light stimulation, but dramatically reduced at high-intensity light stimulation (92). This suggests that synaptic vesicles can fuse but cannot maintain sustained high-rate exocytosis without the ribbon anchored to the plasma membrane. In *Drosophila*, a coiled-coil domain protein Bruchpilot (BRP) was recently identified and found to be required for dense projection (T-bar) assembly. At *brp* mutant active zones, T-bars are entirely lost, and postsynaptic receptor fields identified by the glutamate receptor are enlarged. Consistent with these morphological changes, evoked excitatory junctional current (eEJC) amplitudes were greatly decreased, whereas the amplitude of miniature excitatory junctional currents (mEJCs) resulting from spontaneous release of single synaptic vesicles was increased (93). This study suggests that dense projections facilitate synchronized transmitter release but are not required for synaptic vesicle fusion. In mice, knockout studies of synapsin (a component of the pyramid-like dense projections), suggest that it may not be required for the vesicle fusion step, but rather for the synapsin-dependent cluster of vesicles. This clustering is apparently required to sustain neurotransmitter release in response to high levels of neuronal activity (90).

If the function of dense projections was to tether synaptic vesicles, what would be the physiologic advantage of varying their size and shape? One possibility is that larger dense projections greatly increase the number of synaptic vesicles tethered at the active zone and therefore increase the size of the readily releasable pool. This possibility is favored by observations at ribbon synapses. For example, only 124 vesicles are attached to the active zone but ~400 vesicles are attached to the ribbon at the ribbon synapse of frog saccular hair cells (Fig. 1.1K), and all the vesicles attached to the ribbon may be released upon strong stimulation (94–96). Therefore, these large dense projections allow an increase in the size of the readily releasable pool without necessitating an increase of the active zone size. This feature is particularly important in sensory synapses, where sustained release upon continuous stimulation requires a huge readily releasable pool and a large synaptic vesicle replenishment capacity, but the confined space representation of individual sensory neurons in the visual or auditory field restricts the size of each terminal. In contrast, dense projections are relatively small at many NMJs, where stimulations are not continuous, the size of nerve terminals is not spatially restricted, and the active zone may expand with muscle growth. Interestingly, at *Drosophila* and crustacean NMJs, active zones with prominent T-bars may be observed and are often adjacent to those without T-bars within the same presynaptic nerve terminal (Fig. 1.1C,E). It has been proposed that active zones with prominent T-bars have a stronger output because more synaptic vesicles may be released upon stimulation. In support of this notion, crustacean NMJ terminals of high output have a threefold higher density of dense projections than those of low output in the same excitatory motor axon despite having similar total synaptic surface areas (87,97). Thus, although dense projections vary greatly in morphology in different types of synapses, they may serve the same primary function of tethering synaptic vesicles to the active zone. Larger dense projections tether more synaptic vesicles and therefore increase the size of the readily releasable pool.

Active Zone Assembly and the Regulation
of Active Zone Density and Spacing

Active zone assembly begins upon axon-target recognition and contact, and ends with the establishment of functional neurotransmitter release sites. In cultured hippocampal neurons, active zone assembly takes about 30 minutes (98,99). According to a recently proposed unitary assembly model, active zone-specific proteins are packaged into transport vesicles for delivery to the nascent synaptic contact site. Upon fusion of such vesicles with the plasma membrane, the active zone proteins are deposited and localized (100,101). In cultured hippocampal synapses, one active zone forms from two or three such transport vesicles (101,102). Considering that on average one active zone has 10 to 15 synaptic vesicle release sites or "grid units," each transport vesicle should carry the building material for four or five synaptic vesicle release sites. This model suggests that active zone assembly occurs within 1 hour, which allows rapid synaptogenesis during development and synapse expansion during activity-dependent long-term potentiation.

Genetic analyses in *C. elegans* and *Drosophila* have identified mutations in several genes that affect active zone assembly. In *C. elegans*, the *syd-2* gene and its positive regulator *syd-1* appear to be primary regulators of presynaptic development because they are required for the assembly of numerous presynaptic components (103). In *syd-2* loss-of-function mutants, active zones of NMJ terminals are lengthened but less electron-dense (104). The SYD-2 protein is localized to active zones and is a member of the Liprin protein family. Liprins contain coiled-coil and sterile alpha motif domains, which are important for protein–protein interactions (105). They interact with the Lar family of receptor protein tyrosine phosphatases (RPTPs) and cluster RPTPs (105). Similarly, *Drosophila* Liprin-α is localized to the active zone at NMJs. In Liprin and DLar (*Drosophila* Lar) mutant flies, the active zone is ~2.5-fold larger than normal with a more irregular morphology (106). In *Drosophila*, loss of *wishful thinking* (*wit*) causes a reduced number of boutons, an increased number of active zones per bouton, and freely floating T-bar structures in the cytoplasm (107). Wit is a Bone morphogenetic protein (BMP) type II receptor that is expressed in a subset of neurons, including motor neurons. However, it remains to be determined how Wit regulates active zone assembly (107,108).

Active zones are not static but rather are plastic structures. In tetrad synapses of the *Drosophila* visual system, the number of presynaptic ribbon/T-bars changes with alterations of light stimulation (109,110). In crustacean NMJs, long-term facilitation in response to high-frequency stimulation is associated with an increase in the number of active zones and dense projections (111). In mammalian hippocampal neurons, long-term potentiation correlates with an expansion or division of active zones (112,113). Interestingly, a recent study of *Drosophila* larval NMJs showed that persistent augmentation of synaptic vesicle release relies on the assembly of new active zones rather than an increase of active zone density, resulting in an expansion of the bouton size. The same study also showed that an increase of active zone density without an expansion of the bouton size led to only a transient increase of evoked vesicle release in response to single action potentials but not consolidated enhancement of neurotransmission (114).

Ultrastructural observations from *Drosophila* and *Sarcophaga* have suggested that the density of active zones is tightly regulated and that a minimum spacing may be required between neighboring active zones (115), presumably because each active zone needs sufficient access to synaptic vesicle pools and recycling machinery. Nevertheless, the density of active zones may also change under certain conditions. For example, in *Drosophila* mutants of *synaptojanin*, an inositol phosphatase that promotes synaptic vesicle uncoating during endocytosis, there are more active zones per unit of surface area and more T-bars within these active zones (116). Thus, activity-dependent active zone plasticity may be associated with changes of either active zone density or synaptic bouton size depending on synapses or experimental/physiologic conditions.

Ectopic Release Sites

Vesicular release from neuronal membranes that lack active zone morphology has long been recognized but thought to be restricted to large, dense-core vesicles. This view is changing as accumulating evidence supports ectopic release of small synaptic vesicles at sites distant from morphologically defined synapses (12). Evidence for the ectopic release of small synaptic vesicles first came from freeze-fracture studies of the NMJ, where exocytosis evoked by elevating extracellular potassium concentration resulted in almost uniformly distributed fusion sites along the presynaptic membrane independent of the position of active zones (117). The most direct visual observation of ectopic release of small synaptic vesicles comes from evanescent-wave microscopy of isolated retinal bipolar cell terminals, where stimulated exocytosis of vesicles loaded with the fluorescent dye FM1–43 could be observed in the presynaptic plasma membrane (118,119). Although most of these fusion events (64%) clustered at sites corresponding to active zones, the remaining fusion events were randomly dispersed in the presynaptic membrane, indicating the presence of ectopic exocytosis.

The three SNARE proteins, including the target-SNAREs syntaxin 1 and SNAP-25, and the vesicle-SNARE synaptobrevin are the minimum proteins required for the fusion of synaptic (120). Both SNAP-25 and syntaxin 1 are expressed throughout the plasma membrane (28); therefore, the fusion event can occur wherever the SNARE complex is formed. It remains to be determined how the ectopic sites are organized, which proteins that participate in the synaptic vesicle cycling are present at ectopic sites, and how ectopic release is regulated. Physiologic significance of ectopic release also awaits elucidation.

Conclusion

The active zone in the presynaptic nerve terminal is a complex and highly organized structure. Its morphology dynamically adapts to the rate of neurotransmitter release. Nature has presented elaborate variations of active zones, from the ~30-nm pyramid in vertebrate central neurons to the ~400-nm sphere in vertebrate hair cells. Nevertheless, all active zones share key structural features. Their differences in size and shape appear to have evolved to suit synapse-specific kinetic needs of transmitter release.

References

1. Sherrington CS. The central nervous system. In: Foster M, ed. A textbook of physiology, 7th ed. London: Macmillan, 1897:929.
2. Fulton JF. Physiology of the nervous system. London: Oxford University Press, 1938.
3. Elliott TR. On the action of adrenalin. J Physiol (London) 1904;31:20P.
4. Loewi O. Ueber humorale uebertragbarkeit der Herznervenwirkung (II. Miteilung). Pflugers Arch Gesamte Physiol Menschen Tirer 1921;193:201–213.
5. Dale HH. The action of certain esters and ethers of choline, and their relation to muscarine. J Pharmacol 1914;6:147–190.
6. Tsuji S. Rene Couteaux (1909–1999) and the morphological identification of synapses. Biol Cell 2006;98(8):503–509.
7. Couteaux R. Nouvelles observations sur la structure de la plaque motrice et interprétation des rapports myo-neuraux. C R Soc Biol 1944;138:976–979.
8. Couteaux R. Sur les gouttières synaptiques du muscle strié. C R Soc Biol 1946;140:270–273.
9. Couteaux R, Pecot-Dechavassine M. Synaptic vesicles and pouches at the level of "active zones" of the neuromuscular junction. C R Acad Sci Hebd Seances Acad Sci D 1970;271(25):2346–2349.
10. Heuser JE, Reese TS. Evidence for recycling of synaptic vesicle membrane during transmitter release at the frog neuromuscular junction. J Cell Biol 1973;57(2):315–344.
11. Landis DM, Hall AK, Weinstein LA, Reese TS. The organization of cytoplasm at the presynaptic active zone of a central nervous system synapse. Neuron 1988;1(3):201–209.
12. Matsui K, Jahr CE. Exocytosis unbound. Curr Opin Neurobiol 2006;16(3):305–311.
13. Parsegian VA. Approaches to the cell biology of neurons. Bethesda, MD: Society for Neuroscience, 1977.
14. Stanley EF. The calcium channel and the organization of the presynaptic transmitter release face. Trends Neurosci 1997;20(9):404–409.
15. Bennett MR, Farnell L, Gibson WG. The probability of quantal secretion near a single calcium channel of an active zone. Biophys J 2000;78(5):2201–2221.
16. Atwood HL, Karunanithi S. Diversification of synaptic strength: presynaptic elements. Nat Rev Neurosci 2002;3(7):497–516.
17. Kawasaki F, Zou B, Xu X, Ordway RW. Active zone localization of presynaptic calcium channels encoded by the cacophony locus of Drosophila. J Neurosci 2004;24(1):282–285.
18. Robitaille R, Adler EM, Charlton MP. Strategic location of calcium channels at transmitter release sites of frog neuromuscular synapses. Neuron 1990;5(6):773–779.
19. Zhang L, Volknandt W, Gundelfinger ED, Zimmermann H. A comparison of synaptic protein localization in hippocampal mossy fiber terminals and neurosecretory endings of the neurohypophysis using the cryo-immunogold technique. J Neurocytol 2000;29(1): 19–30.
20. Ellisman MH, Rash JE, Staehelin LA, Porter KR. Studies of excitable membranes. II. A comparison of specializations at neuromuscular junctions and nonjunctional sarcolemmas of mammalian fast and slow twitch muscle fibers. J Cell Biol 1976;68(3):752–774.
21. Heuser JE, Reese TS, Landis DM. Functional changes in frog neuromuscular junctions studied with freeze-fracture. J Neurocytol 1974;3(1):109–131.
22. Walrond JP, Reese TS. Structure of axon terminals and active zones at synapses on lizard twitch and tonic muscle fibers. J Neurosci 1985;5(5):1118–1131.
23. Cohen MW, Jones OT, Angelides KJ. Distribution of Ca2+ channels on frog motor nerve terminals revealed by fluorescent omega-conotoxin. J Neurosci 1991;11(4):1032–1039.

24. Pumplin DW, Reese TS, Llinas R. Are the presynaptic membrane particles the calcium channels? Proc Natl Acad Sci U S A 1981;78(11):7210–7213.
25. Haydon PG, Henderson E, Stanley EF. Localization of individual calcium channels at the release face of a presynaptic nerve terminal. Neuron 1994;13(6):1275–1280.
26. Jahn R, Lang T, Sudhof TC. Membrane fusion. Cell 2003;112(4):519–533.
27. Rizo J. SNARE function revisited. Nat Struct Biol 2003;10(6):417–419.
28. Garcia EP, McPherson PS, Chilcote TJ, Takei K, De Camilli P. rbSec1A and B colocalize with syntaxin 1 and SNAP-25 throughout the axon, but are not in a stable complex with syntaxin. J Cell Biol 1995;129(1):105–120.
29. Hiesinger PR, Scholz M, Meinertzhagen IA, Fischbach KF, Obermayer K. Visualization of synaptic markers in the optic neuropils of Drosophila using a new constrained deconvolution method. J Comp Neurol 2001;429(2):277–288.
30. Schulze KL, Broadie K, Perin MS, Bellen HJ. Genetic and electrophysiological studies of Drosophila syntaxin-1A demonstrate its role in nonneuronal secretion and neurotransmission. Cell 1995;80(2):311–320.
31. Jarvis SE, Barr W, Feng ZP, Hamid J, Zamponi GW. Molecular determinants of syntaxin 1 modulation of N-type calcium channels. J Biol Chem 2002;277(46):44399–44407.
32. Taverna E, Saba E, Rowe J, Francolini M, Clementi F, Rosa P. Role of lipid microdomains in P/Q-type calcium channel (Cav2.1) clustering and function in presynaptic membranes. J Biol Chem 2004;279(7):5127–5134.
33. Catterall WA. Interactions of presynaptic Ca2+ channels and snare proteins in neurotransmitter release. Ann N Y Acad Sci 1999;868:144–159.
34. Martin-Moutot N, Charvin N, Leveque C, et al. Interaction of SNARE complexes with P/Q-type calcium channels in rat cerebellar synaptosomes. J Biol Chem 1996;271(12):6567–6570.
35. Lang T, Bruns D, Wenzel D, et al. SNAREs are concentrated in cholesterol-dependent clusters that define docking and fusion sites for exocytosis. EMBO J 2001;20(9):2202–2213.
36. Shapiro L, Colman DR. The diversity of cadherins and implications for a synaptic adhesive code in the CNS. Neuron 1999;23(3):427–430.
37. Yagi T, Takeichi M. Cadherin superfamily genes: functions, genomic organization, and neurologic diversity. Genes Dev 2000;14(10):1169–1180.
38. Frank M, Kemler R. Protocadherins. Curr Opin Cell Biol 2002;14(5):557–562.
39. Mizoguchi A, Nakanishi H, Kimura K, et al. Nectin: an adhesion molecule involved in formation of synapses. J Cell Biol 2002;156(3):555–565.
40. Takai Y, Shimizu K, Ohtsuka T. The roles of cadherins and nectins in interneuronal synapse formation. Curr Opin Neurobiol 2003;13(5):520–526.
41. Rougon G, Hobert O. New insights into the diversity and function of neuronal immunoglobulin superfamily molecules. Annu Rev Neurosci 2003;26:207–238.
42. Davis GW, Schuster CM, Goodman CS. Genetic analysis of the mechanisms controlling target selection: target-derived Fasciclin II regulates the pattern of synapse formation. Neuron 1997;19(3):561–573.
43. Mayford M, Barzilai A, Keller F, Schacher S, Kandel ER. Modulation of an NCAM-related adhesion molecule with long-term synaptic plasticity in Aplysia. Science 1992;256(5057):638–644.
44. Schmucker D, Clemens JC, Shu H, et al. Drosophila Dscam is an axon guidance receptor exhibiting extraordinary molecular diversity. Cell 2000;101(6):671–684.
45. Hsueh YP, Sheng M. Regulated expression and subcellular localization of syndecan heparan sulfate proteoglycans and the syndecan-binding protein CASK/LIN-2 during rat brain development. J Neurosci 1999;19(17):7415–7425.
46. Walsh FS, Doherty P. Neural cell adhesion molecules of the immunoglobulin superfamily: role in axon growth and guidance. Annu Rev Cell Dev Biol 1997;13:425–456.
47. Chavis P, Westbrook G. Integrins mediate functional pre- and postsynaptic maturation at a hippocampal synapse. Nature 2001;411(6835):317–321.
48. Missler M, Sudhof TC. Neurexins: three genes and 1001 products. Trends Genet 1998;14(1):20–26.

49. Yamagata M, Sanes JR, Weiner JA. Synaptic adhesion molecules. Curr Opin Cell Biol 2003;15(5):621–632.
50. Yamagata M, Weiner JA, Sanes JR. Sidekicks: synaptic adhesion molecules that promote lamina-specific connectivity in the retina. Cell 2002;110(5):649–660.
51. Gottardi CJ, Gumbiner BM. Adhesion signaling: how beta-catenin interacts with its partners. Curr Biol 2001;11(19):R792–794.
52. Sheng M, Sala C. PDZ domains and the organization of supramolecular complexes. Annu Rev Neurosci 2001;24:1–29.
53. Packard M, Mathew D, Budnik V. FASt remodeling of synapses in Drosophila. Curr Opin Neurobiol 2003;13(5):527–534.
54. Scheiffele P. Cell-cell signaling during synapse formation in the CNS. Annu Rev Neurosci 2003;26:485–508.
55. Ferreira A, Paganoni S. The formation of synapses in the central nervous system. Mol Neurobiol 2002;26(1):69–79.
56. Bloom FE, Aghajanian GK. Fine structural and cytochemical analysis of the staining of synaptic junctions with phosphotungstic acid. J Ultrastruct Res 1968;22(5):361–375.
57. Pfenninger K, Akert K, Moor H, Sandri C. The fine structure of freeze-fractured presynaptic membranes. J Neurocytol 1972;1(2):129–149.
58. Harlow ML, Ress D, Stoschek A, Marshall RM, McMahan UJ. The architecture of active zone material at the frog's neuromuscular junction. Nature 2001;409(6819):479–484.
59. Phillips GR, Huang JK, Wang Y, et al. The presynaptic particle web: ultrastructure, composition, dissolution, and reconstitution. Neuron 2001;32(1):63–77.
60. Burns ME, Augustine GJ. Synaptic structure and function: dynamic organization yields architectural precision. Cell 1995;83(2):187–194.
61. Hirokawa N, Sobue K, Kanda K, Harada A, Yorifuji H. The cytoskeletal architecture of the presynaptic terminal and molecular structure of synapsin 1. J Cell Biol 1989;108(1):111–126.
62. Kistner U, Wenzel BM, Veh RW, et al. SAP90, a rat presynaptic protein related to the product of the Drosophila tumor suppressor gene dlg-A. J Biol Chem 1993;268(7):4580–4583.
63. Muller BM, Kistner U, Veh RW, et al. Molecular characterization and spatial distribution of SAP97, a novel presynaptic protein homologous to SAP90 and the Drosophila discs-large tumor suppressor protein. J Neurosci 1995;15(3 Pt 2):2354–2366.
64. Hata Y, Butz S, Sudhof TC. CASK: a novel dlg/PSD95 homolog with an N-terminal calmodulin-dependent protein kinase domain identified by interaction with neurexins. J Neurosci 1996;16(8):2488–2494.
65. Koulen P, Fletcher EL, Craven SE, Bredt DS, Wassle H. Immunocytochemical localization of the postsynaptic density protein PSD-95 in the mammalian retina. J Neurosci 1998;18(23):10136–10149.
66. Fanning AS, Anderson JM. PDZ domains: fundamental building blocks in the organization of protein complexes at the plasma membrane. J Clin Invest 1999;103(6):767–772.
67. Garner CC, Nash J, Huganir RL. PDZ domains in synapse assembly and signalling. Trends Cell Biol 2000;10(7):274–280.
68. O'Brien RJ, Lau LF, Huganir RL. Molecular mechanisms of glutamate receptor clustering at excitatory synapses. Curr Opin Neurobiol 1998;8(3):364–369.
69. Butz S, Okamoto M, Sudhof TC. A tripartite protein complex with the potential to couple synaptic vesicle exocytosis to cell adhesion in brain. Cell 1998;94(6):773–782.
70. Hsueh YP, Yang FC, Kharazia V, et al. Direct interaction of CASK/LIN-2 and syndecan heparan sulfate proteoglycan and their overlapping distribution in neuronal synapses. J Cell Biol 1998;142(1):139–151.
71. Maximov A, Sudhof TC, Bezprozvanny I. Association of neuronal calcium channels with modular adaptor proteins. J Biol Chem 1999;274(35):24453–24456.
72. Dieck S, Sanmart-Vila L, Langnaese K, et al. Bassoon, a novel zinc-finger CAG/glutamine-repeat protein selectively localized at the active zone of presynaptic nerve terminals. J Cell Biol 1998;142(2):499–509.
73. Fenster SD, Chung WJ, Zhai R, et al. Piccolo, a presynaptic zinc finger protein structurally related to bassoon. Neuron 2000;25(1):203–214.

74. Wang X, Kibschull M, Laue MM, Lichte B, Petrasch-Parwez E, Kilimann MW. Aczonin, a 550–kD putative scaffolding protein of presynaptic active zones, shares homology regions with rim and bassoon and binds profilin. J Cell Biol 1999;147(1):151–162.

75. Wang Y, Liu X, Biederer T, Sudhof TC. A family of RIM-binding proteins regulated by alternative splicing: implications for the genesis of synaptic active zones. Proc Natl Acad Sci U S A 2002;99(22):14464–14469.

76. Wang Y, Okamoto M, Schmitz F, Hofmann K, Sudhof TC. Rim is a putative Rab3 effector in regulating synaptic-vesicle fusion. Nature 1997;388(6642):593–598.

77. Brose N, Hofmann K, Hata Y, Sudhof TC. Mammalian homologues of Caenorhabditis elegans unc-13 gene define novel family of C2–domain proteins. J Biol Chem 1995;270(42): 25273–25280.

78. Dresbach T, Qualmann B, Kessels MM, Garner CC, Gundelfinger ED. The presynaptic cytomatrix of brain synapses. Cell Mol Life Sci 2001;58(1):94–116.

79. Rosenmund C, Rettig J, Brose N. Molecular mechanisms of active zone function. Curr Opin Neurobiol 2003;13(5):509–519.

80. Takao-Rikitsu E, Mochida S, Inoue E, et al. Physical and functional interaction of the active zone proteins, CAST, RIM1, and Bassoon, in neurotransmitter release. J Cell Biol 2004;164(2):301–311.

81. Lagnado L. Ribbon synapses. Curr Biol 2003;13(16):R631.

82. Lenzi D, von Gersdorff H. Structure suggests function: the case for synaptic ribbons as exocytotic nanomachines. Bioessays 2001;23(9):831–840.

83. von Gersdorff H. Synaptic ribbons: versatile signal transducers. Neuron 2001;29(1):7–10.

84. Hallam SJ, Goncharov A, McEwen J, Baran R, Jin Y. SYD-1, a presynaptic protein with PDZ, C2 and rhoGAP-like domains, specifies axon identity in C. elegans. Nat Neurosci 2002;5(11):1137–1146.

85. Meinertzhagen IA. Ultrastructure and quantification of synapses in the insect nervous system. J Neurosci Methods 1996;69(1):59–73.

86. Yasuyama K, Meinertzhagen IA, Schurmann FW. Synaptic organization of the mushroom body calyx in Drosophila melanogaster. J Comp Neurol 2002;445(3):211–226.

87. Govind CK, Meiss DE. Quantitative comparison of low- and high-output neuromuscular synapses from a motoneuron of the lobster (Homarus americanus). Cell Tissue Res 1979;198(3):455–463.

88. Garner CC, Kindler S, Gundelfinger ED. Molecular determinants of presynaptic active zones. Curr Opin Neurobiol 2000;10(3):321–327.

89. Muresan V, Lyass A, Schnapp BJ. The kinesin motor KIF3A is a component of the presynaptic ribbon in vertebrate photoreceptors. J Neurosci 1999;19(3):1027–1037.

90. Hilfiker S, Pieribone VA, Czernik AJ, Kao HT, Augustine GJ, Greengard P. Synapsins as regulators of neurotransmitter release. Philos Trans R Soc Lond B Biol Sci 1999;354(1381):269–279.

91. Brandstatter JH, Fletcher EL, Garner CC, Gundelfinger ED, Wassle H. Differential expression of the presynaptic cytomatrix protein bassoon among ribbon synapses in the mammalian retina. Eur J Neurosci 1999;11(10):3683–3693.

92. Dick O, tom Dieck S, Altrock WD, et al. The presynaptic active zone protein bassoon is essential for photoreceptor ribbon synapse formation in the retina. Neuron 2003;37(5):775–786.

93. Kittel RJ, Wichmann C, Rasse TM, et al. Bruchpilot promotes active zone assembly, Ca2+ channel clustering, and vesicle release. Science 2006;312(5776):1051–1054.

94. Lenzi D, Crum J, Ellisman MH, Roberts WM. Depolarization redistributes synaptic membrane and creates a gradient of vesicles on the synaptic body at a ribbon synapse. Neuron 2002;36(4):649–659.

95. Lenzi D, Runyeon JW, Crum J, Ellisman MH, Roberts WM. Synaptic vesicle populations in saccular hair cells reconstructed by electron tomography. J Neurosci 1999;19(1):119–132.

96. Matthews G. Synaptic mechanisms of bipolar cell terminals. Vision Res 1999;39(15): 2469–2476.

97. Govind CK, Quigley PA, Pearce J. Synaptic differentiation between two phasic motoneurons to a crayfish fast muscle. Invert Neurosci 2001;4(2):77–84.

98. Ahmari SE, Buchanan J, Smith SJ. Assembly of presynaptic active zones from cytoplasmic transport packets. Nat Neurosci 2000;3(5):445–451.
99. Friedman HV, Bresler T, Garner CC, Ziv NE. Assembly of new individual excitatory synapses: time course and temporal order of synaptic molecule recruitment. Neuron 2000;27(1):57–69.
100. Dresbach T, Torres V, Wittenmayer N, et al. Assembly of active zone precursor vesicles: obligatory trafficking of presynaptic cytomatrix proteins Bassoon and Piccolo via a trans-Golgi compartment. J Biol Chem 2006;281(9):6038–6047.
101. Zhai RG, Vardinon-Friedman H, Cases-Langhoff C, et al. Assembling the presynaptic active zone: a characterization of an active one precursor vesicle. Neuron 2001;29(1):131–143.
102. Shapira M, Zhai RG, Dresbach T, et al. Unitary assembly of presynaptic active zones from Piccolo-Bassoon transport vesicles. Neuron 2003;38(2):237–252.
103. Patel MR, Lehrman EK, Poon VY, et al. Hierarchical assembly of presynaptic components in defined C. elegans synapses. Nat Neurosci 2006;9(12):1488–1498.
104. Zhen M, Jin Y. The liprin protein SYD-2 regulates the differentiation of presynaptic termini in C. elegans. Nature 1999;401(6751):371–375.
105. Serra-Pages C, Medley QG, Tang M, Hart A, Streuli M. Liprins, a family of LAR transmembrane protein-tyrosine phosphatase-interacting proteins. J Biol Chem 1998;273(25):15611–15620.
106. Kaufmann N, DeProto J, Ranjan R, Wan H, Van Vactor D. Drosophila liprin-alpha and the receptor phosphatase Dlar control synapse morphogenesis. Neuron 2002;34(1):27–38.
107. Aberle H, Haghighi AP, Fetter RD, McCabe BD, Magalhaes TR, Goodman CS. wishful thinking encodes a BMP type II receptor that regulates synaptic growth in Drosophila. Neuron 2002;33(4):545–558.
108. Marques G, Bao H, Haerry TE, et al. The Drosophila BMP type II receptor Wishful Thinking regulates neuromuscular synapse morphology and function. Neuron 2002;33(4):529–543.
109. Brandstatter JH, Meinertzhagen IA. The rapid assembly of synaptic sites in photoreceptor terminals of the fly's optic lobe recovering from cold shock. Proc Natl Acad Sci U S A 1995;92(7):2677–2681.
110. Rybak J, Meinertzhagen IA. The effects of light reversals on photoreceptor synaptogenesis in the fly Musca domestica. Eur J Neurosci 1997;9(2):319–333.
111. Wojtowicz JM, Marin L, Atwood HL. Activity-induced changes in synaptic release sites at the crayfish neuromuscular junction. J Neurosci 1994;14(6):3688–3703.
112. Harris KM, Fiala JC, Ostroff L. Structural changes at dendritic spine synapses during long-term potentiation. Philos Trans R Soc Lond B Biol Sci 2003;358(1432):745–748.
113. Weeks AC, Ivanco TL, Leboutillier JC, Racine RJ, Petit TL. Sequential changes in the synaptic structural profile following long-term potentiation in the rat dentate gyrus. II. Induction/early maintenance phase. Synapse 2000;36(4):286–296.
114. Reiff DF, Thiel PR, Schuster CM. Differential regulation of active zone density during long-term strengthening of Drosophila neuromuscular junctions. J Neurosci 2002;22(21):9399–9409.
115. Meinertzhagen IA, Govind CK, Stewart BA, Carter JM, Atwood HL. Regulated spacing of synapses and presynaptic active zones at larval neuromuscular junctions in different genotypes of the flies Drosophila and Sarcophaga. J Comp Neurol 1998;393(4):482–492.
116. Dickman DK, Lu Z, Meinertzhagen IA, Schwarz TL. Altered synaptic development and active zone spacing in endocytosis mutants. Curr Biol 2006;16(6):591–598.
117. Ceccarelli B, Fesce R, Grohovaz F, Haimann C. The effect of potassium on exocytosis of transmitter at the frog neuromuscular junction. J Physiol 1988;401:163–183.
118. Zenisek D, Davila V, Wan L, Almers W. Imaging calcium entry sites and ribbon structures in two presynaptic cells. J Neurosci 2003;23(7):2538–2548.
119. Zenisek D, Steyer JA, Almers W. Transport, capture and exocytosis of single synaptic vesicles at active zones. Nature 2000;406(6798):849–854.
120. Sudhof TC. The synaptic vesicle cycle. Annu Rev Neurosci 2004;27:509–47.

Chapter 2
Multiple Modes of Fusion and Retrieval at the Calyx of Held Synapse

Liming He, Benjamin D. McNeil, and Ling-Gang Wu

Contents

Abstract Neurotransmitter in vesicles is released through a fusion pore when vesicles fuse with the plasma membrane. Subsequent retrieval of the fused vesicle membrane is the key step in recycling exocytosed vesicles. Recent application of advanced electrophysiologic techniques to a large nerve terminal, the calyx of Held, has led to direct recordings of endocytosis, individual vesicle fusion and retrieval, and the kinetics of the fusion pore opening process and the fission pore closure process. These studies have revealed three kinetically different forms of endocytosis—rapid, slow, and bulk endocytosis—and two forms of fusion—full collapse and kiss-and-run. These research advancements are reviewed in this chapter.

Keywords Vesicle fusion, vesicle endocytosis, exocytosis, full collapse fusion, kiss-and-run, capacitance recording, calyx of Held, synaptic transmission, quantal response.

Neurons release neurotransmitter through synaptic vesicle exocytosis, a specialized form of vesicle trafficking whereby synaptic vesicles fuse with the presynaptic

Ling-Gang Wu
National Institute of Neurological Disorders and Stroke, National Institute of Health, Bethesda, Maryland 20892
e-mail: wul@ninds.nih.gov

plasma membrane at the active zone and release their contents into the synaptic cleft. Following exocytosis, vesicles are retrieved from the plasma membrane in a process called endocytosis and refilled with neurotransmitter, forming new vesicles that can be used for further release (1). Thus, coordination of the exocytosis of neurotransmitter and the endocytosis of vesicular components sustains the membrane trafficking of synaptic vesicles.

The modes of exocytosis and endocytosis depend on the behavior of the fusion pore, a molecular structure that forms to connect vesicle membrane and presynaptic plasma membrane during synaptic vesicle fusion. The initial fusion pore may expand rapidly, allowing the vesicles to fully collapse into the plasma membrane (2). This mode is called "full collapse" or "full fusion." Alternatively, the initial fusion pore opens for a short time without dilating and then closes again, allowing the vesicle to retain its integrity when it discharges its contents. This process is called "kiss-and-run" fusion (3,4). Full fusion leads to a rapid release of all neurotransmitter in a bolus, while kiss-and-run may regulate the rate of neurotransmitter discharge by opening the fusion pore to different degrees (5). The rate of neurotransmitter release may affect the postsynaptic response, and possibly contribute to synaptic plasticity (6).

The modes of fusion may also determine a vesicle's fate after neurotransmitter release. It is thought that full collapse fusion is followed by compensatory endocytosis, a clathrin-mediated process in which vesicles are reformed from the plasma membrane and severed by the guanosine triphosphatase (GTPase) dynamin (1). The endocytic rate is much slower than kiss-and-run endocytosis, which simply involves closing of the fusion pore. It is plausible that the differing rates of endocytosis may affect synaptic function, as endocytosis is critical for replenishment of various synaptic vesicle pools, which influences the ability of the nerve terminal to maintain transmitter release during repetitive firing (7). Regulation of vesicle availability through the rate of endocytosis, and thus the rate of vesicle cycling, could contribute to the generation of some forms of synaptic plasticity (7). Owing to these potential important roles, the kinetics of endocytosis and its regulation have been intensively studied in the past decade.

Both fusion and retrieval can be monitored in live synapses with imaging and electrophysiologic techniques (8). Compared to imaging techniques, electrophysiologic techniques, including whole-cell and cell-attached capacitance recording techniques, provide faster time resolution and allow for the measurement of the fusion pore opening process and the fission pore closure kinetics. In the past few years, these advanced electrophysiologic techniques have been applied to a large nerve terminal, the calyx of Held, to study the rates and modes of endocytosis. These studies have provided direct recordings of fast endocytosis and individual vesicle fusion and retrieval. Further, the kinetics of the fusion pore opening process and the fission pore closure process have been measured. These results have not been reported at any other synapse, which is at least partly due to the small size of most other synapses that has precluded the application of the electrophysiologic techniques. This chapter discusses what we have learned from electrophysiologic studies of fusion and retrieval at the calyx of Held. We believe that the calyx of Held synapse is an excellent model for the study of vesicle fusion and retrieval, and that the results obtained at this large synapse can provide useful lessons for further studies of fusion and retrieval at most small conventional synapses.

The Calyx of Held Synapse and the Whole-Cell Capacitance Measurement

The calyx of Held is a glutamatergic nerve terminal that forms part of the relay pathway involved in sound localization in the auditory brainstem (Fig. 2.1a) (9). The calyx of Held arises from globular bushy cells in the anterior ventral cochlear nucleus (aVCN), which project onto principal neurons of the contralateral medial nucleus of the trapezoid body (MNTB; Fig. 2.1b) (9). Electron microscopy (EM) reconstruction of the calyx of Held has shown the presence of approximately 300 to 700 individual active zones, each with about two morphologically docked vesicles (10,11). The large number of active zones helps ensure rapid signaling, as a presynaptic action potential (AP) releases hundreds of vesicles, generating a large

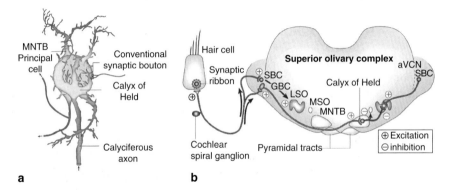

Fig. 2.1 Anatomy of the calyx of Held synapse. **(a)** A diagram of the adult calyx of Held, a glutamatergic synapse in the mammalian auditory brainstem. Note the large-caliber axon (4 to 12 μm in diameter) that gives rise to the calyx. The postsynaptic cell has relatively short dendrites and an axon with a collateral branch. MNTB, medial nucleus of the trapezoid body. **(b)** A diagram of the circuitry of the superior olivary complex (SOC), which is involved in computing sound localization from the auditory inputs from both ears. Auditory information from the cochlea is transmitted to the ipsilateral anterior ventral cochlear nucleus (aVCN) through excitatory synapses onto spherical bushy cells (SBCs) (black arrow) and globular bushy cells (GBCs) (lighter neuron beside "GBC" label). The GBCs synapse onto the contralateral medial nucleus of the trapezoid body (MNTB), which makes an inhibitory synapse onto the lateral superior olive (LSO). The LSO also receives excitatory input from the ipsilateral SBCs. It is at the level of the LSO that discharges evoked by interaural intensity differences are first represented as differences in the timing of excitatory and inhibitory inputs. So, the LSO is thought to function as a coincidence detector of binaural signals, whereas the main role of the MNTB is simply to act as a fast, sign-inverting relay station. The principal cells of the MNTB, however, also receive strong inhibitory input from unknown sources, and are organized in a tonotopic map of characteristic sound frequencies. The MNTB is therefore not a functionally homogeneous nucleus, and its output might be modulated by other brainstem nuclei. MSO, medial superior olive. (Adapted from Von Gersdorff and Borst [9], with permission.)

excitatory postsynaptic current (EPSC) that rapidly depolarizes the postsynaptic neuron to the threshold for generating action potentials (9).

Except for the large size of the terminal and the large quantal synaptic output, the calyx of Held synapse acts in a similar way to a conventional fast synapse in the central nervous system (CNS). For example, the terminal releases glutamate in response to presynaptic action potential stimulation. The terminal contains many spherical, clear-core vesicles with a diameter of about 50 nm (10,12). The delay between the peak of a presynaptic action potential and the onset of the EPSC is less than 1 ms (13). Multiple types of voltage-dependent Ca^{2+} channels control transmitter release at single release sites in the calyx of Held synapse (14,15), as in many other CNS synapses (16). The synapse exhibits short-term synaptic depression and facilitation (9,17). Since the MNTB synapse functionally resembles other fast central synapses in many aspects, the experimental results obtained from this synapse not only may be applied to calyceal synapses, but also may have a more general significance.

Presynaptic patch-clamp measurements of exocytosis and endocytosis rely on the increase in surface membrane area when vesicles fuse with the plasma membrane during exocytosis, and the decrease in area when membrane is retrieved by endocytosis. The changes in surface area can be monitored electrically as changes in membrane capacitance (C_m) (18). Whole-cell capacitance measurement is best achieved in round cells that are electrically equivalent to a membrane capacitance in parallel with a membrane resistance (Fig. 2.2a) (18). Recent studies demonstrated that this technique can also be applied to the calyx of Held (19–21). Although the calyx is connected with an axon, simulation suggests that the axon does not significantly affect the measurement of the capacitance at the calyx when Lindau-Neher's technique is used (20); thus, changes in membrane size at the calyx can be accurately measured. Experimental results have confirmed this simulation result. First, when both the EPSC and the presynaptic capacitance were simultaneously recorded at the same synapse, the EPSC amplitude or the charge increased as the capacitance jump (ΔC_m) increased (Fig. 2.2b). The relation between EPSC amplitude and presynaptic capacitance jump could be fit by a linear regression line with a slope of about 148 picoamperes per femtofarad (pA/fF) (Fig. 2.2c) (19). Furthermore, by averaging about 2.7 million spontaneous miniature EPSCs (mEPSCs) and the corresponding presynatpic capacitance traces from 459 individual synapses, we found that the presynaptic membrane capacitance jumped by about 65 atofarads (aF) within 1 ms before the onset of the mean mEPSC (Fig. 2.2d) (22,23). As the specific membrane capacitance is 9 fF μm^{-2} (24), 65 aF corresponds to a vesicle with a diameter of 48 nm, which is similar to the estimate from EM (10). We concluded that the capacitance jump accurately reflects vesicle fusion.

Whole-cell recordings of fusion have advantages and drawbacks, compared to the more common measurement of postsynaptic currents induced by transmitter binding. The drawbacks are that the signal-to-noise ratio is not as high as postsynaptic current recordings, and recording release during a stimulus is not possible. However, one significant advantage is that capacitance measurements provide a better estimate of total release, since they are independent of the functional state of the postsynaptic receptors, while postsynaptic currents are complicated by the effects of receptor saturation, desensitization, and inactivation that skew the relationship between release

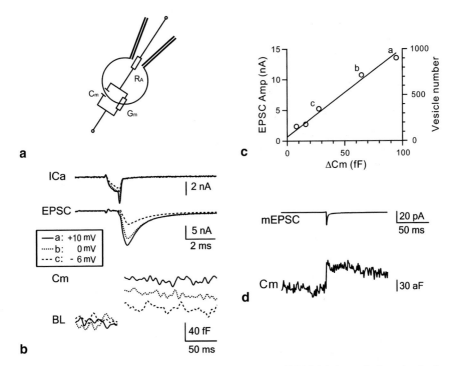

Fig. 2.2 Capacitance jumps reflect exocytosis at the calyx of Held. (**a**) An equivalent circuit of a cell in the whole-cell recording configuration. C_m is the membrane capacitance, R_A is the access resistance, and R_m is the membrane resistance. (**b**) Sample recordings of the presynaptic Ca^{2+} currents and excitatory postsynaptic currents (EPSCs) induced by 1-ms steps to +10 mV, 0 mV, and −6 mV at the calyx. Presynaptic Ca^{2+} currents and EPSCs are plotted at the same time scale, whereas capacitance changes are plotted at a different time scale. BL, baseline capacitance; a, b, c, data points. (**c**) The linear relation between the EPSC amplitude (EPSC Amp, left y axis) and ΔC_m evoked by a series of 1-ms step depolarizations from −80 mV to a voltage ranging from −10 to +20 mV at a synapse. Right y axis is approximate vesicle number, calculated from the ΔC_m, assuming an average vesicle diameter of 50 nm. (B,C: Adapted from Sun and Wu [19], with permission.) (**d**) The mean mEPSC and C_m averaged from 2.66 million fusion events obtained from 459 paired recordings. Traces are shown without filtering. (Adapted from Wu et al [23].)

and postsynaptic response. In addition to its utility in the study of vesicle fusion, time-resolved capacitance measurement at the calyx provides a powerful technique to study synaptic vesicle endocytosis at a central synapse.

A Linear Relation Between the Time Constant of Endocytosis and the Amount of Exocytosis

Synaptic vesicle endocytosis can be detected as the decay of the capacitance jump to baseline levels after a stimulus. At the calyx of Held this decay is exponential, and is described by the time constant (τ) in an exponential equation. The τ is the time at which ~63% of the jump has decayed. Recent studies at the calyx of Held showed that the time course of endocytosis, as measured by whole-cell capacitance recordings, depended on the stimulation intensity. The capacitance change after a single action potential-equivalent (AP-e) stimulus was measured by two labs, using slightly different stimuli. One lab used a 1-ms step depolarization from −80 mV to +7 mV, which induces the release of the same number of vesicles as an action potential (22). After this stimulus, the capacitance jump was about 20 fF, and decayed with a τ of about 2.2 seconds (Fig. 2.3a) (21). Earlier measurements indicated that the decay was much faster, at τ ≈115 ms (22), but it was later shown that they were contaminated by the presence of an artifactual capacitance jump with a decay time in the hundreds of milliseconds, which persists after abolishing exocytosis with botulinum neurotoxin E (25) or C (21). Another lab approximated an AP-e with a 4-ms step depolarization from −80 mV to +80 mV, followed by a 1-ms step to +40 mV (25). This was found to evoke approximately three times the amount of release as an action potential (21), and induced a capacitance jump of about 60 fF. After this stimulus, the decay was fit with a τ of about 10.4 seconds when the first 500 ms after stimulation was ignored (25). The difference in the τ reported by these two labs is at least partly due to the difference in the stimulation intensity and thus the capacitance jump, because when the first lab changed the stimulus protocol and increased the capacitance jump from about 20 fF to about 60 fF, the τ increased from about 2.2 to 4.2 seconds (21).

The τ after short AP-e trains increased in linear proportion to the net capacitance jump at the end of the stimulus (Fig. 2.3b,c) (21,22). This relationship cannot be attributed to an increase in stimulus frequency alone, as similar capacitance jumps elicited by AP-e trains at frequencies from 20 to 333 Hz had similar decay times (21,22). As further evidence, the trend was also seen when longer AP-e trains or continuous step depolarizations from −80 mV to 0 to 10 mV with durations from 2 to 20 ms were used to evoke exocytosis (Fig. 2.3c) (21,22,25). The lengthening of the time constant also cannot be explained by the increase in global calcium influx due to increased stimulation, because ethylene glycol tetraacetic acid (EGTA), a slow-binding calcium chelator that eliminates the residual calcium transient, did not reduce the τ (22). Moreover, clamping presynaptic calcium levels at ~1 μM, which exceeds the peak global calcium concentration after 10 AP-e at 333 Hz, did not lengthen the τ (22). The duration of elevated local calcium domains can also be ruled out, as the τ was similar after 10- and 30-ms step depolarizations from −80 mV to +10 mV, which elicited similar capacitance jumps and similar time courses of endocytosis (22). Thus, it appears that the net accumulation of fused vesicle membrane at the end of a stimulus is itself the cause of the increase in the τ.

This linear relation is also seen at other synapses. Styryl dye uptake studies at the frog neuromuscular junction show that the endocytic τ increases as the duration of a 30-Hz stimulus train of APs increases (26). Similarly, at cultured hippocampal neuron boutons, studies using the genetically encoded exo-/endocytic marker synaptopHluorin demonstrated that the τ increased linearly with the number of APs in a 10-Hz train, from <10 seconds after 20 APs to ~90 seconds after 600 APs (27). There is some question about what happens at very mild stimulation, as another

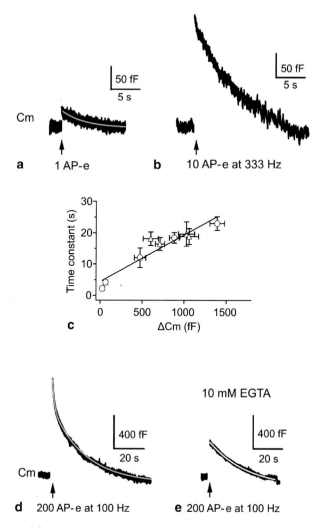

Fig. 2.3 Slow and fast endocytosis at the calyx of Held. (**a**) Sampled whole-cell capacitance (Cm) response to an action potential-equivalent (AP-e) (1-ms step to +7 mV). The capacitance decay, starting from 200 ms after stimulation, was fit with an exponential function with a time constant of 2.9 seconds. (Adapted from Wu et al [21].) (**b**) Sampled Cm response to 10 AP-e at 333 Hz. Note that the retrieval time is significantly longer than after 1 AP-e. (Adapted from Sun et al [22].) (**c**) The relation between the time constant and the amplitude of endocytosis. A plot of endocytosis time constant versus its amplitude after various stimuli. Endocytosis after step depolarizations are indicated by circles, and endocytosis after AP-e is indicated by triangles. Average amount of endocytosis and time constant are as follows: 1-ms step to +7 mV: 20 fF, 2.2 seconds; 1-ms step to +15–30 mV: 57 fF, 4.2 seconds; 20–ms step to +10 mV: 473 fF, 12.0 seconds; ten 20-ms steps to +10 mV at 10 Hz: 880 fF (slow component), 18.4 seconds; ten 20-ms steps to +10 mV at 1 Hz: 1390 fF (slow component), 23.0 seconds; 50 AP-e at 100 Hz: 710 fF, 16.4 seconds; 200 AP-e at 100 Hz: 1025 fF (slow component), 19.6 seconds; 50 AP-e at 100 Hz repeated five times at 1 Hz: 1060 fF (slow component), 18.8 seconds; 50 AP-e at 30 Hz repeated five times at 0.4 Hz: 599 fF (slow component), 18.0 seconds. The data were fit with a linear regression line with a slope of 1.4 seconds/100 fF. (**d**) Sampled Cm response to 200 AP-e at 100 Hz (bars). The capacitance decay was fit with a biexponential function [gray, τ_1 = 1.8 seconds (377 fF), τ_2 = 24.0 seconds (1020 fF)]. (**e**) Sampled Cm response to 200 AP-e at 100 Hz with 10 mM ethyleneglycoltetraacetic acid (EGTA) in the pipette. The capacitance decay was fit with a monoexponential function (gray, τ = 24.7 seconds). (c–e: Adapted from Wu et al [21], with permission.)

study with a similar marker, called sypHy, found that this linearity did not hold for trains of up to 40 APs at a 20-Hz frequency (28). However, the authors did see a lengthening of the τ with stronger stimulation.

A hypothesis to explain this correlation between τ and net exocytosis has been described (27). In this model, the endocytic apparatus has a fixed rate and limited capacity; when the amount of fusion exceeds the capacity for retrieval, membrane accumulates at the plasma membrane and is cleared at a constant rate. Thus, addition of more fused vesicles will lengthen the τ in a linear fashion. This model predicts the observed linear relationship between the τ and the net exocytosis after mild-to-moderate stimulation at the calyx. However, it also predicts a linear decay, while at the calyx (and in cultured hippocampal neurons), membrane retrieval is best fit with an exponential function. Thus, this model may be similar, but not identical, to the physiologic mechanism in the calyx of Held at mild-to-moderate stimulation.

Intense Stimulation Activates Rapid Endocytosis by Increasing the Calcium Influx

Under stronger stimulus conditions at the calyx, the linear relationship between the τ and net exocytosis no longer applies (21). When a 20-ms pulse stimulation is repeated 10 times at 10 Hz, a fast component with a τ of 1 to 2 seconds is evident immediately after the end of stimulation. After several seconds it gives way to slow endocytosis, and the total capacitance decline is fit well with a double exponential. The fast component can also be evoked by a train of 200 AP-e at 100 Hz (Fig. 2.3d), suggesting that it is physiologically important.

Slowing the frequency of the 20-ms pulses to 1 Hz allows capacitance measurements to be made between pulses, enabling an examination of how the fast component develops. Under this condition, the initial rate of endocytosis increased from about 28 fF/s after the first pulse to a plateau of about 208 fF/s after the sixth pulse, which corresponds to about six vesicles per second per active zone (21). It is estimated that this high retrieval rate is mostly (two thirds) due to rapid endocytosis, indicating that the fast component of endocytosis becomes dominant during stimulation.

The trigger for fast endocytosis is calcium. EGTA (10 mM) added to the presynaptic pipette blocked the fast component induction during a train of 200 AP-es at 100 Hz (Fig. 2.3e). Likewise, lowering the depolarization voltage during a train of ten 20-ms pulses at 1 Hz from 90 mV (−80 mV to +10 mV) to 75 mV (−80 mV to −5 mV) reduced the evoked calcium current and eliminated the fast component. Membrane accumulation is not the trigger for fast endocytosis, because 20 pulses at the reduced 75-mV jump at 1 Hz failed to elicit a fast component, though this stimulus caused a net accumulation (~1.5 picofarad [pF]) similar to the control condition (using 90-mV depolarization steps) in which fast endocytosis was observed (21).

The role of calcium in endocytosis has been investigated at several other synapses. At the frog neuromuscular junction, only a slow form of endocytosis is detected, and its rate is not sensitive to raised intracellular calcium levels (26). In cultured hippocampal neurons, experiments using synaptophluorin or sypHy have not detected a fast kinetic component of endocytosis, either (27–29). The rate of the single component is reduced when extracellular calcium is reduced, but raising Ca^{2+} levels above physiologic concentrations does not accelerate the endocytic process (29). At goldfish bipolar cells, endocytosis is fast following a brief depolarization (30,31), and can be slowed by adding EGTA or 1,2-bis(o-aminophenoxy)ethane-N,N,N′,N′-tetraacetic acid (BAPTA), another calcium chelator, to the patch pipette. However, during intensive stimulation, fast endocytosis appears to be slowed down or even blocked (30,32), which may be due to a buildup in intracellular calcium (30). The reasons for this apparent discrepancy have not been discovered, but it has been proposed that intensive stimulation causes nonsynchronous release to occur, far away from central active zones, and that these vesicles can only be retrieved through a slower pathway (32). A flash photolysis study in mouse cochlear inner hair cells has shown that a fast form of endocytosis is activated at internal calcium concentrations above $15\,\mu M$, and that above this level the percentage of total retrieval conducted by the fast component increases with calcium levels, though the τ stays the same (33). Thus, it appears that calcium regulation of endocytosis depends on the type of neuron.

Bulk Endocytosis and the Measurement of the Fission Pore Formation and Closure

An early, pioneering study of endocytosis using EM noted the appearance of large endosome-like structures in the nerve terminal after strong stimulation, from which small vesicles bud off (2). Further studies led to the widely held hypothesis that these endosome-like structures are generated slowly (~1 min) from the plasma membrane, a process called bulk endocytosis (34–39). However, the kinetic evidence indicating the instant of bulk membrane fission was missing at synapses. This section discusses a recent study at the calyx of Held that provides this missing piece of evidence (40).

Bulk membrane uptake could be detected after stimulation by step depolarizations and AP-e trains, and events were characterized by downward capacitance shifts (DCSs) with a 10% to 90% decay time between approximately 30 and 500 ms (Fig. 2.4a). The sizes of the DCSs ranged from the detection limit of ~20 fF up to 500 fF, with an average size of about 131 fF. These values were much larger than the membrane capacitance (~65 aF) of a single vesicle. Their size distribution was eccentric and peaked at the detection limit of ~20 fF, suggesting that there were possibly many more events that were too small to be detected (40).

The occurrence of DCSs increased with stimulation. The DCSs were detected during baseline recordings at a frequency of ~0.003 Hz; after ten 20-ms pulses (from −80 mV to +10 mV) at 10 Hz, the frequency increased to about 0.021 Hz in

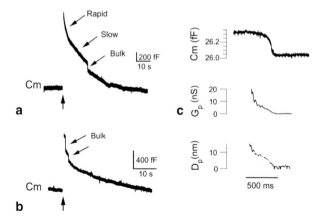

Fig. 2.4 Bulk endocytosis at the calyx of Held. (**a**) Three kinetic forms of endocytosis (arrows)—rapid, slow, and bulk endocytosis—were observed by whole-cell capacitance (Cm) recordings at the calyx of Held. The stimulus (vertical arrow) was 10 depolarizing pulses of 20 ms from −80 to +10 mV at 10 Hz. (**b**) The whole-cell membrane capacitance (Cm) response to 10 depolarizing pulses at 10 Hz (vertical arrow). The arrows indicate bulk endocytosis that occurred within a few seconds after the stimulus. (**c**) The whole-cell membrane capacitance (Cm), the fission pore conductance (G_p), and the fission pore diameter (D_p) during bulk endocytosis. (a–c: Adapted from Wu and Wu [40].)

the first 10 seconds after stimulation (Fig. 2.4b). The frequency decayed to baseline levels within 80 seconds and had a half decay time of <20 seconds. Vesicle fusion was required for this increase, as the increase was not seen after stimulation when exocytosis was blocked by botulinum neurotoxin C. The total amount of retrieval conducted by bulk endocytosis was about ~10% of the net exocytosis. This is likely an underestimate, since, as noted above, events below 20 fF in size could not be detected (40).

The diameter of the fission pore and the rate of closure were determined using the measured pore conductance, and with the assumption that the pore is cylindrical. The initial diameter ranged from approximately 3 to 19 nm, and decreased to undetectable levels within 500 ms (Fig. 2.4c). The slope of the 20% to 80% decrease in diameter was about 39 nm/s (Fig. 2.4c). The slope for each event was not correlated with the DCS size, suggesting that the fission step is separate from the fission pore formation step. Consistent with this suggestion, bulk membrane fission can occur as early as a few seconds after stimulation, and the rate of fission pore closure is much lower than the rate needed to form the fission pore in this time. Thus, bulk endocytosis is composed of two kinetically different steps: a membrane invagination step that forms the fission pore, and the closure of the pore that completes the fission process (40).

It should be noted that the frequency of DCSs peaked in less than 10 seconds after stimulation. Some bulk endocytosis events occurred at only a few seconds after the stimulus (Fig. 2.4b). Such a rapid time course is in sharp contrast to the current view that endosome-like structures are generated on a time scale of minutes (2,38,41,42). This discrepancy is likely due to methodologic differences. Electron microscopy has a low time resolution, whereas the capacitance measurement technique used in the present work provides a time resolution of milliseconds. Electron microscopy measures the lifetime of endosome-like structures, whereas the capacitance measurement indicates the time course of generating endosome-like structures from the plasma membrane. We suggest modifying the current view to a rapid generation of endosome-like structures, followed by the slow budding off of small vesicles from these structures.

Resolving Full Collapse Fusion and Kiss-and-Run with Cell-Attached Capacitance Recordings

We have discovered at least three kinetic forms of endocytosis at the whole-cell configuration at the calyx of Held. These forms are rapid, slow, and bulk endocytosis (Fig. 2.4a). Rapid endocytosis implies a kiss-and-run form of fusion, whereas slow endocytosis is consistent with full collapse fusion (43). However, other interpretations are possible. For example, imaging studies at goldfish retinal bipolar synapses raise the possibility that rapid endocytosis could be a result of full collapse fusion followed by rapid endocytosis (44). The key difference between these two modes of fusion is that kiss-and-run opens a fusion pore and closes the pore rapidly, whereas full collapse fusion fully expands the fusion pore. The only unambiguous way to distinguish these is to record fusion pore kinetics at synapses, which is technically challenging and rarely performed; correspondingly, whether kiss-and-run exists at synapses is currently under intense debate (45). Fusion pore kinetics in nonsynaptic preparations is most commonly measured using the cell-attached technique. When using this technique, the secretory vesicle membrane is modeled as a capacitor C_v, with a conductance G_p that is determined by the fusion pore. Both elements form a $G_p C_v$ series circuit that is added to the cell membrane capacitance C_m upon fusion (Fig. 2.5a). This section describes progress in adapting this technique to synaptic preparations, and a recent study using cell-attached recordings, which has resolved the fusion pore conductance at the calyx (46).

The cell-attached capacitance measurement technique provides a high enough resolution to detect single vesicle fusion events, which appear as unitary capacitance steps directly proportional to the vesicle size. Full vesicle incorporation into the plasma membrane produces an upward capacitance step, whereas kiss-and-run fusion produces an up-step followed within a few seconds by a down-step, called a capacitance flicker (5). In some of these fusion events, fusion pore conductance can be measured, allowing for an estimate of the fusion pore size (5).

Measurements of capacitance steps during large dense core vesicle fusion in endocrine and immune cells have provided a detailed picture of exocytosis of this

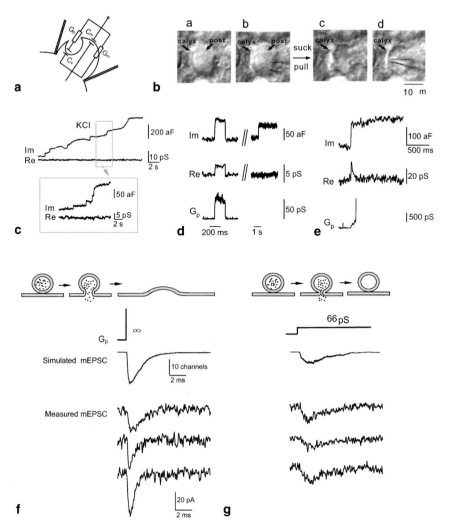

Fig. 2.5 Kiss-and-run and full collapse fusion recorded in the cell-attached mode at the calyx of Held. (**a**) Equivalent circuit of a patch in the cell attached mode, when a vesicle is fused with the plasma membrane and has opened a fusion pore. Double line indicates patch pipette. C_m, G_m, C_v, and G_p are cell membrane capacitance, cell membrane conductance, vesicle capacitance, and fusion pore conductance, respectively. (**b**) The procedure to perform cell-attached recordings at the release face of a calyx. A calyx associated with a postsynaptic neuron was first identified (a). The postsynaptic neuron was sucked and pulled away by a large pipette (b). After the postsynaptic neuron was removed (c), another pipette was positioned at the release face of the calyx membrane (d) for cell-attached recordings. Individual vesicle fusion events, like those shown in c and d, were recorded. (**c**) Im (imaginary component of the admittance, reflecting capacitance), Re (real component of the admittance, reflecting conductance) traces from cell-attached recordings during application of 25 mM KCl. The inset shows discrete capacitance up-steps. (**d**) Im, Re, and G_p during a capacitance flicker. A nonflicker up-step (right) occurring 10 seconds later was not accompanied by detectable Re changes, indicating proper phase adjustment. (**e**) Im, Re, and G_p during a full collapse fusion. Note that G_p was detected in this fusion event. (**f**) Top: Illustration of a full-collapse event. Middle:

vesicle class in nonneuronal cells (5). Extending this approach to synapses has been frustrated by two problems: First, the smaller size of vesicles makes resolving individual vesicle fusion more difficult. Second, the postsynaptic neuron apposing the presynaptic release site might make the release site inaccessible to the patch pipette. These two hurdles can be overcome. First, in pituitary nerve terminals (which do not form synapses), fusion of individual microvesicles similar in size to synaptic vesicles were resolved, demonstrating that these small events can in fact be detected (47,48). About 5% of fusion events were capacitance flickers with a fusion pore conductance of ~19 picosiemens (pS), indicating the existence of kiss-and-run fusion (47). Second, direct patch-clamp recordings of nerve terminals that are not associated with their postsynaptic counterpart have been made at a chick calyx-type synapse (49), synaptosomes (50), and the rat calyx of Held (46).

At the calyx of Held synapse, the release site can be exposed by pulling out the postsynaptic neuron using a large pipette (Fig. 2.5b). At the exposed release sites, cell-attached recordings reveal individual capacitance up-steps reflecting single vesicle fusion during high potassium application (Fig. 2.5c) (46). About 20% of fusion events were capacitance flickers. The capacitance flicker duration ranged from 10 ms to 2 seconds with a mean of ~300 ms (Fig. 2.5d). For most capacitance flickers, the fusion pore conductance was larger than 288 pS. The exact size could not be detected owing to the resolution limit. In a small fraction of capacitance flickers, however, a fusion pore conductance ranging from 15 to 288 pS with a mean of ~66 pS was observed, which might correspond to a fusion pore with a mean diameter of ~1.1 nm (Fig. 2.5d). These results suggest that a minor fraction of fusion events are kiss-and-run during high potassium application (46).

Most capacitance up-steps are not followed in a brief time by an equal size down-step, and thus reflect full-collapse fusion (46). Their initial fusion pores were often too large or too fast to resolve (Fig. 2.5d). However, in a small fraction of up-steps, an initial fusion pore conductance of ~250 pS was resolved, which was followed in approximately 10 to 300 ms by a rapid pore expansion (Fig. 2.5e) (46). These results provide the first kinetic evidence revealing the instant of full collapse fusion at synapses.

Fig. 2.5 (continued) The simulated mEPSC caused by a G_p >288 pS, as observed in 97% of fusion events. This trace was the average of the simulated mEPSC resulting from initial G_p values of ∞ and 288 pS. The scale bars also apply to g. Bottom: Three experimentally observed individual mEPSCs at the calyx of Held with a rapid rise time. The scale bars also apply to panel g. (**g**) Top: Illustration of a kiss-and-run event. Middle: The simulated mEPSC caused by a g_p of 66 pS, as observed in 3% of fusion events. Bottom: Three experimentally observed individual mEPSCs displaying a 10% to 90% rise time slower than 0.8 ms and an amplitude smaller than 25 pA. These represent about 1.1% of all observed events in ref. 46. (Adapted from He et al [46].)

The Impact of Kiss-and-Run Fusion on the Quantal Response

Synapses that are able to use kiss-and-run fusion may have two advantages, compared to those that use only full collapse. First, it allows for rapid and economical vesicle recycling, perhaps preventing some of the rundown in release during strong stimulation. Second, its narrow fusion pore could limit the rate of transmitter discharge out of the vesicle, resulting in a slower and smaller quantal response (Fig. 2.5g) compared to full collapse fusion (Fig. 2.5f). Control over the amplitude and the kinetics of the quantal response by regulation of the two fusion modes may contribute to synaptic plasticity (6). However, whether the fusion pore size is small enough to slow down transmitter diffusion was largely unclear. We have recently attempted to address this issue at the calyx-type synapse.

During capacitance flickers at the calyx-type synapse, the fusion pore conductance of most events was more than 288 pS, whereas the conductance in a minor fraction of events was on average ~66 pS. Knowing the fusion pore conductance (G_p), the fusion pore diameter (D_p) could be estimated by this equation (51,52): $D_p = (4G_p\rho\lambda/\pi)^{0.5}$, where ρ is the saline resistivity (100 Ω cm); and λ, the pore length, is taken as the length of a gap junction channel (15 nm). According to this equation, kiss-and-run fusion with a G_p of 66 pS corresponds to a D_p of 1.1 nm, and kiss-and-run fusion with a G_p more than 288 pS corresponds to a D_d of more than 2.3 nm. The values of the fusion pore diameter can be used to estimate the time constant (τ_{glu_v}) of transmitter diffusion from the vesicle to the synaptic cleft by the equation $\tau_{glu\_v} = (\tau D_v{}^3 / 6)/(\rho K_d G_p)$, where D_v is the vesicle diameter and K_d, the diffusion constant, is 3.3×10^{-6} cm^2 s^{-1} for glutamate in the synaptic cleft. Based on this equation, τ_{glu_v} is 2.3 ms for a G_p of 66 pS, and 0.54 ms for a G_p of 288 pS. These calculations suggest that kiss-and-run with a small fusion pore can slow down the diffusion of transmitter out of the vesicle. This suggestion was further confirmed by Monte Carlo simulations of quantal events with MCell 2.50, a program that models the three-dimensional random walk diffusion and reaction kinetics in complex spatial environments reflecting realistic cellular ultrastructure (53). The simulation shows that kiss-and-run fusion with a D_p of 1.1 nm would cause an mEPSC with a much slower rise and decay (Fig. 2.5g), and a smaller amplitude as compared to full collapse fusion with a D_p that is too large or too fast to resolve (Fig. 2.5f). Since kiss-and-run with a D_p of about 1.1 nm was detected in only ~3% of the total fusion events, small mEPSCs with a slow rise and decay must represent a very minor fraction of mEPSCs. Consistent with this prediction, less than ~1% of the measured mEPSCs were small and slow in both rise and decay (46). These results suggest that kiss-and-run with a small fusion pore may induce small and slow mEPSCs.

It should be pointed out that a small and slow mEPSC is not necessarily the result of kiss-and-run fusion with a small fusion pore. Many other mechanisms may also determine the amplitudes and the kinetics of mEPSCs. These mechanisms include variation in the vesicle size (54–56), the vesicular transmitter content (57–60), the distance between release sites and glutamate receptor clusters (61), differences in receptor subunit compositions (62), and release from boutons other than the calyx that form synapses at the principal cell in the medial nucleus of the trapezoid body (63).

Conclusion

Both whole-cell and cell-attached capacitance measurements have been successfully applied to the calyx of Held synapse in the past few years. Whole-cell recordings reveal three kinetically different forms of endocytosis: rapid, slow, and bulk endocytosis. Intense stimulation triggers rapid endocytosis by increasing the calcium influx, which may speed up vesicle recycling to catch up with the rapid rate of exocytosis. Bulk endocytosis was shown to occur faster than previously estimated, and to carry ~10% of the total endocytic load. Cell-attached recordings show two modes of fusion: kiss-and-run and full collapse fusion. Kiss-and-run fusion is followed by rapid endocytosis, whereas full collapse fusion is not. Kiss-and-run with a small fusion pore is likely to produce a small and slow quantal response. Switch between kiss-and-run and full collapse may thus be a mechanism by which synaptic plasticity can be achieved. Further experiments are needed to determine whether rapid and slow endocytosis observed at the whole-cell level reflect kiss-and-run and full collapse fusion, respectively.

References

1. De Camilli P, Slepnev VI, Shupliakov O, Brodin L. Synaptic vesicle endocytosis. In: Cowan WM, Sudhof TC, Stevens CF, eds. Synapses. Baltimore and London: Johns Hopkins University Press, 2001:217–274.
2. Heuser JE, Reese TS. Evidence for recycling of synaptic vesicle membrane during transmitter release at the frog neuromuscular junction. J Cell Biol 1973;57:315–344.
3. Ceccarelli B, Hurlbut WP, Mauro A. Turnover of transmitter and synaptic vesicles at the frog neuromuscular junction. J Cell Biol 1973;57:499–524.
4. Fesce R, Grohovaz F, Valtorta F, Meldolesi J. Neurotransmitter release, fusion or 'kiss and run'? Trends Cell Biol 1994;4:1–4.
5. Lindau M, Alvarez de Toledo G. The fusion pore. Biochim Biophys Acta 2003;164:167–173.
6. Choi S, Klingauf J, Tsien RW. Fusion pore modulation as a presynaptic mechanism contributing to expression of long-term potentiation. Philos Trans R Soc Lond B Biol Sci 2003;358(1432):695–705.
7. Wu LG. Kinetic regulation of vesicle endocytosis at synapses. Trends Neurosci 2004;27:548–554.
8. Betz WJ, Angleson JK. The synaptic vesicle cycle. Annu Rev Physiol 1998;60:347–363.
9. Von Gersdorff H, Borst JGG. Short-term plasticity at the calyx of Held. Nat Rev Neurosci 2002;3:53–64.
10. Sätzler K, Sohl L, Bollmann JH, et al. Three-dimensional reconstruction of a calyx of Held and its postsynaptic principal neuron in the medial nucleus of the trapezoid body. J Neurosci 2002;22:10567–10579.
11. Taschenberger H, Leao RM, Rowland KC, Spirou GA, Von Gersdorff H. Optimizing synaptic architecture and efficiency for high-frequency transmission. Neuron 2002;36:1127–1143.

12. Lenn NJ, Reese TS. The fine structure of nerve endings in the nucleus of the trapezoid body and the ventral cochlear nucleus. Am J Anat 1966;118:375–390.

13. Borst JGG, Sakmann B. Calcium influx and transmitter release in a fast CNS synapse. Nature 1996;383:431–434.

14. Wu LG, Westenbroek RE, Borst JGG, Catterall WA, Sakmann B. Calcium channel types with distinct presynaptic localization couple differentially to transmitter release in single calyx-type synapses. J Neuorsci 1999;19:726–736.

15. Iwasaki S, Momiyama A, Uchitel OD, Takahashi T. Developmental changes in calcium channel types mediating central synaptic transmission. J Neurosci 2000;20:59–65.

16. Dunlap K, luebke JI, Turner TJ. Exocytotic Ca^{2+} channels in mammalian central neurons. Trends Neurosci 1995;18:89–98.

17. Xu J, He L, Wu LG. Role of Ca(2+) channels in short-term synaptic plasticity. Curr Opin Neurobiol 2007;17(3):352–359.

18. Gillis KD. Techniques for membrane capacitance measurements. In: Sakmann B, Neher E, eds. Single-channel recording. New York: Plenum Press, 1995:155–198.

19. Sun JY, Wu LG. Fast kinetics of exocytosis revealed by simultaneous measurements of presynaptic capacitance and postsynaptic currents at a central synapse. Neuron 2001;30:171–182.

20. Sun JY, Wu XS, Wu W, Jin SX, Dondzillo A, Wu LG. Capacitance measurements at the calyx of Held in the medial nucleus of the trapezoid body. J Neurosci Methods 2004;134(2):121–131.

21. Wu W, Xu J, Wu XS, Wu LG. Activity-dependent acceleration of endocytosis at a central synapse. J Neurosci 2005;25:11676–11683.

22. Sun JY, Wu XS, Wu LG. Single and multiple vesicle fusion induce different rates of endocytosis at a central synapse. Nature 2002;417:555–559.

23. Wu XS, Xue L, Mohan R, Paradiso K, Gillis KD, Wu LG. The origin of quantal size variation: vesicular glutamate concentration plays a significant role. J Neurosci 2007;27(11):3046–3056.

24. Gentet LJ, Stuart GJ, Clements JD. Direct measurement of specific membrane capacitance in neurons. Biophys J 2000;79(1):314–320.

25. Yamashita T, Hige T, Takahashi T. Vesicle endocytosis requires dynamin-dependent GTP hydrolysis at a fast CNS synapse. Science 2005;307:124–127.

26. Wu LG, Betz WJ. Nerve activity but not intracellular calcium determines the time course of endocytosis at the frog neuromuscular junction. Neuron 1996;17:769–779.

27. Sankaranarayanan S, Ryan TA. Real-time measurements of vesicle-SNARE recycling in synapses of the central nervous system. Nat Cell Biol 2000;2(4):197–204.

28. Granseth B, Odermatt B, Royle SJ, Lagnado L. Clathrin-mediated endocytosis is the dominant mechanism of vesicle retrieval at hippocampal synapses. Neuron 2006;51(6):773–786.

29. Sankaranarayanan S, Ryan TA. Calcium accelerates endocytosis of vSNAREs at hippocampal synapses. Nat Neurosci 2001;4(2):129–136.

30. von Gersdorff H, Matthews G. Inhibition of endocytosis by elevated internal calcium in a synaptic terminal. Nature 1994;370:652–655.

31. Neves G, Lagnado L. The kinetics of exocytosis and endocytosis in the synaptic terminal of goldfish retinal bipolar cells. J Physiol 1999;515:181–202.

32. Neves G, Gomis A, Lagnado L. Calcium influx selects the fast mode of endocytosis in the synaptic terminal of retinal bipolar cells. Proc Natl Acad Sci U S A 2001;98(26):15282–15287.

33. Beutner D, Voets T, Neher E, Moser T. Calcium dependence of exocytosis and endocytosis at the cochlear inner hair cell afferent synapse. Neuron 2001;29(3):681–690.

34. Koenig JH, Ikeda K. Disappearance and reformation of synaptic vesicle membrane upon transmitter release observed under reversible blockage of membrane retrieval. J Neurosci 1989;9:3844–3860.

35. Koenig JH, Ikeda K. Synaptic vesicles have two distinct recycling pathways. J Cell Biol 1996;135:797–808.

36. Takei K, Mundigl O, Daniell L, De Camilli P. The synaptic vesicle cycle: a single vesicle budding step involving clathrin and dynamin. J Cell Biol 1996;133(6):1237–1250.

37. Teng H, Wilkinson RS. Clathrin-mediated endocytosis near active zones in snake motor boutons. J Neurosci 2000;20(21):7986–7993.

38. Richards DA, Guatimosim C, Betz WJ. Two endocytic recycling routes selectively fill two vesicle pools in frog motor nerve terminals. Neuron 2000;27(3):551–559.
39. Holt M, Cooke A, Wu MM, Lagnado L. Bulk membrane retrieval in the synaptic terminal of retinal bipolar cells. J Neurosci 2003;23(4):1329–1339.
40. Wu W, Wu LG. Rapid bulk endocytosis and its kinetics of fission pore closure at a central synapse. Proc Natl Acad Sci U S A 2007;104(24):10234–10239.
41. Richards DA, Guatimosim C, Rizzoli SO, Betz WJ. Synaptic vesicle pools at the frog neuromuscular junction. Neuron 2003;39:529–541.
42. de Lange RP, de Roos AD, Borst JG. Two modes of vesicle recycling in the rat calyx of Held. J Neurosci 2003;23(31):10164–10173.
43. Elhamdani A, Azizi F, Artalejo CR. Double patch clamp reveals that transient fusion (kiss-and-run) is a major mechanism of secretion in calf adrenal chromaffin cells: high calcium shifts the mechanism from kiss-and-run to complete fusion. J Neurosci 2006;26(11): 3030–3036.
44. Llobet A, Beaumont V, Lagnado L. Real-time measurement of exocytosis and endocytosis using interference of light. Neuron 2003;40(6):1075–1086.
45. He L, Wu LG. The debate on the kiss-and-run mode of fusion at synapses. Trends Neurosci 2007;30(9):447–455.
46. He L, Wu XS, Mohan R, Wu LG. Two modes of fusion pore opening revealed by cell-attached recordings at a synapse. Nature 2006;444:102–105.
47. Klyachko VA, Jackson MB. Capacitance steps and fusion pores of small and large-dense-core vesicles in nerve terminals. Nature 2002;418:89–92.
48. Debus K, Lindau M. Resolution of patch capacitance recordings and of fusion pore conductances in small vesicles. Biophys J 2000;78:2983–2997.
49. Stanley EF. Single calcium channels and acetylcholine release at a presynaptic nerve terminal. Neuron 1993;11:1007–1011.
50. Smith SM, Bergsman JB, Harata NC, Scheller RH, Tsien RW. Recordings from single neocortical nerve terminals reveal a nonselective cation channel activated by decreases in extracellular calcium. Neuron 2004;41:243–256.
51. Almers W, Breckenridge LJ, Iwata A, Lee AK, Spruce AE, Tse FW. Millisecond studies of single membrane fusion events. Ann N Y Acad Sci 1991;635:318–327.
52. Spruce AE, Breckenridge LJ, Lee AK, Almers W. Properties of the fusion pore that forms during exocytosis of a mast cell secretory vesicle. Neuron 1990;4:643–654.
53. Stiles JR, Bartol TB, Salpeter MM, Salpeter EE, Sejnowski TJ. Synaptic variability. In: Cowan TC, Sudhof TC, Stevens CF, eds. Synapses. Baltimore: Johns Hopkins University Press, 2000:681–732.
54. Bruns D, Riedel D, Klingauf J, Jahn R. Quantal release of serotonin. Neuron 2000;28: 205–220.
55. Zhang B, Koh YH, Beckstead RB, Budnik V, Ganetzky B, Bellen HJ. Synaptic vesicle size and number are regulated by a clathrin adaptor protein required for endocytosis. Neuron 1998;21:1465–1475.
56. Karunanithi S, Marin L, Wong K, Atwood HL. Quantal size and variation determined by vesicle size in normal and mutant Drosophila glutamatergic synapses. J Neurosci 2002;22: 10267–10276.
57. Song HJ, Ming GL, Fon E, Bellocchio E, Edwards RH, Poo MM. Expression of a putative vesicular acetylcholine transporter facilitates quantal transmitter packaging. Neuron 1997;18:815–826.
58. Wojcik SM, Rhee JS, Herzog E, et al. An essential role for vesicular glutamate transporter 1 (VGLUT1) in postnatal development and control of quantal size. Proc Natl Acad Sci U S A 2004;101:7158–7163.
59. Fremeau RT, Jr., Kam K, Qureshi T, et al. Vesicular glutamate transporters 1 and 2 target to functionally distinct synaptic release sites. Science 2004;304:1815–1819.
60. Wilson NR, Kang J, Hueske EV, et al. Presynaptic regulation of quantal size by the vesicular glutamate transporter VGLUT1. J Neurosci 2005;25:6221–6234.

61. Nielsen TA, Digregorio DA, Silver RA. Modulation of glutamate mobility reveals the mechanism underlying slow-rising AMPAR EPSCs and the diffusion coefficient in the synaptic cleft. Neuron 2004;42:757–771.

62. Jonas P. The Time Course of Signaling at Central Glutamatergic Synapses. News Physiol Sci 2000;15:83–89.

63. Hamann M, Billups B, Forsythe ID. Non-calyceal excitatory inputs mediate low fidelity synaptic transmission in rat auditory brainstem slices. Eur J Neurosci 2003;18: 2899–2902.

Chapter 3
Roles of SNARE Proteins in Synaptic Vesicle Fusion

Mark T. Palfreyman and Erik M. Jorgensen

Contents

Abstract Neurotransmitters are stored in small membrane-bound vesicles at synapses. Neurotransmitter release is initiated by depolarization of the neuron, which in turn activates voltage-gated calcium channels. Calcium influx then triggers the fusion of the synaptic vesicles with the plasma membrane. Fusion of the vesicular and plasma membranes is mediated by SNARE (soluble N-ethylmaleimide–sensitive factor attachment receptor) proteins. The SNAREs are now known to be used in all trafficking steps of the secretory pathway, including neurotransmission. This chapter describes the discovery of the SNAREs, their relevant structural features, models for their function, the specificity of interactions, and their interactions with the calcium-sensing machinery.

Keywords SNARE, syntaxin, SNAP-25, synaptobrevin, membrane fusion

Erik M. Jorgensen
Department of Biology and Howard Hughes Medical Institute, University of Utah,
Salt Lake City, UT 84112
e-mail: jorgensen@biology.utah.edu

Z.-W. Wang (ed.) *Molecular Mechanisms of Neurotransmitter Release,*
© Humana Press 2008 a part of Springer Science+Business Media, LLC

SNARE Discovery: A Convergence of Genetics and Biochemistry

To understand the mechanisms of synaptic vesicle fusion, it is useful to think about the evolution of neurotransmission. Eukaryotic cells separate cellular functions into membrane-bound organelles. The content of these organelles are moved between compartments and the extracellular environment by transport vesicles. Cellular compartments must be kept distinct, but membrane-impermeable cargo must be transferred to the target organelle. To transfer cargo the lipid bilayers of the vesicle and the target must merge so that their luminal contents can intermingle. In some cases, cargo must be secreted into the extracellular space via exocytosis. It was perhaps a small step for the cell to develop a mechanism for calcium-dependent regulation of exocytosis, but it was a giant leap for evolution. The nervous system is arguably the universe's greatest invention.

A convergence of independent tracks led to the identification of SNAREs as the central players in membrane fusion. In the late 1980s SNARE proteins were identified in the brain as components of the synapse. Specifically, synaptobrevin (also called vesicle-associated membrane protein [VAMP]) was purified from synaptic vesicles (1). Subsequently, two additional SNAREs, syntaxin and SNAP-25 (synaptosome-associated protein of 25 kDa), were found localized to the plasma membrane of neurons (2–4). The identification of homologues among the yeast *sec* genes linked the mechanisms of synaptic function to vesicular trafficking (5,6) and hinted at the universality of membrane fusion. Although the SNARE proteins were well placed to mediate synaptic vesicle fusion and were related to proteins required for trafficking, there was at this point no evidence that these proteins functioned in calcium-dependent exocytosis of synaptic vesicles.

The groups of Heiner Niemann, Reinhard Jahn, and Cesare Montecucco were looking for the targets of the clostridial toxins. The clostridial toxins from the anaerobic bacteria *Clostridium botulinum* and *Clostridium tetani* can potently inhibit neurotransmission (7). Thus, it was reasoned that their targets would identify essential proteins in synaptic transmission. Botulinum and tetanus toxins cleave the SNARE proteins, demonstrating the central role of the SNAREs in synaptic vesicle release (8–11). These were the first functional data that the SNAREs were involved in neurotransmission (12,13). The central role of the SNAREs in neurotransmission would later be confirmed from electrophysiologic studies on null mutants in the SNARE proteins in *Drosophila*, mice, and *Caenorhabditis elegans* (14–19). Thus, the functional data identified the SNAREs as perpetrators but their association had not been described.

The discovery that these proteins formed a complex was demonstrated soon after. Jim Rothman's group was taking a biochemical approach to understand trafficking in the Golgi apparatus. The toxin *N*-ethylmaleimide (NEM) potently inhibits Golgi trafficking (20). Wilson *et al* (21) found that the target of NEM was the mammalian homologue of a previously cloned yeast gene *SEC18* (22). Rothman's group named this new protein the NEM-sensitive factor (NSF) (23), and NSF was found to bind, via the action of the soluble NSF adaptors (SNAPs) (24), to a set of proteins from brain detergent extracts that came to be collectively known as the soluble *N*-ethylmaleimide–sensitive factor attachment receptor proteins (SNAREs). The evidence for SNARE involvement in synaptic vesicle exocytosis was now overwhelming, but a list of names in a complex did not constitute a model.

The first coherent model, called the SNARE hypothesis, would arise from the melding of the genetic and biochemical observations described above. Although wrong in detail, it would catalyze a number of hypothesis-driven experiments that would lead to more accurate models. Based on the finding that unique SNAREs are found at each of the trafficking steps (25,26), Thomas Söllner and Jim Rothman proposed that SNARE interactions provided the specificity for vesicular trafficking by tethering the vesicle to its target membrane (27,28). The SNAREs would then be acted on by the adenosine triphosphatase (ATPase) NSF which, by disassembling the SNAREs, would drive fusion (27,29).

Further experiments from Bill Wickner's lab, using a purified vacuole fusion assay, demonstrated that NSF acted not at the final fusion step of fusion, but rather to recover monomeric SNAREs for use in further rounds of fusion (30,31). NSF was acting as a chaperone to separate the embracing SNAREs on the plasma membrane to reactivate the system for further fusion (32,33). Thus assembly of the SNAREs, not disassembly, catalyzes fusion.

Finally, Rothman's group demonstrated that the SNAREs alone could fuse membranes. The SNAREs were incorporated into vesicles composed of artificial lipid bilayers. Donor vesicles containing synaptobrevin were capable of fusion with acceptor vesicles containing syntaxin and SNAP-25 (34). This experiment was extended to native membranes by engineering SNAREs to face out of the cell; in this configuration the SNAREs could induce fusion of whole cells (35). Thus, the current thinking is that the SNAREs function in the final steps in fusion and represent the minimal fusion machinery.

In the following sections we briefly define the steps leading to fusion, introduce the structure of the SNARE proteins, present a model for fusion, discuss SNARE specificity, and finally touch on the regulation of the SNARE complex by other proteins.

Definitions: The World Turned Upside Down and Given a Good Shake

In the past, synaptic vesicles were thought to dock with the plasma membrane, and then undergo a maturation step in which they became release ready. Depolarization activated a calcium sensor that then allowed the vesicle to fuse with the plasma membrane. Only a subset of docked vesicles were considered to be in the readily releasable pool (36). Thus, the life of a vesicle could be divided into four steps: docking, maturing to release-ready, calcium sensing, and fusing. The definition of these stages in vesicle fusion relied on morphologic and electrophysiologic criteria.

Current studies have sought to associate these pools with particular molecular interactions and thereby more precisely define these states.

Paradoxically, recent studies have tended to confuse rather than clarify the states of a vesicle. Although some have argued that very few docked vesicles are in the readily releasable pool (36,37), others suggest that docked vesicles are equivalent to the readily releasable pool (38–41). Studies of SNARE proteins have also muddied our previously clean definitions of these pools. The assembly of SNARE proteins between synaptic vesicle and plasma membrane is defined as vesicle "priming." Initial studies suggested that priming occurred after docking (15). However, recent studies suggest that the primed state may correspond to "docked" vesicles as observed in electron micrographs (14). Thus, the morphologic, electrophysiologic, and molecular definitions have seemingly converged on a single state. It is hoped that as the actions of various proteins are more precisely understood, we will once again refine synaptic vesicle fusion into discrete steps.

There is one last sorry note concerning our attempts to define steps in vesicle fusion: the terminology used for synaptic vesicle fusion is at odds with the terminology used in yeast. In yeast, *priming"* refers to the generation of free SNAREs rather than the formation of the SNARE complex, *tethering* rather than *docking* describes the initial membrane association, and *docking* includes SNARE engagement. Only the word *fusion* seems to mean the same thing in these different languages.

Molecular Characteristics of the SNAREs

The SNARE proteins are characterized by a conserved 60- to 70-amino-acid SNARE motif. Phylogenetic analysis indicates that SNARE proteins can be divided into four families (25,42,43). The individual SNARE motifs are largely unstructured in solution, but when all four family members are mixed, the SNARE motifs come together to form a four-helix parallel bundle known as the core complex (Fig. 3.1A,B) (44). The SNARE complex is remarkably stable and can only be separated by boiling in the presence of sodium dodecyl sulfate (SDS) (45,46). The hydrophobic residues of the alpha-helical SNARE motifs are oriented inward to form layers like those in the coiled coil domains of classical leucine zippers. However, the layer in the middle of the complex, called the "0" layer, is formed by ionic interactions between an arginine (R-SNARE) and three glutamines (Qa, Qb, and Qc SNAREs) (Fig. 3.1B,C). The role for these conserved residues buried in the hydrophobic core is briefly discussed in the next section. At each fusion site a unique SNARE complex consisting of all four flavors is formed. While other complexes have been observed *in vitro*, the only complexes that have been shown to efficiently support fusion are QabcR complexes (47–52).

The SNAREs that are used for synaptic vesicle exocytosis are synaptobrevin (R-SNARE, also called VAMP2), syntaxin 1a (Qa SNARE), and SNAP-25 (contains both the Qb and Qc SNARE motifs) (Fig. 3.1) (1–4,53).

In addition to the SNARE motifs, all three SNAREs contain sequences that anchor them to the membrane (Fig. 3.1A). Syntaxin and synaptobrevin are anchored

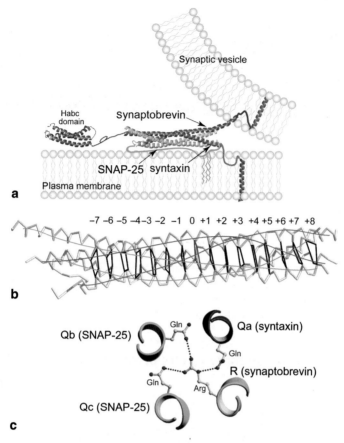

Fig. 3.1 Molecular description of the SNAREs. By assembling into a four-helix parallel bundle, the SNAREs bridge the gap between the two membranes destined to fuse. (**a**) In the case of the neuronal SNAREs, syntaxin (red) and SNAP-25 (green) are found on the plasma membrane and synaptobrevin (blue) is associated with the synaptic vesicle. The 60- to 70-amino-acid SNARE motifs form a four-helix bundle. Syntaxin and synaptobrevin contribute one SNARE motif and SNAP-25 contributes two. Syntaxin contains an additional regulatory domain composed of three alpha-helices called the Habc domain. Syntaxin and synaptobrevin are transmembrane proteins, while SNAP-25 is attached to the membrane via palmitoylation of the linker region. (**b**) The wire frame model shows the backbone of the SNARE motifs. The N-termini are at the left and the C-termini are at the right, matching the illustration in (A). The amino acids facing toward the center of this helix (denoted as layers −7 to +8) are largely hydrophobic in nature with the notable exception of the zero layer. (**c**) In the zero layer charged residues are oriented toward the center of the helix. Syntaxin contributes one glutamine (Qa), SNAP-25 contributes two glutamines (Qb and Qc), and synaptobrevin contributes one arginine (R). (A: Courtesy of Enfu Hui and Edwin R. Chapman. B: Adapted from Fasshauer et al [42]. C: Adapted from Bracher et al [195].)

via transmembrane domains. SNAP-25 is anchored via the palmitoylation of cysteines in the linker region connecting the two SNARE motifs. In all SNARE-based fusion reactions, each of the two membranes destined to fuse must contain a SNARE with a transmembrane domain; otherwise fusion will not occur (54).

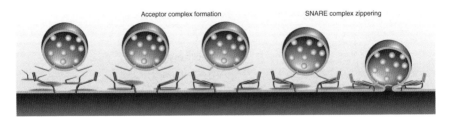

Fig. 3.2 Acceptor complex and zipper model for SNARE assembly. The Q SNAREs syntaxin and SNAP-25 assemble on the plasma membrane. This Qabc acceptor complex then contacts the distal N-terminus of synaptobrevin on the synaptic vesicle. This conformation is known as a "loose" SNARE complex. The "zippering" of the rest of the SNAREs into the complex serves two potential functions. First, full assembly of the SNAREs leads to close proximity between the membranes destined to fuse. Second, the zippering might provide torque that is transferred to the transmembrane domain leading to full fusion

Synaptobrevin is located on synaptic vesicles, while syntaxin and SNAP-25 are on the plasma membrane. The assembly of synaptobrevin, syntaxin, and SNAP-25 into the SNARE complex would thus bridge the vesicle and plasma membrane, forming what is known as a *trans* SNARE complex (Fig. 3.1A).

Assembly and Disassembly Cycles in SNARE Function

The steps in the assembly of the *trans* SNARE complex are still in dispute. Based on biochemical experiments using the yeast SNAREs, it was proposed that homologues of syntaxin (Sso1p) and SNAP-25 (Sec9p) might form an "acceptor complex" (55) (Fig. 3.2). A syntaxin–SNAP-25 complex was also subsequently proposed for the neuronal SNAREs (56). This acceptor complex greatly speeds up the assembly of the core complex (57). However, it is not known whether this complex exists *in vivo*. It has been shown that SNAP-25 and syntaxin can stably associate in cells (58). Specifically, a fluorescently tagged SNAP-25 generated an intramolecular fluorescence resonance energy transfer (FRET) signal upon assembly with syntaxin in PC12 cells.

This acceptor complex comprising one SNAP-25 molecule and one syntaxin molecule is highly reactive and will rapidly incorporate a second syntaxin molecule to form a dead-end Qaabc complex (55–58). This dead-end complex might be prevented *in vivo* by the action of tomosyn, a molecule with an R-SNARE domain (59,60). By occupying the synaptobrevin position in the complex, tomosyn might prevent the accumulation of the nonproductive Qaabc complexes and thus promote SNARE complex formation (60,61). However, this model is not consistent with the largely inhibitory role for tomosyn; genetic knockouts yield large increases in synaptic vesicle release (62,63). Tomosyn is thus more likely to bind to the acceptor complexes and, just like the Qaabc complexes, might form inactive complexes (62–64).

A second protein family that might serve to stabilize the acceptor complex is the SM (Sec1/Munc-18) family. At the synapse these proteins are called Unc18 proteins (UNC-18 in *C. elegans*, Munc18 in mammals, and ROP in *Drosophila*). It was originally thought that Unc18 exclusively bound to syntaxin monomers (65–69). However, more recent experiments have suggested alternative modes of binding (70–73). When reconstituted into lawns of plasma membrane, Unc18 was displaced from syntaxin by synaptobrevin but only when SNAP-25 was also present (70). Unc18 might therefore stabilize a syntaxin/SNAP-25 acceptor complex awaiting synaptobrevin (70). Nonetheless, it is still at present unclear how acceptor complexes are maintained or even whether they are true intermediates in core complex assembly. Indeed, synaptobrevin and syntaxin have been shown to assemble *in vitro* in the absence of SNAP-25 (74–76), suggesting that SNAP-25 might join the complex last. It has even been suggested that syntaxin might be the last molecule to enter the core complex *in vivo* (77). Until SNARE assembly can be monitored *in vivo*, we are forced to rely on these studies of *in vitro* SNARE interactions.

Once synaptobrevin enters the complex it is proposed to make contact at the N-terminal portion of the SNARE domain distal from the membrane. This conformation of the SNAREs is termed a loose configuration and is then thought to zipper down to a tight conformation (Fig. 3.2). Synaptic vesicles are held in a release-ready state in which the *trans* SNARE complex is likely to be arrested in a partially zippered state. Calcium binding to synaptotagmin would release arrest so that the SNARE complex could fully zipper to the tight conformation. This transition to the tight conformation would pull the transmembrane domains of the SNAREs, and hence the membranes, into close proximity and induce fusion (78,79). Models for the action of SNAREs in membrane fusion are described below.

Once the two membranes have merged, the core complex is now located in a single membrane and is referred to as a *cis* SNARE complex. To undergo further rounds of fusion, this *cis* complex must be disassembled and the SNAREs repartitioned to their appropriate compartments. Disassembly is mediated by the action of NSF and the SNAPs. Together NSF and the SNAPs are able to disassemble all SNARE complexes thus far tested (80). The ATPase NSF itself does not directly bind SNAREs; instead, it binds SNAREs through the action of the SNAPs. The SNAPs bind to the surface of the *cis* SNAREs around the central zero layer, which contains the conserved Q and R residues (81). The disassembly of the mammalian core complexes in PC12 cells is inhibited by mutation in these conserved residues (82). However, the disassembly of the *C. elegans* core complex is not affected by the same mutations (83). An alternative model for the function of these conserved residues is that they have a role before fusion in getting the four helixes to align in register to ensure that their transmembrane domains are directly opposed at their C-terminal ends (42,78). It has also been proposed that they might function in the prevention of full SNARE zippering (77). The next section explores how the formation of these SNARE complexes might catalyze fusion.

A Model for Membrane Fusion

Membranes do not spontaneously fuse, because of the high repulsive forces between two phospholipid bilayers 1 to 2 nm apart. How might the SNAREs fuse membranes? Three characteristics of the SNAREs are central to the current models for their function in fusing membranes. First, the assembled SNARE complex is remarkably stable. The formation of the SNARE complex is therefore an energy source that can be used to overcome barriers to fusion. Second, the SNARE complex must consist of at least two SNARE molecules with transmembrane domains (84). The transmembrane domains must be inserted into both of the membranes destined to fuse (54). Third, the SNAREs assemble in a parallel orientation (44,78,79,85). Due to the parallel orientation of the SNARE motifs, SNARE assembly leads to the close apposition of the transmembrane domains and hence the membranes themselves. This section describes how the assembly of the SNARE complexes might lead the membranes through the sequential intermediates of a lipid stalk, a hemifusion diaphragm, an initial fusion pore, and finally full fusion (Fig. 3.3).

The stability of the SNARE complexes combined with their parallel orientation led to the idea that their formation might provide the driving force for fusion. By first assembling at their N-terminals and subsequently "zippering" down to their membrane proximal C-terminals, the assembly of the SNAREs would bring the transmembrane domains of synaptobrevin and syntaxin into close proximity (77–79, 86–88) (Fig. 3.2). Evidence for zippering comes from two complementary experiments. First, biochemical and structural studies have shown that the membrane proximal domain of syntaxin becomes sequentially more ordered upon binding synaptobrevin in a directed N- to C-terminal fashion (55,57,87,89). The temperatures for assembly and disassembly of SNARE complex differ by as much as 10°C. Thus, assembly and dissociation follow different reaction pathways. This hysteresis suggests a kinetic barrier between folded and unfolded states (45). Mutations in the N-terminal hydrophobic core of the SNARE complex selectively slowed SNARE assembly, while those in the C-terminal did not slow assembly (56,87), suggesting that the N-terminal nucleates SNARE assembly. The kinetic barrier to assembly also suggests that loose SNARE complexes could be an intermediate.

The second line of evidence for zippering comes from *in vivo* disruption studies using clostridial toxins, antibodies directed toward the SNARE motifs, and mutations in the hydrophobic core of the SNARE complex (77,86–88,90). The toxin and antibody disruption studies demonstrated that the N-termini of SNAREs become resistant to cleavage or antibody block at early stages, while C-termini are only resistant to disruptions at late stages. As a specific example, Hua *et al* injected either botulinum toxin D, which cleaves free synaptobrevin at the N-terminal side of the SNARE motif, or botulinum toxin B, which cleaves synaptobrevin toward the C-terminal side of the SNARE motif (86). SNAREs cannot be cleaved once they have assembled into the four helix SNARE complex (46). Exocytosis from the crayfish neuromuscular junction was not sensitive to cleavage at the N-terminus of the SNARE motif, suggesting that this region was protected, presumably by the SNARE complex. By contrast, neurotransmitter release was blocked by cleavage at the C-terminus of the

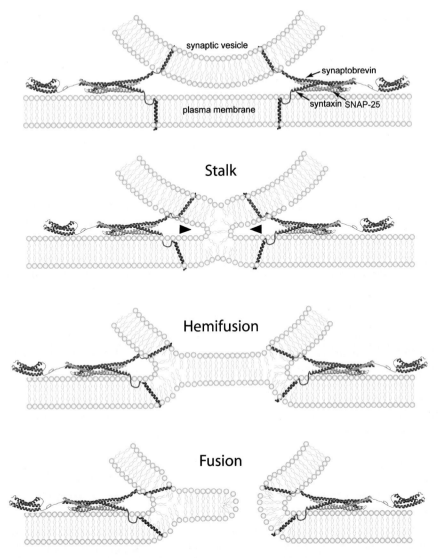

Fig. 3.3 A model for SNARE-mediated membrane fusion. The high repulsive forces between lipid membranes prevent them from fusing. The SNAREs are thought to provide the energy that enables the lipid rearrangements required for fusion. Pairing of the SNAREs brings the membranes into close proximity and leads to the merger of the proximal leaflet of the membranes to form a lipid stalk. The lipid stalk can then expand into a hemifusion diaphragm. Fusion is likely to require the transfer of energy from the SNARE motif to the transmembrane domains. It is thought that the weakest points lie at the edge of the hemifusion diaphragm. A rupture in the membrane at one of these points leads to fusion of the distal leaflet of the membranes and completes the fusion process. Regions of negative lipid curvature are indicated by arrowheads in the stalk. (Courtesy of Enfu Hui and Edwin R. Chapman.)

SNARE motif (86). Importantly, once the neuromuscular junction was electrically stimulated, botulinum toxin B was able to block exocytosis, demonstrating that the crayfish synaptobrevin monomers were indeed targets for the toxin. Thus, these data suggested that the N-terminus, but not the C-terminus, of synaptobrevin, is zippered into a SNARE complex in primed vesicles; presumably, calcium influx stimulates full zippering and membrane fusion.

As a second example, the mutations in the hydrophobic core of the SNARE complex have been expressed in neurosecretory chromaffin cells (87,90). Mutations in the C-terminal hydrophobic core incrementally reduced the kinetics of the rapid component of secretion, while those in the N-terminal reduced the sustained component of release, which is thought to correspond to engagement of new SNARE complexes (87). Importantly, the N-terminal mutants did not change the kinetics of the fast or slow components of release, only the amplitude of the response. Thus, it was interpreted that the C-terminal mutations were slowing "zippering" while those in the N-terminal were disrupting nucleation of the SNARE complexes (87). By contrast, when SNAREs bearing mutations in the hydrophobic core were introduced into the neurosecretory PC12 cells, there was no gradient in the efficacy of mutations in the kinetics of exocytosis (90).

The zippering of the membrane proximal portion of the SNARE complex likely serves two functions. First, the SNAREs are thought to catalyze the formation of a "hemifusion" transition state in which the proximal membrane leaflets have merged. This state can be achieved with comparatively low-energy requirements (91–94) and might simply need the SNAREs to bring the membranes into close proximity (95). Second, the SNAREs have been proposed to open up a fusion pore. This step requires the transmembrane domains of the SNAREs and likely involves the transfer of energy from the zippering of the SNARE cytoplasmic domains being passed to the transmembrane domain in order to locally disrupt lipid membranes (96).

Inspired by experiments in viral fusion and modeling of lipid bilayers, it is proposed that the initial steps of membrane merger result in a lipid stalk (97,98). The stalk corresponds to an hourglass-like structure that may contain as few as a dozen lipid molecules (98–100). The expansion of the stalk then results in a hemifusion diaphragm (91,101). These steps are not as highly energetically unfavorable as later steps and can be experimentally observed by dehydration of planar lipid bilayers, even in the absence of SNAREs (92,93,100,102). Direct evidence for lipid stalks has come from x-ray–scattering experiments that have given us a structure of this intermediate (100). The hemifusion state has been shown to be a metastable intermediate *in vivo* and can be observed for extensive periods of time in certain fusion reactions (103). Importantly, *in vitro* liposome fusion experiments have shown that hemifusion is an intermediate in the fusion pathway mediated by the synaptic vesicle SNAREs (104–106). Hemifusion intermediates have also been seen at central synapses using conical electron tomography; hemifused vesicles corresponded to those vesicles that were docked at the active zone (107).

Aside from the tomography and x-ray–scattering experiments, the evidence for stalk intermediates and hemifusion diaphragms comes from two observations:

the sensitivity of the fusion reaction to lipids of different intrinsic curvature (108), and the exchange of lipid membrane without luminal content mixing (103,109–111). The intrinsic curvature of lipids is determined by the ratio of the size of the lipid head group to their acyl chain tails. For example, a lipid with a single acyl chain would promote a positive intrinsic curvature (convex). At stalk structures and hemifusion diaphragms the outer, nonfused monolayer must adopt a negative curvature (concave) (arrowheads in Fig. 3.3) compared to the fused proximal monolayer, which adopts a net positive curvature (Fig. 3.3). This model predicts that, when added at the final steps of fusion, lipids with negative curvature would stimulate fusion while those with positive curvature would hinder fusion. Indeed, for all fusion reactions thus far tested, this prediction has been borne out (112). The application of lipids with altered curvature has been particularly useful in determining at which step fusion is arrested in various experimental manipulations (91,95,112).

When the SNARE transmembrane domain is replaced by artificial lipid anchors or when the transmembrane domain is truncated, fusion no longer proceeds (95,96,113). However, these perturbations do lead to a state in which lipids can exchange—a hallmark of hemifusion (91). Interestingly, replacement of the membrane anchor of the influenza hemagglutinin with an artificial membrane anchor, a glycosylphosphatidylinositol (GPI) tail, traps influenza viral fusion at a hemifusion stage (111). This observation demonstrates that membrane fusion events as varied as synaptic vesicle exocytosis and viral fusion might use a common mechanism to catalyze fusion. Importantly, the fusion arrest that results from the replacement of the transmembrane domain in both SNARE-based fusion and viral fusion can be bypassed by the addition of lipids with intrinsic negative curvature to the outer membrane or lipids that induce positive curvature to the inner membrane (95,114,115). This demonstrates that the proximity resulting from the SNARE pairing might be enough to achieve a hemifusion state, but that full fusion requires the transmembrane domains of the respective fusion proteins (95,111,114).

The dependence on the transmembrane domains for full fusion also suggests that the zippering of the SNAREs might result in the transduction of force to the transmembrane domain. The domain linking the SNARE motif to the membrane may be rather rigid; when synaptobrevin and syntaxin are placed in planar bilayers, they stand straight up from the membrane (116,117). Disrupting this rigidity by the addition of flexible linkers of incremental lengths, between the SNARE motif and the transmembrane domain, incrementally reduces fusion to complete elimination (50,96,113,118). In addition, mutations in the linker domain do not disrupt liposome fusion, while those in the SNARE motif have dramatic effects (119). This experiment favors the model of the linker as largely a force transducer (119). By contrast, mutations in the linker domain of yeast syntaxin (Sso1p) do cause dramatic decreases in fusion (120). Nonetheless, these results suggest that the winding of the SNARE proteins during core complex assembly transduces force to the transmembrane domains (96,116). Torque on the transmembrane domains might force dimples in the lipid bilayer at regions of *trans* SNARE complex formation (84) (Fig. 3.3).

It is likely that more than one core complex is required to catalyze fusion. Like viral fusion proteins, the SNAREs used in exocytosis also seem to work as higher order multimers (121). Thus, a ring of SNAREs could induce a controlled local disruption of lipids. One possibility is that the hemifusion diaphragm would be delineated by a ring of SNARE transmembrane domains (84,121). Alternatively, it has been suggested that the transmembrane domains of the SNAREs might serve as a proteinaceous pore (122). Though the interactions are quite weak (123), it has been shown that both syntaxin and synaptobrevin form higher order multimers via conserved regions located in their transmembrane domains (124–127). Electron microscopy has provided images of these multimers and shows that they form star-shaped structures with the transmembrane domains at the vertex (128). *In vivo* evidence for the existence of such multimers comes from the cooperative action of the SNAREs and dose dependency of inhibition by botulinum neurotoxins and SNARE peptide blockers (121,129–132). Together, the evidence has suggested multimers containing from between three and 15 complexes (121). Nonetheless, working models for multimerization are currently quite preliminary; it will remain to be seen how these multimers might aid in catalyzing fusion.

The Reliable Opposition: Protein Models for the Fusion Pore

Despite the appeal and considerable evidence for a lipidic fusion pore, there remain data suggesting that the fusion pore could be proteinaceous (133). First, it has been proposed that the SNAREs are the fusogen but that the pore is lined by the transmembrane of the five to eight syntaxin molecules rather than by lipids (122). This model derived from the observation that the replacement of residues in the transmembrane domain of syntaxin with bulky amino acids slowed the conductance of the initial fusion pore. Second, some data indicate that SNAREs were not involved in the fusion step. NSF disassembles SNARE complexes, yet in yeast overexpression of NSF (Sec18p) did not block vacuole fusion (134). Third, techniques that can detect early stages of pore formation, amperometry, and capacitance measurements indicate that the fusion pore in chromaffin cells might be formed by a protein. In these experiments the initial fusion pore was found to have a pore size equivalent to a large ion channel (approximately 1 to 2 nm in diameter) (135). In addition, these initial fusion pores "flickered" like ion channel fusion pores (132,135,136). Fourth, it has been proposed that the V_o sector of the vacuolar ATPase could act as a protein-aceous fusion pore (137,138). In yeast, calcium and calmodulin might be required in a step after SNARE complex formation in the process of fusion (139). The target of calcium-calmodulin in this late step in fusion was identified as the V_o sector of the vacuolar ATPase (137). Furthermore, analysis of *Drosophila* mutants indicated that the vacuolar ATPase was important for fusion of synaptic vesicles (140).

Nonetheless, several points are difficult to reconcile with a protein pore–based model for fusion. First, *trans* SNARE complexes are resistant to the action of NSF, suggesting that functional SNAREs were still present in yeast experiments (141).

Second, fusion pore sizes have been found to vary considerably in different fusion reactions, an observation more consistent with a lipid-based pore (142). Third, null mutants in many of the SNAREs proteins have been shown to have a stronger phenotype—often they are completely inviable—than respective mutants in the vacuolar ATPase (143). Fourth, lysophosphatidyl choline, a lipid that induces positive membrane curvature, is able to block all fusion reactions so far tested (112). Finally, the observed fusion pore flickering has been seen in pure lipid bilayers induced to fuse by polyethylene glycol (PEG) (144). PEG dehydrates the spaces between lipid bilayers and drives lipid mixing. Flickering is therefore not a hallmark solely of proteinaceous fusion pores.

Other observations that are apparently inconsistent with the lipid-based model for fusion have arisen from liposome fusion assays. For example, NSF and other proteins can catalyze the fusion of liposomes (145). However, the liposome fusion assay can be problematic (146). First, the lipid composition is critical in these assays and can produce misleading results; NSF could no longer fuse membranes when more physiologic lipid mixes were used (147). Second, many liposome fusion assays have used excessive and nonphysiologic concentrations of the SNARE molecules. Third, in most instances the speed of neurotransmitter release has not been replicated in this assay. Thus, results from liposome fusion assays must be interpreted cautiously and be supported by *in vivo* or genetic experiments.

SNAREs Encode Specificity

The original SNARE hypothesis proposed that compartmental specificity of fusion was encoded by SNARE proteins. Each intracellular fusion would be mediated by a specific set of SNARE proteins and thereby provide an addressing system for vesicle trafficking (27,28). This model makes several predictions. First, SNAREs should only bind their cognate SNARE partners. Second, SNAREs should only catalyze fusion when mixed with their SNARE partners. Third, SNAREs should be required for docking of vesicles to the correct target membrane. Fourth, the removal of a SNARE should selectively and completely eliminate fusion in one and only one fusion reaction. All of these hypotheses have been tested.

In vitro, the binding between cytoplasmic SNARE motifs is surprisingly promiscuous (148–150). However, these same SNAREs exhibited specificity in catalyzing fusion reactions when inserted into artificial lipid bilayers (151, 152). Specifically, only cognate SNARE complexes could catalyze fusion reaction. To date, out of the 275 pairwise combinations of yeast SNAREs tried, only nine are functional in the liposome fusion assay. Eight of these nine SNARE combinations represented interactions that occur *in vivo*, thus the specificity of fusion is greater than 99% (274/275) accurate (151). This specificity is preserved among the neuronal SNAREs; after cleavage of SNAP-25 in PC12 cells, secretion could only be rescued by SNAP-25 itself and not other SNAP-25 homologues (153). Thus, the SNAREs can encode the specificity of fusion.

Morphologic docking of synaptic vesicles long appeared to be independent of SNAREs. Genetic or pharmacologic disruption of SNAREs did not perturb synaptic vesicle docking (12,13,15,154). However, more recent experiments indicate that docking of synaptic vesicles (14) and dense core vesicles requires syntaxin (155–157). Importantly, if syntaxin is required for docking, experiments claiming roles for syntaxin in fusion must be interpreted with caution since fusion is downstream of docking. Docking defects will lead by necessity to defects in fusion. The discrepancy for syntaxin's role in docking could be due to different morphologic definitions of docking, which has been defined as everything from direct contact with the plasma membrane to vesicles 50 nm from the plasma membrane. Alternatively, additional docking factors might be present in some cell types to ensure the specificity of fusion (155). For example, syntaxin is required for docking in neurosecretory cells but not neurons in mice (155,157). Perhaps tethering factors also contribute to docking of synaptic vesicles at the active zone (158–162). Overlapping roles for SNAREs and docking factors have been observed in yeast (163,164). Specifically, *sec35* encodes a tethering protein for Golgi trafficking in yeast; *sec35* mutants can be partially bypassed by overexpression of the relevant SNARE proteins (165). Similarly, overexpression of SNAREs can bypass mutations in the tethering complex for plasma membrane fusion (166,167). It is likely that these overlapping redundant functions are necessary to achieve the high level of fidelity seen in membrane trafficking.

Thus far *in vivo* perturbations of the SNAREs have mostly been shown to selectively eliminate single trafficking steps. However, in all cases fusion was not completely eliminated. There are two possible explanations. First, it is possible that the SNAREs are not executing fusion—an unlikely interpretation given the wealth of data described above. Second, the SNAREs might be partially redundant. Evidence so far points to the latter interpretation. Knockout mice in synaptobrevin II were found to retain some synaptic activity in hippocampal neurons (16). In chromaffin cells, this remnant activity could be attributed to the synaptobrevin paralog cellubrevin (168). Redundancy can also explain the remaining fusion events in synaptobrevin null *Drosophila* mutants. Syb, the *Drosophila* equivalent of cellubrevin, can functionally substitute for n-Syb, the *Drosophila* equivalent of synaptobrevin, when overexpressed in neurons (169). Redundancy is also seen in the Q SNAREs. SNAP-23, SNAP-47, and SNAP-24 can provide partial function when SNAP-25 is absent (19,170,171). Finally, redundancy might also explain the almost complete lack of phenotype in syntaxin 1a knockout mice (172), where it is likely that syntaxin 1b is sufficient to almost entirely replace syntaxin 1a action. These observations are supported by experiments in yeast where redundancy between SNAREs has also been conclusively demonstrated in numerous trafficking reactions (173–175). By contrast, loss of syntaxin (*unc-64*) in *C. elegans* neurons results in a 500-fold reduction in neurotransmitter release with no apparent developmental defects (14); UNC-64 is committed to synaptic vesicle fusion and is unlikely to have a redundant syntaxin, like in mice; nor is it involved in other cellular functions, like in flies (176). In summary, the SNAREs do encode specificity; nonetheless, in some instances it is likely that other factors can provide overlapping functions to ensure that fusion happens with the appropriate target membrane.

SNARE Regulation

We will only touch on SNARE regulation briefly in this chapter, since other chapters will cover this topic in greater depth. SNARE regulation can roughly be divided into two forms: before and after initiation of complex formation. Before core complex formation, regulation involves occlusion of the SNARE motif of syntaxin to prevent the assembly of SNARE core complexes. After the initiation of SNARE assembly regulation likely takes place at the level of complex zippering. The calcium-sensing machinery works at these later steps.

Syntaxin itself has its own regulatory domain; the N-terminal Habc domain can fold over and occlude the SNARE motif (Fig. 3.1). Syntaxin can adopt two conformations: a closed form, in which the SNARE motif is occluded, and an open form, in which the SNARE motif is available to interact with SNAP-25 and synaptobrevin. At least two synaptic proteins, Unc13 and Unc18 proteins, have been proposed to act directly on this N-terminal extension of syntaxin (65,177). In *C. elegans, unc-13* mutants can be partially bypassed by an open form of syntaxin, demonstrating a direct or indirect role of UNC-13 in the conversion of syntaxin from a closed to an open form (14,62,178). Several additional proteins may regulate SNARE complex assembly by directly occluding the SNARE motif of syntaxin. These molecules include tomosyn, amisyn, and syntaphilin (59,62–64,179–181).

At steps after core complex assembly, regulation might take place at the level of preventing full zippering of the SNARE proteins. Three proteins—Unc18, complexin, and synaptotagmin—may act at this late stage. The precise function of the SM superfamily of proteins, which include the Unc18 synaptic proteins, is not yet known (see Chapter 7), but Unc18 proteins might function in these later stages (70–73,182–184). Sec1p, the yeast SM homologue that acts at the plasma membrane, binds to the SNARE complex rather than syntaxin monomers (185). Recent data suggest that Unc18 also uses this mode of interaction (70–73).

Complexin and synaptotagmin serve as part of the calcium-sensing machinery. The coupling of fusion to calcium influx is the key evolutionary modifications of SNARE function to adapt it for neurotransmission. At synapses, the time delay between the elevation in calcium concentration and the postsynaptic response can be as little as 60 to 200 μs (186). Though calcium is needed for fusion in other membrane trafficking steps, it usually serves as a facilitator of fusion rather than directly functioning as a signal in triggering fusion (187,188). The addition of complexin and synaptotagmin appear to impart the calcium trigger to SNARE-mediated fusion (189, 190). Complexin appears to act as a fusion clamp—a brake preventing constitutive fusion from occurring (191–194).

Interestingly, recent experiments have shown that the complexin clamp holds the SNAREs in a state where the membranes are hemifused (193). This observation demonstrates that the transition from hemifusion to full fusion can be regulated at the cytoplasmic SNARE motifs. Complexin sits in a groove between syntaxin and synaptobrevin, potentially preventing the full zippering of the core SNARE complex (195,196). The calcium sensor is synaptotagmin (197–201). Synaptotagmin binds to lipids and to syntaxin and SNAP-25 in a calcium-dependent manner (200–204). Importantly, synaptotagmin appears to compete with complexin for SNARE complex binding and relieves the clamp when calcium is present (reviewed in ref. 194). One possibility is that calcium binding allows synaptotagmin to actively displace complexin from the SNARE complex, which is then free to fully wind and to break the membrane of the hemifused intermediate. In this model the SNAREs could function like a wheel, with complexin the stick in the spokes preventing the wheel from turning. Calcium binding to synaptotagmin would pull the stick from the spokes and allow the wheel to turn and drive fusion. This model, however, remains speculative, and several pieces of data are currently incompatible with the above model. First, complexin knockout in mice do not have elevated synaptic vesicle fusion, as would be predicted (205). In addition, synaptotagmin when reconstituted with the neuronal SNAREs in the liposome fusion assay, can act alone as both a fusion clamp in the absence of calcium as well as an accelerator of fusion in the presence of calcium (206). However, a second group did not observe calcium sensitivity in SNARE-mediated liposome fusion assays by the addition of synaptotagmin; instead, synaptotagmin simply accelerated the rate of liposome fusion independent of calcium (207). Since subsequent chapters will delve further into the murky depths of calcium regulation, here we will suffice to stay in the shallow end of the pool.

Conclusion

Rounds of SNARE assembly and disassembly lie at the center of all vesicular trafficking. Assembly of the SNAREs into a four-helix bundle drives fusion of synaptic vesicles with the plasma membrane and thereby mediates the release of neurotransmitter. The entwined SNAREs are then pulled apart by the ATPase NSF, which reenergizes the system for further rounds of fusion. This model is widely accepted, yet its details are in considerable dispute. So far, reconstitution experiments have examined interactions between only a very few of the proteins involved in what is undoubtedly a complex and highly regulated fusion machine. As such, they have given us largely static images of the complex. Thus, the overarching challenge in the coming years will be to understand the regulation of the SNAREs and how the assembly of SNAREs catalyzes fusion.

Several questions must be resolved. First, is a preassembled Q-SNARE acceptor complex present on the plasma membrane *in vivo*, and if so how is it stabilized? Second, how is assembly of the SNAREs regulated? SNARE regulators, including MUN domain proteins such as Unc13, SM proteins, and Tomosyn, have been identified, yet their mechanism of action is unclear. Third, are SNAREs fully zippered prior to or during fusion? Fourth, is SNARE complex zippering arrested in the readily releasable pool of synaptic vesicles? Fifth, does formation of the SNARE complex generate a hemifusion intermediate? And finally, what rearrangements occur in the SNARE complex when synaptotagmin binds calcium and phospholipids?

Acknowledgments We thank Enfu Hui and Edwin R. Chapman for providing versions of Figures 3.1 and 3.3. Thanks also to Winfried Weissenhorn, Dirk Fasshauer, and Reinhard Jahn for allowing us to use and modify their images for Figure 3.1. Michael Ailion, Eric Bend, M. Wayne Davis, and Robert Hobson were instrumental in reading early versions of the manuscript.

References

1. Trimble WS, Cowan DM, Scheller RH. VAMP-1: a synaptic vesicle-associated integral membrane protein. Proc Natl Acad Sci U S A 1988;85(12):4538–4542.
2. Inoue A, Obata K, Akagawa K. Cloning and sequence analysis of cDNA for a neuronal cell membrane antigen, HPC-1. J Biol Chem 1992;267(15):10613–10619.
3. Bennett MK, Calakos N, Scheller RH. Syntaxin: a synaptic protein implicated in docking of synaptic vesicles at presynaptic active zones. Science 1992;257(5067):255–259.
4. Oyler GA, Higgins GA, Hart RA, et al. The identification of a novel synaptosomal-associated protein, SNAP-25, differentially expressed by neuronal subpopulations. J Cell Biol 1989; 109(6 pt 1):3039–3052.
5. Brennwald P, Kearns B, Champion K, Keranen S, Bankaitis V, Novick P. Sec9 is a SNAP-25–like component of a yeast SNARE complex that may be the effector of Sec4 function in exocytosis. Cell 1994;79(2):245–258.
6. Novick P, Field C, Schekman R. Identification of 23 complementation groups required for post-translational events in the yeast secretory pathway. Cell 1980;21(1):205–215.
7. Burgen AS, Dickens F, Zatman LJ. The action of botulinum toxin on the neuro-muscular junction. J Physiol 1949;109(1–2):10–24.
8. Blasi J, Chapman ER, Link E, et al. Botulinum neurotoxin A selectively cleaves the synaptic protein SNAP-25. Nature 1993;365(6442):160–163.
9. Blasi J, Chapman ER, Yamasaki S, Binz T, Niemann H, Jahn R. Botulinum neurotoxin C1 blocks neurotransmitter release by means of cleaving HPC-1/syntaxin. EMBO J 1993;12(12):4821–4828.
10. Link E, Edelmann L, Chou JH, et al. Tetanus toxin action: inhibition of neurotransmitter release linked to synaptobrevin proteolysis. Biochem Biophys Res Commun 1992;189(2): 1017–1023.
11. Schiavo G, Benfenati F, Poulain B, et al. Tetanus and botulinum-B neurotoxins block neurotransmitter release by proteolytic cleavage of synaptobrevin. Nature 1992;359(6398):832–835.
12. Marsal J, Ruiz-Montasell B, Blasi J, et al. Block of transmitter release by botulinum C1 action on syntaxin at the squid giant synapse. Proc Natl Acad Sci U S A 1997;94(26):14871–14876.
13. O'Connor V, Heuss C, De Bello WM, et al. Disruption of syntaxin-mediated protein interactions blocks neurotransmitter secretion. Proc Natl Acad Sci U S A 1997;94(22):12186–12191.
14. Hammarlund M, Palfreyman MT, Watanabe S, Olsen S, Jorgensen EM. Open syntaxin docks synaptic vesicles. PLoS Biol 2007;5(8):e198.
15. Broadie K, Prokop A, Bellen HJ, O'Kane CJ, Schulze KL, Sweeney ST. Syntaxin and synaptobrevin function downstream of vesicle docking in *Drosophila*. Neuron 1995;15(3):663–673.
16. Schoch S, Deak F, Konigstorfer A, et al. SNARE function analyzed in synaptobrevin/VAMP knockout mice. Science 2001;294(5544):1117–1122.
17. Washbourne P, Thompson PM, Carta M, et al. Genetic ablation of the t-SNARE SNAP-25 distinguishes mechanisms of neuroexocytosis. Nat Neurosci 2002;5(1):19–26.
18. Deitcher DL, Ueda A, Stewart BA, Burgess RW, Kidokoro Y, Schwarz TL. Distinct requirements for evoked and spontaneous release of neurotransmitter are revealed by mutations in the *Drosophila* gene neuronal-synaptobrevin. J Neurosci 1998;18(6):2028–2039.
19. Vilinsky I, Stewart BA, Drummond JA, Robinson IM, Deitcher DL. A *Drosophila* SNAP-25 null mutant reveals context-dependent redundancy with SNAP-24 in neurotransmission. Genetics 2002;162(1):259–271.

20. Balch WE, Glick BS, Rothman JE. Sequential intermediates in the pathway of intercompartmental transport in a cell-free system. Cell 1984;39(3 Pt 2):525–536.

21. Wilson DW, Wilcox CA, Flynn GC, et al. A fusion protein required for vesicle-mediated transport in both mammalian cells and yeast. Nature 1989;339(6223):355–359.

22. Eakle KA, Bernstein M, Emr SD. Characterization of a component of the yeast secretion machinery: identification of the SEC18 gene product. Mol Cell Biol 1988;8(10): 4098–4109.

23. Block MR, Glick BS, Wilcox CA, Wieland FT, Rothman JE. Purification of an N-ethylmaleimide-sensitive protein catalyzing vesicular transport. Proc Natl Acad Sci U S A 1988;85(21):7852–7856.

24. Clary DO, Griff IC, Rothman JE. SNAPs, a family of NSF attachment proteins involved in intracellular membrane fusion in animals and yeast. Cell 1990;61(4):709–721.

25. Bock JB, Matern HT, Peden AA, Scheller RH. A genomic perspective on membrane compartment organization. Nature 2001;409(6822):839–841.

26. Jahn R, Lang T, Südhof TC. Membrane fusion. Cell 2003;112(4):519–533.

27. Söllner T, Whiteheart SW, Brunner M, et al. SNAP receptors implicated in vesicle targeting and fusion. Nature 1993;362(6418):318–324.

28. Söllner T, Bennett MK, Whiteheart SW, Scheller RH, Rothman JE. A protein assembly-disassembly pathway in vitro may correspond to sequential steps of synaptic vesicle docking, activation, and fusion. Cell 1993;75(3):409–418.

29. Rothman JE. Intracellular membrane fusion. Adv Second Messenger Phosphoprotein Res 1994;29:81–96.

30. Mayer A, Wickner W, Haas A. Sec18p (NSF)-driven release of Sec17p (alpha-SNAP) can precede docking and fusion of yeast vacuoles. Cell 1996;85(1):83–94.

31. Nichols BJ, Ungermann C, Pelham HR, Wickner WT, Haas A. Homotypic vacuolar fusion mediated by t- and v-SNAREs. Nature 1997;387(6629):199–202.

32. Littleton JT, Chapman ER, Kreber R, Garment MB, Carlson SD, Ganetzky B. Temperature-sensitive paralytic mutations demonstrate that synaptic exocytosis requires SNARE complex assembly and disassembly. Neuron 1998;21(2):401–413.

33. Grote E, Carr CM, Novick PJ. Ordering the final events in yeast exocytosis. J Cell Biol 2000;151(2):439–452.

34. Weber T, Zemelman BV, McNew JA, et al. SNAREpins: minimal machinery for membrane fusion. Cell 1998;92(6):759–772.

35. Hu C, Ahmed M, Melia TJ, Söllner TH, Mayer T, Rothman JE. Fusion of cells by flipped SNAREs. Science 2003;300(5626):1745–1749.

36. Wickelgren WO, Leonard JP, Grimes MJ, Clark RD. Ultrastructural correlates of transmitter release in presynaptic areas of lamprey reticulospinal axons. J Neurosci 1985;5(5):1188–1201.

37. Xu-Friedman MA, Harris KM, Regehr WG. Three-dimensional comparison of ultrastructural characteristics at depressing and facilitating synapses onto cerebellar Purkinje cells. J Neurosci 2001;21(17):6666–6672.

38. Satzler K, Sohl LF, Bollmann JH, et al. Three-dimensional reconstruction of a calyx of Held and its postsynaptic principal neuron in the medial nucleus of the trapezoid body. J Neurosci 2002;22(24):10567–10579.

39. Schneggenburger R, Meyer AC, Neher E. Released fraction and total size of a pool of immediately available transmitter quanta at a calyx synapse. Neuron 1999;23(2):399–409.

40. Stevens CF, Tsujimoto T. Estimates for the pool size of releasable quanta at a single central synapse and for the time required to refill the pool. Proc Natl Acad Sci U S A 1995;92(3):846–849.

41. Rosenmund C, Stevens CF. Definition of the readily releasable pool of vesicles at hippocampal synapses. Neuron 1996;16(6):1197–1207.

42. Fasshauer D, Sutton RB, Brunger AT, Jahn R. Conserved structural features of the synaptic fusion complex: SNARE proteins reclassified as Q- and R-SNAREs. Proc Natl Acad Sci U S A 1998;95(26):15781–15786.

43. Kloepper TH, Nickias Kienle C, Fasshauer D. An elaborate classification of SNARE proteins sheds light on the conservation of the eukaryotic endomembrane system. Mol Biol Cell 2007;18(9):3463–3471.

44. Sutton RB, Fasshauer D, Jahn R, Brunger AT. Crystal structure of a SNARE complex involved in synaptic exocytosis at 2.4 A resolution. Nature 1998;395(6700):347–353.
45. Fasshauer D, Antonin W, Subramaniam V, Jahn R. SNARE assembly and disassembly exhibit a pronounced hysteresis. Nat Struct Biol 2002;9(2):144–151.
46. Hayashi T, McMahon H, Yamasaki S, et al. Synaptic vesicle membrane fusion complex: action of clostridial neurotoxins on assembly. EMBO J 1994;13(21):5051–5061.
47. Fratti RA, Collins KM, Hickey CM, Wickner W. Stringent 3Q.1R composition of the SNARE 0–layer can be bypassed for fusion by compensatory SNARE mutation or by lipid bilayer modification. J Biol Chem 2007;282(20):14861–14867.
48. Ossig R, Schmitt HD, de Groot B, et al. Exocytosis requires asymmetry in the central layer of the SNARE complex. EMBO 2000;19(22):6000–6010.
49. Wei S, Xu T, Ashery U, et al. Exocytotic mechanism studied by truncated and zero layer mutants of the C-terminus of SNAP-25. EMBO J 2000;19(6):1279–1289.
50. Wang Y, Dulubova I, Rizo J, Südhof TC. Functional analysis of conserved structural elements in yeast syntaxin Vam3p. J Biol Chem 2001;276(30):28598–28605.
51. Dilcher M, Kohler B, von Mollard GF. Genetic interactions with the yeast q-SNARE vti1 reveal novel functions for the r-snare ykt6. J Biol Chem 2001;276(37):34537–34544.
52. Gil A, Gutierrez LM, Carrasco-Serrano C, Alonso MT, Viniegra S, Criado M. Modifications in the C terminus of the synaptosome-associated protein of 25 kDa (SNAP-25) and in the complementary region of synaptobrevin affect the final steps of exocytosis. J Biol Chem 2002;277(12):9904–9910.
53. Baumert M, Maycox PR, Navone F, De Camilli P, Jahn R. Synaptobrevin: an integral membrane protein of 18,000 daltons present in small synaptic vesicles of rat brain. EMBO J 1989;8(2):379–384.
54. Parlati F, McNew JA, Fukuda R, Miller R, Söllner TH, Rothman JE. Topological restriction of SNARE-dependent membrane fusion. Nature 2000;407(6801):194–198.
55. Fiebig KM, Rice LM, Pollock E, Brunger AT. Folding intermediates of SNARE complex assembly. Nat Struct Biol 1999;6(2):117–123.
56. Fasshauer D, Margittai M. A transient N-terminal interaction of SNAP-25 and syntaxin nucleates SNARE assembly. J Biol Chem 2004;279(9):7613–7621.
57. Pobbati AV, Stein A, Fasshauer D. N- to C-terminal SNARE complex assembly promotes rapid membrane fusion. Science 2006;313(5787):673–676.
58. An SJ, Almers W. Tracking SNARE complex formation in live endocrine cells. Science 2004;306(5698):1042–1046.
59. Fujita Y, Shirataki H, Sakisaka T, et al. Tomosyn: a syntaxin-1–binding protein that forms a novel complex in the neurotransmitter release process. Neuron 1998;20(5):905–915.
60. Widberg CH, Bryant NJ, Girotti M, Rea S, James DE. Tomosyn interacts with the t-SNAREs syntaxin4 and SNAP23 and plays a role in insulin-stimulated GLUT4 translocation. J Biol Chem 2003;278(37):35093–35101.
61. Hatsuzawa K, Lang T, Fasshauer D, Bruns D, Jahn R. The R-SNARE motif of tomosyn forms SNARE core complexes with syntaxin 1 and SNAP-25 and down-regulates exocytosis. J Biol Chem 2003;273(33):31159–31166.
62. McEwen JM, Madison JM, Dybbs M, Kaplan JM. Antagonistic Regulation of Synaptic Vesicle Priming by Tomosyn and UNC-13. Neuron 2006;51(3):303–315.
63. Gracheva EO, Burdina AO, Holgado AM, et al. Tomosyn inhibits synaptic vesicle priming in *Caenorhabditis elegans*. PLoS Biol 2006;4(8):e261
64. Pobbati AV, Razeto A, Boddener M, Becker S, Fasshauer D. Structural basis for the inhibitory role of tomosyn in exocytosis. J Biol Chem 2004;279(45):47192–47200.
65. Hata Y, Slaughter CA, Südhof TC. Synaptic vesicle fusion complex contains *unc-18* homologue bound to syntaxin. Nature 1993;366(6453):347–351.
66. Garcia EP, Gatti E, Butler M, Burton J, De Camilli P. A rat brain Sec1 homologue related to Rop and UNC18 interacts with syntaxin. Proc Natl Acad Sci U S A 1994;91(6):2003–2007.
67. Pevsner J, Hsu SC, Scheller RH. n-Sec1: a neural-specific syntaxin-binding protein. Proc Natl Acad Sci U S A 1994;91(4):1445–1449.

68. Misura KM, Scheller RH, Weis WI. Three-dimensional structure of the neuronal-Sec1–syntaxin 1a complex. Nature 2000;404(6776):355–362.
69. Gallwitz D, Jahn R. The riddle of the Sec1/Munc-18 proteins—new twists added to their interactions with SNAREs. Trends Biochem Sci 2003;28(3):113–116.
70. Zilly FE, Sorensen JB, Jahn R, Lang T. Munc18–bound syntaxin readily forms SNARE complexes with synaptobrevin in native plasma membranes. PLoS Biol 2006;4(10):e330.
71. Shen J, Tareste DC, Paumet F, Rothman JE, Melia TJ. Selective activation of cognate SNAREpins by Sec1/Munc18 proteins. Cell 2007;128(1):183–195.
72. Rickman C, Medine CN, Bergmann A, Duncan RR. Functionally and spatially distinct modes of MUNC18–syntaxin 1 interaction. J Biol Chem 2007;282(16):12097–12103.
73. Dulubova I, Khvotchev M, Liu S, Huryeva I, Südhof TC, Rizo J. Munc18–1 binds directly to the neuronal SNARE complex. Proc Natl Acad Sci U S A 2007;104(8):2697–2702.
74. Liu T, Tucker WC, Bhalla A, Chapman ER, Weisshaar JC. SNARE-driven, 25-millisecond vesicle fusion *in vitro*. Biophys J 2005;89(4):2458–2472.
75. Bowen ME, Weninger K, Brunger AT, Chu S. Single molecule observation of liposome-bilayer fusion thermally induced by soluble *N*-ethyl maleimide sensitive-factor attachment protein receptors (SNAREs). Biophys J 2004;87(5):3569–3584.
76. Fix M, Melia TJ, Jaiswal JK, et al. Imaging single membrane fusion events mediated by SNARE proteins. Proc Natl Acad Sci U S A 2004;101(19):7311–7316.
77. Chen YA, Scales SJ, Scheller RH. Sequential SNARE assembly underlies priming and triggering of exocytosis. Neuron 2001;30:161–170.
78. Hanson PI, Roth R, Morisaki H, Jahn R, Heuser JE. Structure and conformational changes in NSF and its membrane receptor complexes visualized by quick-freeze/deep-etch electron microscopy. Cell 1997;90(3):523–535.
79. Lin RC, Scheller RH. Structural organization of the synaptic exocytosis core complex. Neuron 1997;19(5):1087–1094.
80. Zhao C, Slevin JT, Whiteheart SW. Cellular functions of NSF: not just SNAPs and SNAREs. FEBS Lett 2007;581(11):2140–2149.
81. Marz KE, Lauer JM, Hanson PI. Defining the SNARE complex binding surface of α-SNAP: implications for SNARE complex disassembly. J Biol Chem 2003;278(29):27000–27008.
82. Scales SJ, Yoo BY, Scheller RH. The ionic layer is required for efficient dissociation of the SNARE complex by α-SNAP and NSF. Proc Natl Acad Sci U S A 2001;98(25):14262–14267.
83. Lauer JM, Dalal S, Marz KE, Nonet ML, Hanson PI. SNARE complex zero layer residues are not critical for *N*-ethylmaleimide-sensitive factor-mediated disassembly. J Biol Chem 2006;281(21):14823–14832.
84. Langosch D, Hofmann M, Ungermann C. The role of transmembrane domains in membrane fusion. Cell Mol Life Sci 2007;64(7–8):850–864.
85. Poirier MA, Xiao W, Macosko JC, Chan C, Shin YK, Bennett MK. The synaptic SNARE complex is a parallel four-stranded helical bundle. Nat Struct Biol 1998;5(9):765–769.
86. Hua SY, Charlton MP. Activity-dependent changes in partial VAMP complexes during neurotransmitter release. Nat Neurosci 1999;2(12):1078–1083.
87. Sorensen JB, Wiederhold K, Muller EM, et al. Sequential N- to C-terminal SNARE complex assembly drives priming and fusion of secretory vesicles. EMBO J 2006;25(5):955–966.
88. Xu T, Rammner B, Margittai M, Artalejo AR, Neher E, Jahn R. Inhibition of SNARE complex assembly differentially affects kinetic components of exocytosis. Cell 1999;99(7):713–722.
89. Melia TJ, Weber T, McNew JA, et al. Regulation of membrane fusion by the membrane-proximal coil of the t-SNARE during zippering of SNAREpins. J Cell Biol 2002;158(5):929–940.
90. Han X, Jackson MB. Structural transitions in the synaptic SNARE complex during Ca2+-triggered exocytosis. J Cell Biol 2006;172(2):281–293.
91. Chernomordik LV, Kozlov MM. Membrane hemifusion: crossing a chasm in two leaps. Cell 2005;123(3):375–382.
92. Kasson PM, Kelley NW, Singhal N, Vrljic M, Brunger AT, Pande VS. Ensemble molecular dynamics yields submillisecond kinetics and intermediates of membrane fusion. Proc Natl Acad Sci U S A 2006;103(32):11916–11921.

93. Cohen FS, Melikyan GB. The energetics of membrane fusion from binding, through hemifusion, pore formation, and pore enlargement. J Membr Biol 2004;199(1):1–14.
94. Kuzmin PI, Zimmerberg J, Chizmadzhev YA, Cohen FS. A quantitative model for membrane fusion based on low-energy intermediates. Proc Natl Acad Sci U S A 2001;98(13): 7235–7240.
95. Grote E, Baba M, Ohsumi Y, Novick PJ. Geranylgeranylated SNAREs are dominant inhibitors of membrane fusion. J Cell Biol 2000;151(2):453–466.
96. McNew JA, Weber T, Parlati F, et al. Close is not enough: SNARE-dependent membrane fusion requires an active mechanism that transduces force to membrane anchors. J Cell Biol 2000;150(1):105–117.
97. Earp LJ, Delos SE, Park HE, White JM. The many mechanisms of viral membrane fusion proteins. Curr Top Microbiol Immunol 2005;285:25–66.
98. Kozlov MM, Markin VS. [Possible mechanism of membrane fusion]. Biofizika 1983;28(2):242–247.
99. Knecht V, Mark AE, Marrink SJ. Phase behavior of a phospholipid/fatty acid/water mixture studied in atomic detail. J Am Chem Soc 2006;128(6):2030–2034.
100. Yang L, Huang HW. Observation of a membrane fusion intermediate structure. Science 2002;297(5588):1877–1879.
101. Jahn R, Südhof TC. Membrane fusion and exocytosis. Annu Rev Biochem 1999; 68:863–911.
102. Efrat A, Chernomordik LV, Kozlov MM. Point-like protrusion as a prestalk intermediate in membrane fusion pathway. Biophys J 2007;92(8):L61–63.
103. Wong JL, Koppel DE, Cowan AE, Wessel GM. Membrane hemifusion is a stable intermediate of exocytosis. Dev Cell 2007;12(4):653–659.
104. Xu Y, Zhang F, Su Z, McNew JA, Shin YK. Hemifusion in SNARE-mediated membrane fusion. Nat Struct Mol Biol 2005;12(5):417–422.
105. Lu X, Zhang F, McNew JA, Shin YK. Membrane fusion induced by neuronal SNAREs transits through hemifusion. J Biol Chem 2005;280(34):30538–30541.
106. Yoon TY, Okumus B, Zhang F, Shin YK, Ha T. Multiple intermediates in SNARE-induced membrane fusion. Proc Natl Acad Sci U S A 2006;103(52):19731–19736.
107. Zampighi GA, Zampighi LM, Fain N, Lanzavecchia S, Simon SA, Wright EM. Conical electron tomography of a chemical synapse: vesicles docked to the active zone are hemifused. Biophys J 2006;91(8):2910–2918.
108. Melia TJ, You D, Tareste DC, Rothman JE. Lipidic antagonists to SNARE-mediated fusion. J Biol Chem 2006;281(40):29597–29605.
109. Reese C, Heise F, Mayer A. Trans-SNARE pairing can precede a hemifusion intermediate in intracellular membrane fusion. Nature 2005;436(7049):410–414.
110. Jun Y, Wickner W. Assays of vacuole fusion resolve the stages of docking, lipid mixing, and content mixing. Proc Natl Acad Sci U S A 2007;104(32):13010–13015.
111. Kemble GW, Danieli T, White JM. Lipid-anchored influenza hemagglutinin promotes hemifusion, not complete fusion. Cell 1994;76(2):383–391.
112. Chernomordik LV, Zimmerberg J, Kozlov MM. Membranes of the world unite! J Cell Biol 2006;175(2):201–207.
113. McNew JA, Weber T, Engelman DM, Söllner TH, Rothman JE. The length of the flexible SNAREpin juxtamembrane region is a critical determinant of SNARE-dependent fusion. Mol Cell 1999;4(3):415–421.
114. Melikyan GB, Brener SA, Ok DC, Cohen FS. Inner but not outer membrane leaflets control the transition from glycosylphosphatidylinositol-anchored influenza hemagglutinin-induced hemifusion to full fusion. J Cell Biol 1997;136(5):995–1005.
115. Razinkov VI, Melikyan GB, Epand RM, Epand RF, Cohen FS. Effects of spontaneous bilayer curvature on influenza virus-mediated fusion pores. J Gen Physiol 1998;112(4):409–422.
116. Knecht V, Grubmüller H. Mechanical coupling via the membrane fusion SNARE protein syntaxin 1A: a molecular dynamics study. Biophys J 2003;84(3):1527–1547.

117. Kiessling V, Tamm LK. Measuring distances in supported bilayers by fluorescence interference-contrast microscopy: polymer supports and SNARE proteins. Biophys J 2003;84(1): 408–418.

118. Deak F, Shin OH, Kavalali ET, Südhof TC. Structural determinants of synaptobrevin 2 function in synaptic vesicle fusion. J Neurosci 2006;26(25):6668–6676.

119. Siddiqui TJ, Vites O, Stein A, Heintzmann R, Jahn R, Fasshauer D. Determinants of synaptobrevin regulation in membranes. Mol Biol Cell 2007;18(6):2037–2046.

120. Van Komen JS, Bai X, Rodkey TL, Schaub J, McNew JA. The polybasic juxtamembrane region of Sso1p is required for SNARE function in vivo. Eukaryot Cell 2005; 4(12):2017–2028.

121. Montecucco C, Schiavo G, Pantano S. SNARE complexes and neuroexocytosis: how many, how close? Trends Biochem Sci 2005;30(7):367–372.

122. Han X, Wang CT, Bai J, Chapman ER, Jackson MB. Transmembrane segments of syntaxin line the fusion pore of Ca2+-triggered exocytosis. Science 2004;304(5668):289–292.

123. Bowen ME, Engelman DM, Brunger AT. Mutational analysis of synaptobrevin transmembrane domain oligomerization. Biochemistry 2002;41(52):15861–15866.

124. Roy R, Laage R, Langosch D. Synaptobrevin transmembrane domain dimerization-revisited. Biochemistry 2004;43(17):4964–4970.

125. Roy R, Peplowska K, Rohde J, Ungermann C, Langosch D. Role of the Vam3p transmembrane segment in homodimerization and SNARE complex formation. Biochemistry 2006;45(24):7654–7660.

126. Laage R, Rohde J, Brosig B, Langosch D. A conserved membrane-spanning amino acid motif drives homomeric and supports heteromeric assembly of presynaptic SNARE proteins. J Biol Chem 2000;275(23):17481–17487.

127. Margittai M, Otto H, Jahn R. A stable interaction between syntaxin 1a and synaptobrevin 2 mediated by their transmembrane domains. FEBS Lett 1999;446(1):40–44.

128. Rickman C, Hu K, Carroll J, Davletov B. Self-assembly of SNARE fusion proteins into star-shaped oligomers. Biochem J 2005;388(1):75–79.

129. Raciborska DA, Trimble WS, Charlton MP. Presynaptic protein interactions in vivo: evidence from botulinum A, C, D and E action at frog neuromuscular junction. Eur J Neurosci 1998;10(8):2617–2628.

130. Stewart BA, Mohtashami M, Trimble WS, Boulianne GL. SNARE proteins contribute to calcium cooperativity of synaptic transmission. Proc Natl Acad Sci U S A 2000;97(25): 13955–13960.

131. Hua Y, Scheller RH. Three SNARE complexes cooperate to mediate membrane fusion. Proc Natl Acad Sci U S A 2001;98(14):8065–8070.

132. Keller JE, Cai F, Neale EA. Uptake of botulinum neurotoxin into cultured neurons. Biochemistry 2004;43(2):526–532.

133. Almers W, Tse FW. Transmitter release from synapses: does a preassembled fusion pore initiate exocytosis? Neuron 1990;4(6):813–818.

134. Ungermann C, Sato K, Wickner W. Defining the functions of trans-SNARE pairs. Nature 1998;396(6711):543–548.

135. Spruce AE, Breckenridge LJ, Lee AK, Almers W. Properties of the fusion pore that forms during exocytosis of a mast cell secretory vesicle. Neuron 1990;4(5):643–654.

136. Monck JR, Fernandez JM. The fusion pore and mechanisms of biological membrane fusion. Curr Opin Cell Biol 1996;8(4):524–533.

137. Peters C, Bayer MJ, Buhler S, Andersen JS, Mann M, Mayer A. Trans-complex formation by proteolipid channels in the terminal phase of membrane fusion. Nature 2001;409 (6820):581–588.

138. Israel M, Morel N, Lesbats B, Birman S, Manaranche R. Purification of a presynaptic membrane protein that mediates a calcium-dependent translocation of acetylcholine. Proc Natl Acad Sci U S A 1986;83(23):9226–9230.

139. Peters C, Mayer A. Ca2+/calmodulin signals the completion of docking and triggers a late step of vacuole fusion. Nature 1998;396(6711):575–580.

140. Hiesinger PR, Fayyazuddin A, Mehta SQ, et al. The v-ATPase V0 subunit a1 is required for a late step in synaptic vesicle exocytosis in *Drosophila*. Cell 2005;121(4):607–620.
141. Weber T, Parlati F, McNew JA, et al. SNAREpins are functionally resistant to disruption by NSF and alphaSNAP. J Cell Biol 2000;49(5):1063–1072.
142. Klyachko VA, Jackson MB. Capacitance steps and fusion pores of small and large-dense-core vesicles in nerve terminals. Nature 2002;418(6893):89–92.
143. Giaever G, Chu AM, Ni L, et al. Functional profiling of the *Saccharomyces cerevisiae* genome. Nature 2002;418(6896):387–391.
144. Chanturiya A, Chernomordik LV, Zimmerberg J. Flickering fusion pores comparable with initial exocytotic pores occur in protein-free phospholipid bilayers. Proc Natl Acad Sci U S A 1997;94(26):14423–14428
145. Otter-Nilsson M, Hendriks R, Pecheur-Huet E, Hoekstra D, Nilsson T. Cytosolic ATPases, p97 and NSF, are sufficient to mediate rapid membrane fusion. EMBO J 1999;18(8): 2074–2083.
146. Rizo J, Chen X, Araç D. Unraveling the mechanisms of synaptotagmin and SNARE function in neurotransmitter release. Trends Cell Biol 2006;16(7):339–350.
147. Brugger B, Nickel W, Weber T, et al. Putative fusogenic activity of NSF is restricted to a lipid mixture whose coalescence is also triggered by other factors. EMBO J 2000;19(6):1272–1278.
148. Yang B, Gonzalez LJ, Prekeris R, Steegmaier M, Advani RJ, Scheller RH. SNARE interactions are not selective. Implications for membrane fusion specificity. J Biol Chem 1999;274(9):5649–5653.
149. Tsui MM, Banfield DK. Yeast Golgi SNARE interactions are promiscuous. J Cell Sci 2000;113(1):145–152.
150. Fasshauer D, Antonin W, Margittai M, Pabst S, Jahn R. Mixed and non-cognate SNARE complexes. Characterization of assembly and biophysical properties. J Biol Chem 1999;274(22):15440–15446.
151. Parlati F, Varlamov O, Paz K, et al. Distinct SNARE complexes mediating membrane fusion in Golgi transport based on combinatorial specificity. Proc Natl Acad Sci U S A 2002;99(8): 5424–5429.
152. McNew JA, Parlati F, Fukuda R, et al. Compartmental specificity of cellular membrane fusion encoded in SNARE proteins. Nature 2000;407(6801):153–159.
153. Scales SJ, Chen YA, Yoo BY, Patel SM, Doung YC, Scheller RH. SNAREs contribute to the specificity of membrane fusion. Neuron 2000;26(2):457–464.
154. Hunt JM, Bommert K, Charlton MP, et al. A post-docking role for synaptobrevin in synaptic vesicle fusion. Neuron 1994;12(6):1269–1279.
155. de Wit H, Cornelisse LN, Toonen RF, Verhage M. Docking of secretory vesicles is syntaxin dependent. PLoS ONE 2006;1(1):e126.
156. Toonen RF, Kochubey O, de Wit H, et al. Dissecting docking and tethering of secretory vesicles at the target membrane. EMBO J 2006;25(16):3725–3737.
157. Ohara-Imaizumi M, Fujiwara T, Nakamichi Y, et al. Imaging analysis reveals mechanistic differences between first- and second-phase insulin exocytosis. J Cell Biol 2007;177(4):695–705.
158. Sztul E, Lupashin V. Role of tethering factors in secretory membrane traffic. Am J Physiol Cell Physiol 2006;290(1):C11–26.
159. Whyte JR, Munro S. Vesicle tethering complexes in membrane traffic. J Cell Sci 2002;115(13):2627–2637.
160. Zerial M, McBride H. Rab proteins as membrane organizers. Nat Rev Mol Cell Biol 2001;2(2):107–117.
161. Waters MG, Pfeffer SR. Membrane tethering in intracellular transport. Curr Opin Cell Biol 1999;11(4):453–459.
162. Guo W, Sacher M, Barrowman J, Ferro-Novick S, Novick P. Protein complexes in transport vesicle targeting. Trends Cell Biol 2000;10(6):251–255.
163. Wiederkehr A, Du Y, Pypaert M, Ferro-Novick S, Novick P. Sec3p is needed for the spatial regulation of secretion and for the inheritance of the cortical endoplasmic reticulum. Mol Biol Cell 2003;14(12):4770–4782.

164. Finger FP, Hughes TE, Novick P. Sec3p is a spatial landmark for polarized secretion in budding yeast. Cell 1998;92(4):559–571.

165. VanRheenen SM, Cao X, Lupashin VV, Barlowe C, Waters MG. Sec35p, a novel peripheral membrane protein, is required for ER to Golgi vesicle docking. J Cell Biol 1998;141(5): 1107–1119.

166. Wiederkehr A, De Craene JO, Ferro-Novick S, Novick P. Functional specialization within a vesicle tethering complex: bypass of a subset of exocyst deletion mutants by Sec1p or Sec4p. J Cell Biol 2004;167(5):875–887.

167. Novick P, Medkova M, Dong G, Hutagalung A, Reinisch K, Grosshans B. Interactions between Rabs, tethers, SNAREs and their regulators in exocytosis. Biochem Soc Trans 2006;34(5):683–686.

168. Borisovska M, Zhao Y, Tsytsyura Y, et al. v-SNAREs control exocytosis of vesicles from priming to fusion. EMBO J 2005;24(12):2114–2126.

169. Bhattacharya S, Stewart BA, Niemeyer BA, et al. Members of the synaptobrevin/vesicle-associated membrane protein (VAMP) family in *Drosophila* are functionally interchangeable in vivo for neurotransmitter release and cell viability. Proc Natl Acad Sci U S A 2002;99(21):13867–13872.

170. Sorensen JB, Nagy G, Varoqueaux F, et al. Differential control of the releasable vesicle pools by SNAP-25 splice variants and SNAP-23. Cell 2003;114(1):75–86.

171. Holt M, Varoqueaux F, Wiederhold K, et al. Identification of SNAP-47, a novel Qbc-SNARE with ubiquitous expression. J Biol Chem 2006;281(25):17076–17083.

172. Fujiwara T, Mishima T, Kofuji T, et al. Analysis of knock-out mice to determine the role of HPC-1/syntaxin 1A in expressing synaptic plasticity. J Neurosci 2006;26(21):5767–5776.

173. Liu Y, Barlowe C. Analysis of Sec22p in endoplasmic reticulum/Golgi transport reveals cellular redundancy in SNARE protein function. Mol Biol Cell 2002;13(9):3314–3324.

174. Fischer von Mollard G, Stevens TH. The *Saccharomyces cerevisiae* v-SNARE Vti1p is required for multiple membrane transport pathways to the vacuole. Mol Biol Cell 1999;10 (6):1719–1732.

175. Darsow T, Rieder SE, Emr SD. A multispecificity syntaxin homologue, Vam3p, essential for autophagic and biosynthetic protein transport to the vacuole. J Cell Biol 1997;138b (11):517–529.

176. Burgess RW, Deitcher DL, Schwarz TL. The synaptic protein syntaxin1 is required for cellularization of *Drosophila* embryos. J Cell Biol 1997;138(4):861–875.

177. Betz A, Okamoto M, Benseler F, Brose N. Direct interaction of the rat *unc-13* homologue Munc13-1 with the N terminus of syntaxin. J Biol Chem 1997;272(4):2520–2526.

178. Richmond JE, Weimer RM, Jorgensen EM. An open form of syntaxin bypasses the requirement for UNC-13 in vesicle priming. Nature 2001;412(6844):338–341.

179. Scales SJ, Hesser BA, Masuda ES, Scheller RH. Amisyn, a novel syntaxin-binding protein that may regulate SNARE complex assembly. J Biol Chem 2002;277(31):28271–28279.

180. Masuda ES, Huang BC, Fisher JM, Luo Y, Scheller RH. Tomosyn binds t-SNARE proteins via a VAMP-like coiled coil. Neuron 1998;21(3):479–480.

181. Lao G, Scheuss V, Gerwin CM, et al. Syntaphilin: a syntaxin-1 clamp that controls SNARE assembly. Neuron 2000;25(1):191–201.

182. Fisher RJ, Pevsner J, Burgoyne RD. Control of fusion pore dynamics during exocytosis by Munc18. Science 2001;291(5505):875–878.

183. Latham CF, Lopez JA, Hu SH, et al. Molecular dissection of the munc18c/syntaxin4 interaction: implications for regulation of membrane trafficking. Traffic 2006;7(10):1408–1419.

184. Hu SH, Latham CF, Gee CL, James DE, Martin JL. Structure of the Munc18c/Syntaxin4 N-peptide complex defines universal features of the N-peptide binding mode of Sec1/Munc18 proteins. Proc Natl Acad Sci U S A 2007;104(21):8773–8778.

185. Togneri J, Cheng YS, Munson M, Hughson FM, Carr CM. Specific SNARE complex binding mode of the Sec1/Munc-18 protein, Sec1p. Proc Natl Acad Sci U S A 2006;103 (47):17730–17735.

186. Sabatini BL, Regehr WG. Timing of neurotransmission at fast synapses in the mammalian brain. Nature 1996;384(6605):170–172.
187. Flanagan JJ, Barlowe C. Cysteine-disulfide cross-linking to monitor SNARE complex assembly during endoplasmic reticulum-Golgi transport. J Biol Chem 2006;281 (4):2281–2288.
188. Starai VJ, Thorngren N, Fratti RA, Wickner W. Ion regulation of homotypic vacuole fusion in *Saccharomyces cerevisiae*. J Biol Chem 2005;280(17):16754–16762.
189. McMahon HT, Missler M, Li C, Südhof TC. Complexins: cytosolic proteins that regulate SNAP receptor function. Cell 1995;83(1):111–119.
190. Perin MS, Fried VA, Mignery GA, Jahn R, Südhof TC. Phospholipid binding by a synaptic vesicle protein homologous to the regulatory region of protein kinase C. Nature 1990;345(6272):260–263.
191. Giraudo CG, Eng WS, Melia TJ, Rothman JE. A clamping mechanism involved in SNARE-dependent exocytosis. Science 2006;313(5787):676–680.
192. Tang J, Maximov A, Shin OH, Dai H, Rizo J, Südhof TC. A complexin/synaptotagmin 1 switch controls fast synaptic vesicle exocytosis. Cell 2006;126(6):1175–1187.
193. Schaub JR, Lu X, Doneske B, Shin YK, McNew JA. Hemifusion arrest by complexin is relieved by Ca2+-synaptotagmin I. Nat Struct Mol Biol 2006;13(8):748–750.
194. Melia TJ. Putting the clamps on membrane fusion: How complexin sets the stage for calcium-mediated exocytosis. FEBS Lett 2007;581(11):2131–2139.
195. Bracher A, Kadlec J, Betz H, Weissenhorn W. X-ray structure of a neuronal complexin-SNARE complex from squid. J Biol Chem 2002;277(29):26517–26523.
196. Chen X, Tomchick DR, Kovrigin E, et al. Three-Dimensional Structure of the Complexin/SNARE Complex. Neuron 2002;33(3):397–409.
197. Bai J, Wang CT, Richards DA, Jackson MB, Chapman ER. Fusion Pore Dynamics Are Regulated by Synaptotagmin t-SNARE Interactions. Neuron 2004;41(6):929–942.
198. Fernandez-Chacon R, Konigstorfer A, Gerber SH, et al. Synaptotagmin I functions as a calcium regulator of release probability. Nature 2001;410(6824):41–49.
199. Chapman ER. Synaptotagmin: A Ca(2+) sensor that triggers exocytosis? Nat Rev Mol Cell Biol 2002;3(7):498–508.
200. Davis AF, Bai J, Fasshauer D, Wolowick MJ, Lewis JL, Chapman ER. Kinetics of synaptotagmin responses to Ca2+ and assembly with the core SNARE complex onto membranes. Neuron 1999;24(4):363–376.
201. Brose N, Petrenko AG, Südhof TC, Jahn R. Synaptotagmin: a calcium sensor on the synaptic vesicle surface. Science 1992;256(5059):1021–1025.
202. Bennett MK, Calakos N, Kreiner T, Scheller RH. Synaptic vesicle membrane proteins interact to form a multimeric complex. J Cell Biol 1992;116(3):761–775.
203. Chapman ER, Hanson PI, An S, Jahn R. Ca2+ regulates the interaction between synaptotagmin and syntaxin 1. J Biol Chem 1995;270(40):23667–23671.
204. Schiavo G, Stenbeck G, Rothman JE, Söllner TH. Binding of the synaptic vesicle v-SNARE, synaptotagmin, to the plasma membrane t-SNARE, SNAP-25, can explain docked vesicles at neurotoxin-treated synapses. Proc Natl Acad Sci U S A 1997;94(3):997–1001.
205. Reim K, Mansour M, Varoqueaux F, et al. Complexins regulate a late step in Ca2+-dependent neurotransmitter release. Cell 2001;104(1):71–81.
206. Tucker WC, Weber T, Chapman ER. Reconstitution of Ca2+-regulated membrane fusion by synaptotagmin and SNAREs. Science 2004;304(5669):435–438.
207. Mahal LK, Sequeira SM, Gureasko JM, Söllner TH. Calcium-independent stimulation of membrane fusion and SNAREpin formation by synaptotagmin I. J Cell Biol 2002;158 (2):273–283.

Chapter 4
Roles and Sources of Calcium in Synaptic Exocytosis

Zhao-Wen Wang, Bojun Chen, and Qian Ge

Contents

Abstract Ca^{2+} triggers neurotransmitter release. The release rate is supralinearly related to Ca^{2+} concentration. The sources of Ca^{2+} triggering synaptic vesicle fusion include influx through voltage-sensitive Ca^{2+} channels in the plasma membrane and release from the endoplasmic reticulum through ryanodine receptors. Mitochondria may also play a role in regulating presynaptic Ca^{2+} concentration. This chapter addresses the roles of Ca^{2+} in evoked and spontaneous neurotransmitter release, the relationship between neurotransmitter release rate and Ca^{2+} concentration, the sources of Ca^{2+} at the presynaptic nerve terminal, and the mechanisms by which the Ca^{2+} concentrations necessary for triggering synaptic exocytosis are achieved at the presynaptic site.

Keywords Calcium, exocytosis, neurotransmitter release, calcium channel, ryanodine receptor, mitochondrion.

Zhao-Wen Wang
Department of Neuroscience, University of Connecticut Health Center, Farmington,
CT 06030-3401, USA
e-mail: zwwang@uchc.edu

Ca^{2+} is remarkable for its diverse functions in biology. One of the best known functions of Ca^{2+} is to trigger neurotransmitter release at the presynaptic nerve terminal. More than a century ago, Locke (1) observed that neuromuscular transmission is greatly affected by Ca^{2+} in the surrounding medium. Subsequent studies by many others showed that extracellular Ca^{2+} is essential to evoked neurotransmitter release, and its concentration affects the amplitude of end-plate potentials (2–5).

Neurotransmitters may be released both spontaneously and in response to action potentials. Generally, spontaneous release results from the exocytosis of individual synaptic vesicles, whereas action potential–evoked release reflects synchronized exocytosis of multiple synaptic vesicles. The role of Ca^{2+} in action potential–evoked release is well established. When an action potential invades the nerve terminal, depolarization opens voltage-sensitive Ca^{2+} channels (VSCCs) in the plasma membrane, resulting in Ca^{2+} influx. Ca^{2+} may also come from the endoplasmic reticulum (ER) through a coupling between VSCCs in the plasma membrane and ryanodine receptors (RYRs) in the ER membrane (6,7). Ca^{2+} binds to a Ca^{2+}-sensing protein(s) to trigger synaptic exocytosis (details are provided in Chapter 6). The released neurotransmitter acts on specific postsynaptic receptors to cause either excitatory or inhibitory postsynaptic currents in the postsynaptic cell (depending on the types of neurotransmitter and postsynaptic receptor). The temporal relationships among the presynaptic action potential, presynaptic Ca^{2+} current, excitatory postsynaptic current (EPSC) and postsynaptic action potential are shown in Figure 4.1. Ca^{2+} release from the ER is not included in this figure because its kinetics is poorly defined. As shown in the figure, Ca^{2+} influx begins approximately at the peak of the action

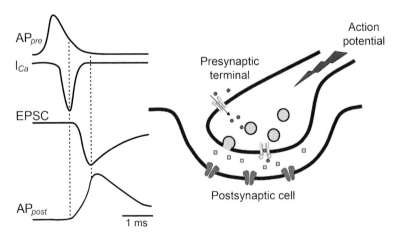

Fig. 4.1 Pre- and postsynaptic events in response to a presynaptic action potential. Depolarization of the presynaptic terminal by the action potential (AP$_{pre}$) causes Ca^{2+} influx (I_{Ca}) through voltage-sensitive Ca^{2+} channels in the plasma membrane. Ca^{2+} triggers the release of a neurotransmitter, which causes excitatory postsynaptic currents (EPSCs) by activating ionotropic postsynaptic receptors. An action potential may occur in the postsynaptic cell (AP$_{post}$) if the cell is depolarized beyond a threshold by the EPSC. (Based on data from Meinrenken et al [129] and Xu and Wu [130].)

potential, and ends before the nerve terminal is fully repolarized. Neurotransmitter release, as reflected by the postsynaptic currents, occurs with a further delay.

Neurotransmitter Release Rate is Supralinearly Related to Ca^{2+} Concentration

The rate of neurotransmitter release is quantitatively related to Ca^{2+} concentration ($[Ca^{2+}]$). Dodge and Rahamimoff (4) showed that neurotransmitter release rate at the frog neuromuscular junction (NMJ) increased with elevations of extracellular $[Ca^{2+}]$ ($[Ca^{2+}]_o$). However, the relationship was not a linear one. When $[Ca^{2+}]_o$ was relatively low, a small change of the concentration resulted in a large change of neurotransmitter release, as reflected by the amplitude of end-plate potentials. Plotting the results in double-logarithmic coordinates yielded a straight line with a slope of approximately 4, which led to the conclusion that neurotransmitter release rate is proportional to $[Ca^{2+}]_o$ raised to the fourth power (release rate $\propto [Ca^{2+}]_o{}^4$).

The work of Dodge and Rahamimoff showed the quantitative relationship between neurotransmitter release rate and $[Ca^{2+}]_o$. However, the Ca^{2+} sensor of the synaptic release machinery is located inside the presynaptic nerve terminal. Thus, intracellular rather than extracellular Ca^{2+} directly contributes to neurotransmitter release. What would be the relationship between neurotransmitter release rate and cytoplasmic $[Ca^{2+}]$ ($[Ca^{2+}]_i$)? This relationship has been analyzed with a technique called Ca^{2+}-uncaging. In this technique, a photolysable Ca^{2+}-chelator such as DM-nitrophen is introduced into the presynaptic nerve terminal through a whole-cell patch pipette. Ca^{2+} is released from the photolysable Ca^{2+}-chelator upon flash of the ultraviolet light, resulting in a rapid and uniform increase of $[Ca^{2+}]_i$ at the presynaptic nerve terminal. The level of $[Ca^{2+}]_i$ at the presynaptic nerve terminal may be controlled by varying the light intensity and measured by imaging with a low-affinity fluorescent Ca^{2+} indictor. The rate of neurotransmitter release is evaluated by measuring either membrane capacitance of the presynaptic terminal, which increases when the plasma membrane area enlarges with synaptic vesicle fusion, or the amplitude of excitatory postsynaptic potential or current, which reflects postsynaptic responses to the released neurotransmitter. This Ca^{2+}-uncaging technique is apparently suitable for analyzing the relationship between release rate and $[Ca^{2+}]_i$ because it triggers release of the same pool of synaptic vesicles as action potentials do (8). Analyses of several nerve terminals, including the goldfish retinal bipolar cell synaptic terminal (Fig. 4.2) (9), crayfish motor neuron terminal (10), and rat calyx of Held nerve terminal (Fig. 4.2) (8,11), reveal a nonlinear dependence of the release rate on $[Ca^{2+}]_i$ with a slope of approximately 3 to 4 in plots with double-logarithmic coordinates, which resembles the relationship between the release rate and $[Ca^{2+}]_o$ (4).

Two kinetically distinct components may be identified in action potential–induced neurotransmitter release: an early fast component representing synchronous release, and a delayed slow component representing asynchronous release (12). It is thought that the fast component is triggered by Ca^{2+} binding to a low-affinity Ca^{2+} sensor,

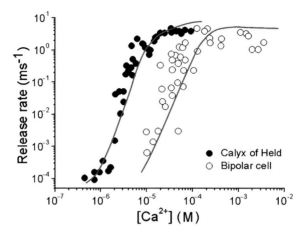

Fig. 4.2 Neurotransmitter release rate is proportional to Ca^{2+} concentration raised to the fourth power, and the sensitivity to Ca^{2+} differs by approximately one order of magnitude between the calyx of Held and goldfish retinal bipolar cell presynaptic terminals. (Based on data from Heidelberger et al [9] and Bollmann et al [11].)

whereas the slow component results from Ca^{2+} binding to a high-affinity Ca^{2+} sensor. Nevertheless, the two components appear to have similar Ca^{2+} cooperativity despite of their differences in Ca^{2+} sensitivity (12).

It is unclear why neurotransmitter release rate is supralinearly related to $[Ca^{2+}]_i$. Several mechanisms have been proposed as the basis for the apparent Ca^{2+} cooperativity. First, Ca^{2+} binding properties of synaptotagmin might determine the cooperativity (13). Fitting of the flash-photolysis data from the calyx of Held synapse with a minimal kinetic model suggests that five identical Ca^{2+}-binding steps are needed prior to synaptic vesicle fusion (8,11). The total number of Ca^{2+} binding sites in synaptotagmin I (three in the C2A domain and two in the C2B domain) matches the number of Ca^{2+} binding steps in the proposed Ca^{2+} binding kinetic model (13). Furthermore, Ca^{2+} cooperativity for the fast synchronous release component is abolished in *Drosophila* synaptotagmin null or C2B domain-deletion mutant (14,15). Second, soluble N-ethylmaleimide–sensitive factor attachment receptor (SNARE) proteins might be the basis for Ca^{2+} cooperativity because mutations of either syntaxin 1A or synaptobrevin reduces Ca^{2+} cooperativity at the *Drosophila* NMJ (16). Third, overlapping of Ca^{2+} micro- or nanodomains (defined later) at the active zone might contribute to the Ca^{2+} cooperativity (17). Fourth, saturation of cytoplasmic Ca^{2+} buffer(s) might contribute to the supralinearity (18). Fifth, the apparent Ca^{2+} cooperativity might reflect the mean number of SNARE complexes that mediate a vesicle fusion because SNARE complexes have the intrinsic ability to form oligomers of 3 to 4 (19). Sixth, the apparent Ca^{2+} cooperativity may be affected by the function of presynaptic BK channels, as shown by analyses of NMJ transmission in wild-type and the *slo-1* BK channel mutant of

Fig. 4.3 The apparent Ca^{2+} cooperativity is decreased in *slo-1* BK channel mutants. (**a**) The amplitude of evoked postsynaptic currents (EPSCs) was significantly reduced at the *C. elegans* neuromuscular junction in a *slo-1* null mutant at 250 or 500 μM but not 1 or 5 mM $[Ca^{2+}]_o$. The asterisk indicates a statistically significant difference compared with the wild-type (WT). (**b**) The same data as in (A) but plotted using logarithmic coordinates showing that the apparent Ca^{2+} cooperativity, as indicated by the slope factor from a linear fit, was decreased in the *slo-1* mutant. (Based on data from Liu et al [20].)

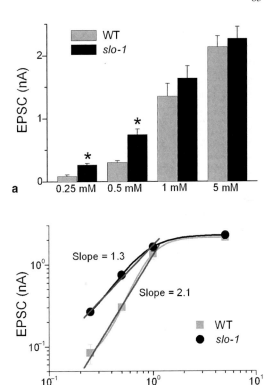

Caenorhabditis elegans (Fig. 4.3). The apparent Ca^{2+} cooperativity is decreased in the *slo-1* mutant because SLO-1 dysfunction increases neurotransmitter release at low but not high $[Ca^{2+}]_o$ (20). The diversity of the models implies that the molecular basis of Ca^{2+} cooperativity is still poorly understood, and could be attributable to more than one mechanism.

Although an approximately 4th power relationship often exists between neurotransmitter release rate and $[Ca^{2+}]$, there are exceptions. For example, at the squid giant synapse (17) and chick ciliary ganglion synapse (21), the apparent Ca^{2+} cooperativity is approximately 1. At the excitatory synapse between sensory afferent fibers and motoneurons in rat lumbar spinal cord, the apparent Ca^{2+} cooperativity is 1.6 (22). At the *C. elegans* NMJ, the apparent Ca^{2+} cooperativity is 2.1, which is changed to 1.3 when the *slo-1* BK channel is mutated (20) (Fig. 4.3). One interpretation for the ~1 apparent Ca^{2+} cooperativity is that synaptic vesicle exocytosis may be triggered by Ca^{2+} nanodomains (see below) at some synapses (17).

Another divalent cation, Mg^{2+}, has also been implicated in controlling neurotransmitter release under experimental conditions. Unlike Ca^{2+}, however, Mg^{2+} is an inhibitor of the release. An increase of Mg^{2+} concentration reduces the Ca^{2+} sensitivity of neurotransmitter release (4). It has been suggested that Mg^{2+} antagonizes the function of Ca^{2+} through a competitive effect (22,23). However, the exact mechanism is unclear. One possibility is that Mg^{2+} blocks Ca^{2+} entry through membrane Ca^{2+} channels (24,25). Mg^{2+} has been shown to activate the BK channel when applied to the cytoplasmic side in inside-out membrane patches (26). Because the BK channel is an important negative regulator of neurotransmitter release (27,28), an elevation of $[Mg^{2+}]$ could potentially downregulate neurotransmitter release via the BK channel. However, it is questionable whether an elevation of $[Mg^{2+}]_o$ will lead to increased $[Mg^{2+}]_i$ in neurons.

Ca^{2+} Concentrations Required for Neurotransmitter Release Vary from Synapse to Synapse

Relatively high Ca^{2+} concentrations are needed to trigger the fast phase of action potential–induced neurotransmitter release. At the squid giant synapse terminal, analyses of the inhibitory effects of intraterminally injected Ca^{2+} chelators with different Ca^{2+} affinities suggest that a Ca^{2+} concentration of several hundred micromolars may be needed to trigger neurotransmitter release (29). At the goldfish retinal bipolar neuron synaptic terminal, Ca^{2+}-uncaging experiments suggest that ~$10\,\mu M$ Ca^{2+} is the minimum to trigger neurotransmitter release, and ~$200\,\mu M$ Ca^{2+} is needed for release at half maximal rate (9). In permeabilized synaptosomes prepared from rat cerebral cortex, glutamate release has a threshold of ~$50\,\mu M$ Ca^{2+}, with half-maximal and maximal release at 200 to $300\,\mu M$ and $1\,mM$ Ca^{2+}, respectively (30). These studies suggest that hundreds of micromolar Ca^{2+} is needed for action potential–evoked neurotransmitter release at these synapses. However, at the calyx of Held glutamatergic terminal, Ca^{2+}-uncaging experiments suggest that 10 to $25\,\mu M$ Ca^{2+} is sufficient to cause the peak release rate (31) or to mimic the release induced by action potentials (8,11). Thus, Ca^{2+} concentrations required for fast neurotransmitter release could vary as much as one order of magnitude in different synapses (Fig. 4.2).

Ca^{2+} Forms High Concentration Domains at the Presynaptic Terminal

In response to an action potential, the presynaptic nerve terminal only shows a small increase in spatially averaged $[Ca^{2+}]_i$. For example, presynaptic $[Ca^{2+}]_i$ increases by $5\,nM$ from a resting level of approximately 50 to $100\,nM$ at the squid giant synapse (17). The spatially averaged $[Ca^{2+}]_i$ following an action potential is much lower than that required for fast neurotransmitter release. Mathematical modeling in the 1980s suggests $[Ca^{2+}]_i$ in the presynaptic terminal does not change uniformly in response to action potentials but forms hemispheric high-concentration domains (<$50\,nm$ in radius) around the mouth of open Ca^{2+} channels (32–34). A focal Ca^{2+} domain resulting from Ca^{2+} entry through a single Ca^{2+} channel is defined

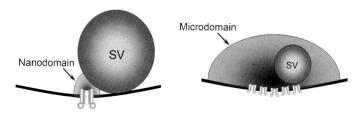

Fig. 4.4 Ca^{2+} accumulates at the inner mouth of voltage-sensitive Ca^{2+} channels to form Ca^{2+} nanodomains and microdomains. A Ca^{2+} nanodomain results from the opening of one Ca^{2+} channel, whereas a Ca^{2+} microdomain results from the opening of a cluster of Ca^{2+} channels (32,131)

as a Ca^{2+} nanodomain (32) (Fig. 4.4). The modeling experiments suggest that the Ca^{2+} nanodomain is restricted within tens of nanometers from the channel; $[Ca^{2+}]$ in the nanodomain peaks within 1 ms upon channel opening, and quickly diminishes upon channel closing; and $[Ca^{2+}]$ can be as high as a few hundreds of micromolar in the center of the nanodomain but drops steeply with increasing distance from the channel (34). Mathematical modeling also suggests that Ca^{2+} domains of larger radii and higher concentrations may result from simultaneous opening of clustered Ca^{2+} channels (35), and such Ca^{2+} domains are called Ca^{2+} microdomains (32) (Fig. 4.4).

The concentration of Ca^{2+} in Ca^{2+} microdomains has been evaluated by analyzing "hot spots," which are putative Ca^{2+} microdomains, in Ca^{2+} imaging experiments. At the presynaptic terminal of squid giant synapse, $[Ca^{2+}]$ in the Ca^{2+} microdomain is 200 to 300 μM (36), which is consistent with the estimate made by analyzing the inhibitory effects of different Ca^{2+}-chelating agents on neurotransmitter release (29). At the presynaptic terminal of goldfish retinal bipolar cells, the Ca^{2+} microdomain has a spatially averaged concentration of ~2 μM and a peak concentration of ~7 μM in the center of the microdomain (37). Besides Ca^{2+} imaging techniques, the activity of presynaptic BK channels has been used to measure local $[Ca^{2+}]$ resulting from Ca^{2+} entry through VSCCs. This approach takes advantages of the Ca^{2+}-dependent property of the BK channel and the physical colocalization of the BK channel with VSCCs at the presynaptic terminal. The analyses show that local $[Ca^{2+}]$ reaches over 100 μM at the presynaptic terminal of cultured *Xenopus* NMJ (38). The Ca^{2+} concentrations determined using either the Ca^{2+} imaging or BK channel sensor approach are in agreement with those needed to trigger fast neurotransmitter release at these synapses.

The spatial and temporal properties of Ca^{2+} microdomains at several presynaptic terminals have been analyzed using imaging techniques. At the presynaptic terminal of the squid giant synapse, imaging with *n*-aequorin-J shows that a stable set of quantum emission domains (QEDs) develop in response to sustained stimulation at 10 Hz. These QEDs are 0.25 to 0.6 μm² in size and have an average lifetime of 200 ms (36). The measured lifetime of QEDs is much longer than what would be expected for the transient Ca^{2+} signal in the microdomain, probably due to technical limitations (36). At the presynaptic terminal of a cultured frog NMJ preparation, confocal imaging with the low-affinity Ca^{2+} indicator Oregon Green 488 shows that action potentials induce spot-like fluorescent transients. The fluorescent spot peaks within ~1 ms, decays with one rapid (τ_1 = 1.7 ms) and two slow (τ_2 = 16 ms, τ_3 = 78 ms) components, and is 0.6 to 3.0 μm in full width at maximum (39).

More recently, total internal reflection fluorescence microscopy (TIRFM) has been adapted to measure Ca^{2+} signals in the Ca^{2+} nano- or microdomains. This technique offers excellent spatial and temporal resolutions because fluorescent excitation is restricted to a very thin (~100 nm) layer at the refractive boundary between the microscope cover glass and the cell (40). Using this technique, fluorescent "hot spots" are observed near the plasma membrane at the presynaptic terminal of goldfish bipolar neurons in response to membrane depolarization (41). The fluorescent hot spot has two components, including a fast component that rises and declines abruptly with membrane depolarization and repolarization, and a slow component that rises steadily during depolarization and declines rather slowly after repolarization. Interestingly, the slow component is also observed outside of the fluorescent hot spots, suggesting that it likely reflects the global cytoplasmic $[Ca^{2+}]$ changes that are also observed using standard fluorescence microscopy (42–44). Another recent study using the TIRFM technique in goldfish retinal bipolar cells (37) shows that depolarization generates Ca^{2+} microdomains that appear within 20 to 40 ms and disappear within 20 to 40 ms. The apparent width of these Ca^{2+} microdomains shows an inverse relationship with the concentration of cytoplasmic ethylene glycol-bis(2-aminoethylether)-N,N,N′,N′-tetraacetic acid (EGTA) (37).

What is the distance between the Ca^{2+} nano- or microdomain and the Ca^{2+} sensor for synaptic vesicle exocytosis? The distance is often estimated by comparing the inhibitory effects of the Ca^{2+}-chelating agents BAPTA [1,2-Bis(2-aminophenoxy)ethane-N′, N′, N′, N′-tetraacetic acid] and EGTA on neurotransmitter release. Although BAPTA and EGTA have similar equilibrium affinities for Ca^{2+}, BAPTA binds Ca^{2+} several hundred times faster than EGTA. Both BAPTA and EGTA would inhibit the release if the Ca^{2+} domain is hundreds of nanometers away from the Ca^{2+} sensor. Conversely, only BAPTA inhibits the release if the Ca^{2+} domain is tens of nanometers away from the Ca^{2+} sensor. Analyses of this kind have led to the conclusion that the distance between presynaptic VSCCs and the Ca^{2+} sensor for synaptic release varies from synapse to synapse, ranging from hundreds of nanometers at the presynaptic terminals of squid giant synapse (29) and goldfish retinal bipolar neurons (45) to tens of nanometers at the calyx of Held presynaptic terminal (46). In addition, a kinetic model simulating Ca^{2+} influx, buffered Ca^{2+} diffusion, and Ca^{2+} binding to the release sensor at the calyx of Held terminal suggests that one to a few clusters of Ca^{2+} channels control the release of synaptic vesicles, and that the distance of a vesicle to the Ca^{2+} channel cluster(s) varies from 30 to 300 nm with an average of ~100 nm (47).

There is debate about whether the release of synaptic vesicles is controlled by Ca^{2+} nano- or microdomains. Two different approaches have been used to address this problem. One approach is to analyze the inhibitory effects of BAPTA and EGTA on neurotransmitter release (32). Synaptic release is probably mediated by Ca^{2+} nanodomains if only BAPTA inhibits the release. Conversely, synaptic release is probably mediated by Ca^{2+} microdomains if both BAPTA and EGTA inhibit the release. This kind of analysis suggests that the release at the squid giant synapse, the chick ciliary ganglion synapse, and the goldfish retinal bipolar synapse is controlled by Ca^{2+} nanodomains, whereas that at the mammalian calyx of Held synapse, the cerebellar parallel fiber-Purkinje cell synapse, and the frog auditory hair cell synapse is controlled by Ca^{2+} microdomains (32). Another approach is to analyze the relationship between the release rate and the number of functional Ca^{2+} channels (48). A linear relationship would be observed if the release was triggered by Ca^{2+} nanodomains. Conversely, a supralinear relationship would be observed if the release was triggered by Ca^{2+} microdomains. Analyses of this kind suggest that the release at the squid giant synapse and chick ciliary synapse is mediated by Ca^{2+} nanodomains, whereas that at the calyx of Held synapse is triggered by Ca^{2+} microdomains (48). There are potential limitations with both approaches. For example, it might be difficult to distinguish between the contribution from one Ca^{2+} nanodomain and that from a Ca^{2+} microdomain formed by just a few Ca^{2+} channels simply by comparing the inhibitory effects of BAPTA and EGTA on neurotransmitter release. The relationship between neurotransmitter release rate and $[Ca^{2+}]$ might be affected by a variety of other factors, as described above. Thus, it is technically challenging to determine whether synaptic exocytosis is triggered by Ca^{2+} nano- or microdomains.

Voltage-Sensitive Ca^{2+} Channels are the Primary Source of Ca^{2+} for Neurotransmitter Release

Neuronal VSCCs generally consist of four subunits: α_1, β, α_2, and δ (49). The α_2 and δ subunits are also collectively called the $\alpha_2\delta$ subunit because they are formed from cleavage of a single translational product. The α_1 subunit is a large (190 to 250 kDa) transmembrane protein consisting of four repeat domains. The membrane topology of each repeat domain resembles that of the α subunit of a typical voltage-gated K^+ channel, with six membrane spanning segments (S1 to S6), a P (pore) loop between S5 and S6, cytoplasmic amino and carboxyl terminals, and positively charged residues in the S4 segment. The δ subunit is also a membrane-associated protein with a single membrane-spanning domain. The β and α_2 subunits have no integral membrane spanning domains. The β subunit interacts with the intracellular loop between the first and second repeat domains of the α_1 subunit, whereas the α_2 subunit associates with the δ subunit on the extracellular side through a disulfide linkage. In skeletal muscle and some other tissues, VSCCs may include an additional γ-subunit, which is an integral membrane protein with four membrane-spanning domains. A schematic diagram of these subunits and their physical relationships is shown in Figure 4.5.

Ca^{2+} channels are encoded by multiple genes and have diverse functional and pharmacologic properties. Several methods have been used to classify Ca^{2+} channels. They are classified into high voltage-activated (HVA) and low voltage-activated (LVA) channels according to the degree of membrane depolarization needed for

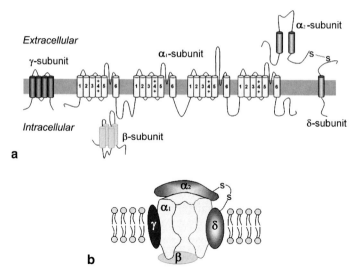

Fig. 4.5 Schematic diagrams showing the membrane topology and organization of Ca²⁺ channel subunits. (**a**) Membrane topology of Ca²⁺ channel subunits. The α_1-subunit consists of four repeat domains (I, II, III, and IV). Each repeat domain has six membrane-spanning segments (S1 to S6) with a P (pore) loop between S5 and S6. The β-subunit interacts with the α_1-subunit at the intracellular loop between the first and second repeating domains. The δ-subunit has a single membrane-spanning segment. The α_2-subunit associates with the δ-subunit through a disulfide linkage on the extracellular side. The γ-subunit has four putative membrane-spanning segments. (**b**) Overall structure of a voltage-sensitive Ca²⁺ channel (VSCC)

activation. The LVA channels activate at a threshold of −70 mV, whereas HVA channels activate at a threshold of −20 mV (49). Ca²⁺ channels are classified into L-, N-, P/Q-, R-, and T-types according to biophysical/pharmacologic properties and tissue distribution. The L-type channel was named for its relatively *l*arge single channel conductance and *l*ong open duration (slow inactivation). The T-type channel was named for its *t*iny conductance and *t*ransient opening. The N-type channel was named because it was first identified in *n*eurons. The P-type was first described in *P*urkinje cells. The Q-type was named because it was blocked by the same toxin that blocks the P-type (ω-agatoxin IVA) but with a lower sensitivity to the toxin and distinct inactivation kinetics, and because the letter Q follows P in the English alphabet. P- and Q-type channels are often collectively called the P/Q-type. The R-type was named for being *r*esistant to organic calcium channel antagonists available at the time (49–51).

With the molecular cloning of the different subunits of Ca²⁺ channels, a nomenclature system based on compositions of the α_1 subunit was suggested in 1994 (52). The α_1-subunit of skeletal muscle Ca²⁺ channels was named as α_{1S}, and subsequently cloned α_1-subunits as α_{1A} through α_{1I}. However, this nomenclature system cannot conveniently accommodate newly identified Ca²⁺ channels, and does not reflect the evolutionary relationship among the different α_1 subunits. As a result, a new nomen-

Table 4.1 Classification of voltage-sensitive Ca^{2+} channels (VSCCs)

Activation voltage	Pharmacologic and biophysical properties	α_1-Subunit composition	α_1-Subunit sequence	Most commonly used blockers
HVA	L-type	$\alpha1S$	$Ca_V1.1$	Dihydropyridine antagonists
		$\alpha1C$	$Ca_V1.2$	
		$\alpha1D$	$Ca_V1.3$	
		$\alpha1F$	$Ca_V1.4$	
	P/Q-type	$\alpha1A$	$Ca_V2.1$	ω-Agatoxin IVA
	N-type	$\alpha1B$	$Ca_V2.2$	ω-Conotoxin GVIA
	R-type	$\alpha1E$	$Ca_V2.3$	SNX-482
LVA	T-type	$\alpha1G$	$Ca_V3.1$	Mibefradil
		$\alpha1H$	$Ca_V3.2$	
		$\alpha1I$	$Ca_V3.3$	

Note: VSCCs are classified into high-voltage–activated (HVA) and low-voltage–activated (LVA) channels according to the degree of membrane depolarization needed for activation, into L-, P/Q-, N-, R-, and T-type channels according to biophysical/pharmacologic properties and tissue distribution, into α_{1S}, α_{1A-I} according to the α_1 subunit composition, and into $Ca_V1.1$–1.4, $Ca_V2.1$–2.3, and $Ca_V3.1$–3.3 according to the primary sequence of the α_1 subunit.
Based on Lacinova (49) and Catterall et al (50).

clature system based on amino acid sequence was adopted in 2000 (53). Ca^{2+} channels are named $Ca_Vx.y$, where *Ca* indicates the principal permeating ion, *v* indicates the principal physiologic regulator (voltage), *x* is a numerical identifier of the α_1 subunit subfamily, and *y* is a number indicating the order of discovery of the α_1 subunit within that subfamily. In this new nomenclature system, primary sequences of α_1 subunits are >70% identical within the same subfamily, but <40% between different subfamilies. Table 4.1shows the relationships among the different nomenclatures, and commonly used blockers specific to the Ca^{2+} channels. It is worth noting that the α_1-subunits of the P- and Q-type channels are encoded by the same gene. The distinct biophysical and pharmacologic properties of P- and Q-type channels are caused by different splice forms of the α_1 subunit and different β-subunits (50).

Many studies have been performed to identify Ca^{2+} channels triggering neurotransmitter release at the presynaptic nerve terminal. Generally, they are identified by analyzing the effects of specific Ca^{2+} channel blockers on the amplitude of evoked postsynaptic currents or potentials, or on the amplitude or slope of field excitatory postsynaptic potentials. These analyses revealed that $Ca_V2.1$ (P/Q-type) and $Ca_V2.2$ (N-type) channels play prominent roles in neurotransmitter release at many synapses examined, such as excitatory synapses in the hippocampus (54–57), inhibitory synapses in the cerebellum and spinal cord (56), and dopaminergic synapses in the striatum (58). At some synapses, only one type of channels appears to be responsible for Ca^{2+} influx at the presynaptic terminal. For example, neurotransmitter release at mature NMJs is triggered by Ca^{2+} influx through $Ca_V2.1$ alone (59–63). At other synapses, such as the glutamatergic synapse between hippocampal CA1 and CA3 neurons, neurotransmitter release is triggered by Ca^{2+} influx through both $Ca_V2.1$ and $Ca_V2.2$ (54). At still other synapses, such as the calyx of Held synapse, $Ca_V2.3$ (R-type) as well as $Ca_V2.1$ and $Ca_V2.2$ channels contributes to the release (64). Thus, members of the Ca_V2 subfamily play important roles in triggering neurotransmitter release. However, their relative contributions may vary from synapse to synapse.

Ca_V1 (L-type) and Ca_V3 (T-type) generally do not contribute to Ca^{2+} influx at the presynaptic nerve terminal. However, unusual examples have been reported. At the presynaptic terminal of rat retinal bipolar cells, both Ca_V1 and Ca_V3 contribute to neurotransmitter release (65). At the presynaptic terminal of goldfish retinal bipolar cells, Ca_V1 appears to be exclusively responsible for mediating neurotransmitter release (66). It is unclear why Ca_V2 channels are more suited to control neurotransmitter release than Ca_V1 and Ca_V3 channels. One hint came from analyses of the effects of exogenously introduced α_1-subunits in superior cervical ganglion neurons (SCGNs). In SCGNs, acetylcholine release is normally mediated by $Ca_V2.2$. When different α_1-subunits were expressed in these neurons, $Ca_V2.1$ and $Ca_V2.3$ were localized to nerve terminals and could mediate synaptic transmission, whereas $Ca_V1.2$ showed no presynaptic localization and no effect on synaptic transmission (67). The results of this study suggest that trafficking to nerve terminals may be a factor in determining whether a particular Ca^{2+} channel may contribute to neurotransmitter release.

The types of Ca^{2+} channels mediating neurotransmitter release at the presynaptic terminal are developmentally regulated and could change when the predominant channel is mutated. For example, at thalamic and cerebellar inhibitory synapses, the predominant Ca^{2+} channel for neurotransmitter release is $Ca_V2.2$ in immature neurons but $Ca_V2.1$ in mature neurons (68). At the rat calyx of Held synapse, neurotransmitter release is triggered by Ca^{2+} influx through $Ca_V2.1$, $Ca_V2.2$, and $Ca_V2.3$ (R-type) during postnatal days 4 to 9 (64,69). However, the contributions from $Ca_V2.2$ and $Ca_V2.3$ gradually decrease after postnatal day 7. By postnatal day 10, the release is mediated almost exclusively by $Ca_V2.1$ (69). At wild-type mouse NMJ, neurotransmitter release relies on $Ca_V2.1$ (70). However, in $Ca_V2.1$ knockout mice, $Ca_V2.2$ and $Ca_V2.3$ mediate neurotransmitter release at the NMJ (70). Similarly, at the NMJ of tottering mice, which carries a mutation in the α_1 subunit of $Ca_V2.1$, the predominant Ca^{2+} channels mediating neurotransmitter release are $Ca_V2.2$ and/or $Ca_V2.3$ (71,72). The developmental switch from $Ca_V2.2$ to $Ca_V2.1$ is potentially of physiologic significance. In $Ca_V2.1$ knockout mice, paired-pulse facilitation, which is observed at wild-type synapses, is often absent at the calyx of Held synapse (73) and NMJ (70); furthermore, synaptic depression in response to high-frequency (100 Hz) stimulation is more severe in the knockout mice than wild-type (74). Thus, the developmental switch from $Ca_V2.2$ to $Ca_V2.1$ may serve to increase synaptic efficacy.

Ryanodine Receptor-Mediated Ca^{2+} Release May Contribute to Neurotransmitter Release

The ER exists as an extensive network inside the neuron. It exists not only in the soma, but also in dendrites and axons, including the presynaptic nerve terminal (75). Such an extensive network of ER inside the neuron has led to the opinion that the ER is a neuron-within-a-neuron (7). The ER is a primary intracellular Ca^{2+}

store. Ca^{2+} inside the ER may be released through two kinds of ionotropic receptors in the ER membrane: inositol 1,4,5-trisphosphate receptor ($InsP_3R$) and RYR. The $InsP_3R$ is activated by $InsP_3$, and its sensitivity to $InsP_3$ is enhanced by Ca^{2+} (7). The RYR is mainly activated by Ca^{2+}-induced Ca^{2+} release (CICR), a process that links Ca^{2+} influx through VSCCs or receptor-operated Ca^{2+} channels in the plasma membrane to Ca^{2+} release from the ER (7). The RYR might also be activated through Ca^{2+} influx-independent coupling with VSCCs in the plasma membrane (76). The ER Ca^{2+} store is replenished through Ca^{2+} uptake by sarco(endo)plasmic reticulum Ca^{2+} adenosine triphosphatase (ATPase) (SERCA) (6). Although a large amount of Ca^{2+} is contained in the ER, its concentration is maintained within the range of 100 to 500 μM due to buffering by Ca^{2+}-binding proteins (77).

The RYR is a homomeric complex of four ~565-kDa subunits surrounding a central pore. Each subunit probably has six to eight transmembrane domains with the amino- and carboxyl-termini facing the cytoplasmic side. The amino terminal of the RYR subunit is very long, accounting for ~90% of the entire protein (78). In mammals, there are three isoforms of RYRs (RYR1, RYR2, and RYR3) encoded by three different genes. The predominant RYR isoforms in skeletal and cardiac muscles are RYR1 and RYR2, respectively (78). In contrast, all three isoforms are expressed in the nervous system (75). It was previously thought that Ca^{2+} influx through VSCCs is the sole source of Ca^{2+} mediating neurotransmitter release. However, a number of recent studies suggest that presynaptic RYRs may also play important roles in the release.

Presynaptic RYRs may control several aspects of neurotransmitter release. One reported function of presynaptic RYRs is that they regulate the frequency and amplitude of miniature postsynaptic currents (minis). In rat cerebellum, the frequency of inhibitory minis recorded from Purkinje cells was increased by 10 μM ryanodine but decreased by 100 μM ryanodine. The higher concentration of ryanodine also reduced the proportion of large-amplitude minis, whereas the lower concentration of ryanodine showed no effect on the amplitude (79). These opposite effects of ryanodine were thought to be due to activation and blockade of RYRs, respectively (79), because ryanodine locks RYR in a subconductance state at low micromolar or submicromolar concentrations but blocks it at higher micromolar concentrations (80). In rat hippocampus, nicotine increased the frequency of glutamatergic minis and the fraction of large-amplitude events. These effects of nicotine were mimicked by the RYR activator caffeine but blocked by 100 μM ryanodine (81). At the *C. elegans* NMJ, cholinergic and γ–aminobutyric acid (GABA)ergic minis occur at a relatively high frequency with many large-amplitude (>50 picoampere [pA]) events. In null mutants of *unc-68*, which encodes the only RYR of *C. elegans*, the frequency of minis was greatly reduced and large-amplitude events essentially disappeared, although postsynaptic receptor sensitivities to acetylcholine and GABA remained normal (82). All these observations suggest that presynaptic RYRs function to increase the frequency of minis and to promote the occurrence of large-amplitude events.

Minis are generally thought to result from sporadic exocytosis of individual synaptic vesicles. The amplitude of minis could potentially be affected by a variety of factors. How might presynaptic RYRs increase the occurrence of large-amplitude minis? One hypothesis is that presynaptic RYRs may promote synchronized multivesicular exocytosis. This hypothesis was mainly based on the results of two studies. In one study (79), large-amplitude minis were thought to be due to multi-vesicular release because their proportion could be reduced by prolonged exposure to a Ca^{2+}-free extracellular solution. In the other study (81), a similar conclusion was reached because a positive correlation was observed between the rise time and mean amplitude of minis. It was reasoned that when multiple synaptic vesicles exocytose at the same time, a lack of absolute synchrony would result in an increase of the rise time. An alternative hypothesis is that presynaptic RYRs may increase the quantal size (the amount of neurotransmitter released from a vesicle in a single exo-cytotic event). This hypothesis was mainly based on analyses of synaptic transmis-sion at the *C. elegans* NMJ. Several lines of evidence suggest that RYR-dependent large-amplitude minis at the *C. elegans* NMJ were not due to multivesicular release. First, the proportion of large-amplitude events did not decrease in syntaxin or SNAP-25 (synaptosome-associated protein of 25 kilodaltons) mutants, which are deficient in synchronizing synaptic vesicle exocytosis. Second, the rise time of minis was constant regardless of the amplitude. Third, the proportion of large-amplitude events did not decrease when $[Ca^{2+}]_o$ was changed from 5 mM to zero(82). Given the existence of these two competing hypotheses, further studies are needed to deter-mine whether RYR-mediated large-amplitude minis are mono- or multiquantal.

Presynaptic RYRs may be also important to evoked neurotransmitter release and to synaptic plasticity. At the *C. elegans* NMJ, the amplitude of evoked postsynaptic currents decreased by ~40% in *unc-68* null mutants compared with the wild-type, and this defect could be rescued by expressing a wild-type *unc-68* transgene in neurons but not muscle cells (82). At inhibitory synapses between cerebellar basket and Purkinje neurons, blocking RYRs with ryanodine decreased the mean ampli-tude of evoked inhibitory postsynaptic currents by ~30%, and this effect of ryanod-ine appeared to be presynaptic because ryanodine also increased paired-pulse ratio and failure rate (83). At the presynaptic terminal of hippocampal pyramidal neu-rons, blocking RYRs with ryanodine inhibited the paired-pulse facilitation of evoked EPSCs, suggesting that presynaptic RYRs play a role in short-term synaptic plasticity (84). At excitatory synapses between hippocampal CA3 neurons, block-ing RYRs with ryanodine during the induction period but not afterward abolished *N*-methyl-D-aspartate (NMDA) receptor-dependent long-term depression (LTD), suggesting that presynaptic RYR-sensitive stores are required for LTD induction but not expression (85).

The function of RYRs in regulating presynaptic Ca^{2+} signal has been examined by Ca^{2+} imaging in several studies. Two-photon laser scanning fluorescence micros-copy with Oregon Green-1 shows that ryanodine (100 μM) inhibits action potential-evoked Ca^{2+} transients by ~50% at the presynaptic terminal of rat cerebellar basket cells (79). Confocal laser scanning microscopy with Oregon Green 488 BAPTA-1 shows that ryanodine (20 μM) inhibits paired-pulse facilitation of Ca^{2+} transients at presynaptic boutons of hippocampal CA3 neurons (84). Ca^{2+} imaging with fluo-3 and a signal mass approach shows that 10 μM ryanodine increases whereas 100 μM ryanodine decreases the frequency of syntillas, which are brief and highly localized

Ca²⁺ transients, at isolated mouse hypothalamic magnocellular nerve terminals (86). These results show that presynaptic RYRs indeed mobilize Ca^{2+}.

Skeletal muscle contractions are triggered by Ca^{2+} release from the sarcoplasmic reticulum (SR). Ca^{2+} release from the SR is mediated by a functional coupling between dihydropyridine receptors (DHPRs or $Ca_V1.1$) in the plasma membrane and RYR1 in the SR membrane. A voltage-dependent conformational change of the DHPR rather than Ca^{2+} influx through the channel is required for RYR activation (87). A recent study (76) shows that depolarization (from −80 to −60 mV) increased the frequency of RYR-mediated Ca^{2+} syntillas or diffuse Ca^{2+} transients in the absence of extracellular Ca^{2+} at the presynaptic terminal of mouse hypothalamic magnocellular neurons, and this effect of depolarization was blocked by the DHPR antagonist nifedipine. These observations suggest that membrane depolarization may activate RYRs through functional coupling between Ca_V1 and RYRs without the need of Ca^{2+} influx. Consistent with this notion, the same study shows that RYR1, the isoform of RYRs expressed in skeletal muscle, is expressed at these nerve terminals. However, it is unclear whether this kind of functional coupling between Ca_V1 and RYRs is of general importance because blocking Ca_V1 does not have a detectable effect on neurotransmitter release in the majority of synapses examined.

In spite of the evidence presented above, the function of presynaptic RYRs in controlling neurotransmitter release remains elusive for several reasons. First, some studies show that blocking RYRs has little or no effect on synaptic transmission (88–91). Second, the effect of ryanodine on neurotransmitter release is often highly variable even in studies reporting that presynaptic RYRs play a role in spontaneous or evoked release. For example, application of ryanodine (10 μM) increased the frequency of inhibitory minis in only four of 10 rat cerebellar Purkinje neurons (79) and four of 12 mouse cerebellar Purkinje neurons (88). Ryanodine (100 μM) showed a highly variable and often weak effect on evoked neurotransmitter release from rat cerebellar basket cell terminals (83). Third, while the use of 100 μM ryanodine to inhibit RYRs reduced the proportion of large-amplitude minis at cerebellar inhibitory synapses, the use of 10 μM ryanodine to activate of RYRs did not show an opposite effect (79). Fourth, ryanodine is used as a key pharmacologic tool in the majority of previous studies. However, ryanodine is a bidirectional modulator of RYRs with the boundary of concentrations needed for activation and inhibition poorly defined. For example, 10 to 20 μM ryanodine has been used either to activate (79,81,88) or to block (84,89,92,93) RYRs. Thus, additional analyses with more specific pharmacologic agents, which are currently unavailable, or with RYR mutants are needed to better understand the function of presynaptic RYRs in neurotransmitter release.

Much less is known about the function of presynaptic InsP₃Rs in neurotransmitter release. In rat barrel cortex, blocking InsP₃Rs using 2-aminoethoxydiphenylborane reduced the frequency of minis recorded from layer II pyramidal neurons (93). At the *C. elegans* NMJ, however, synaptic transmission appeared normal in a hypomorphic mutant of *itr-1*, which encodes the only InsP₃R of *C. elegans* (82).

Presynaptic Mitochondria May Play a Role in Sustained Neurotransmitter Release

Mitochondria are enriched at the presynaptic nerve terminal and perform at least two important functions. First, they provide the energy need of the presynaptic nerve terminal, which may account for up to 10% of the total energy required for neuronal signaling (94). Second, they may regulate neurotransmitter release by modulating $[Ca^{2+}]_i$ at the presynaptic nerve terminal.

The inside of mitochondrion is ~200 mV more negative than the outside, which creates a substantial driving force for Ca^{2+} influx. Ca^{2+} may enter mitochondria through undefined uniporter(s) in the inner membrane and leave mitochondria through Na^+/Ca^{2+} and H^+/Ca^{2+} antiporters (95). During sustained high-frequency nerve stimulation, $[Ca^{2+}]$ inside the mitochondrion ($[Ca^{2+}]_m$) elevates due to increased uptake activity. There are debates about what levels $[Ca^{2+}]_m$ can rise to, with estimates ranging from as low as a few micromolars to as high as several hundred micromolars (95). Ca^{2+} uptake into the mitochondrion may occur even when cytoplasmic $[Ca^{2+}]$ is as low as a few hundred nanomolars (96,97).

The function of presynaptic mitochondria in neurotransmitter release has been analyzed in several synapses using pharmacologic agents that either depolarize the mitochondrial membrane or inhibit the uniporter. These analyses suggest that presynaptic mitochondria play several roles in synaptic transmission. First, presynaptic mitochondria may accelerate the recovery from short-term presynaptic depression. At the rat calyx of Held synapse, a train of stimuli at 200 Hz quickly leads to synaptic depression, as indicated by diminishing amplitudes of EPSCs. After a resting period of 500 ms, the amplitude of EPSCs in response to a single stimulus recovered to ~80% of the first EPSC in the train. Pharmacologic agents that either depolarize mitochondria or inhibit the uniporter reduced the recovery of EPSC amplitude as a result of deficient mitochondrial Ca^{2+} sequestration (98). Second, presynaptic mitochondria may alleviate synaptic depression in response to sustained nerve stimulation. At the lizard NMJ, the amplitude of end-plate potentials gradually decrease in response to a train of 500 stimuli at 50 Hz. Treatments that depolarize mitochondria aggravated the synaptic depression (99). Third, mitochondria may contribute to posttetanic potentiation. At the crayfish NMJ, tetanus stimulation of the motor axon for 7 to 10 minutes at 20 to 33 Hz potentiated subsequent responses to nerve stimulation, which were blocked by pharmacologic perturbation of mitochondrial Ca^{2+} handling (100). These observations suggest that regulation of Ca^{2+} by mitochondria may be important to the control of neurotransmitter release during sustained nerve stimulation.

Are minis Ca^{2+}-dependent?

Traditionally, minis were considered resulting from full-collapse fusion of individual synaptic vesicles, being the elementary events of action potential–evoked postsynaptic responses, and having no physiologic significance. In the last decade, however, our understanding of minis has grown considerably with several findings that represent notable progress. First, minis may occur not only from full-collapse fusion but also from kiss-and-run exocytosis. In the latter case, neurotransmitters in the synaptic vesicle might be released partially (see Chapter 2). Second, minis may be needed for several important physiologic functions, including postsynaptic receptor clustering (101), shift of NMDA receptor subunit compositions during development (102), regulation of dendritic protein synthesis (103,104), maintenance of dendritic spines (105), and action potential firing (81,106). Third, minis appear to be distinct from evoked responses in several ways: minis and evoked responses could be due to the release of distinct populations of synaptic vesicles (107); minis and evoked responses could depend on the function of different synaptotagmins, with synaptotagmins 1 and 2 important to evoked neurotransmitter release (13,108,109) and synaptotagmin 12, which does not bind Ca^{2+}, important to minis (110); minis and evoked responses might be mediated by different Ca^{2+} channels in the plasma membrane (111–113); minis and evoked responses are differentially affected by mutations of synaptobrevin (114), SNAP-25 (82,115), and synaptotagmins (108,109,116).

In spite of the physiologic importance of minis and their usefulness to the analysis of synaptic transmission, it is unsettled whether the occurrence of minis requires Ca^{2+}. Minis are frequently referred as "Ca^{2+}-independent" events in the scientific literature because they may occur in the presence of Ca^{2+}-free or nominally Ca^{2+}-free extracellular solutions. However, a significant amount of Ca^{2+} may be contained in the water used to make the nominally Ca^{2+}-free solution. Moreover, RYR-mediated Ca^{2+}-release from the ER may contribute to minis. Thus, the so-called "Ca^{2+} independence" is not a precise description about minis. Indeed, there seems no convincing evidence that minis may occur in the complete absence of Ca^{2+}, with the possible exceptions of minis induced by hypertonic solutions (117) and α-latrotoxin (118,119),

The roles of extracellular Ca^{2+} and RYRs in minis have been examined in a number of previous studies. Extracellular Ca^{2+} appeared to play a variable role in minis at different synapses. For example, changing $[Ca^{2+}]_o$ from 5 mM to zero reduced the frequency of minis by ~80% at the *C. elegans* NMJ (82,120). Application of ionomycin, a Ca^{2+} ionophore, increased the frequencies of both excitatory and inhibitory minis in hippocampal brain slices (119). These observations suggest that Ca^{2+} influx may cause minis. However, application of the Ca^{2+} channel blocker cadmium or a Ca^{2+}-free solution did not affect the frequency of minis at several synapses examined (121–125), suggesting that Ca^{2+} influx may not be a trigger of minis. At the frog NMJ, changing $[Ca^{2+}]_o$ showed variable effects on the frequency of minis (126).

Similarly, manipulating the function of RYRs showed variable effects on minis. Block of RYRs with ryanodine (20–100 μM) reduced the frequency of minis recorded from rat barrel cortex layer II pyramidal neurons (93), cerebellar Purkinje neurons (79), and hippocampal CA3 neurons (81), while activation of RYRs using caffeine or ryanodine (10 μM) increased the frequency of minis recorded from the pyramidal (93) and Purkinje (79) neurons. These observations suggest that

RYR-mediated Ca^{2+} release from the ER is important to minis. However, blocking RYRs with ryanodine (30 or 100 µM) did not show a significant effect on the frequencies of glycinergic minis in rat auditory brainstem nuclei (90) and GABAergic minis in rat hippocampus (91), suggesting that RYRs do not mediate minis at these synapses.

It is unclear why manipulations of $[Ca^{2+}]_o$ and RYR function appeared to have variable effects on minis from synapse to synapse. It is impossible to tell from the results described above whether Ca^{2+} is required for the occurrence of minis because a significant number of minis always existed when either $[Ca^{2+}]_o$ or RYR function was eliminated or inhibited. In a recent study, the combined effects of a Ca^{2+}-free extracellular solution and RYR dysfunction on synaptic transmission were analyzed in *C. elegans*. A null mutation of the RYR gene *unc-68* reduced the frequency of minis by more than 75% at the NMJ in the presence of 5 mM $[Ca^{2+}]_o$; the remaining minis were almost completely eliminated by applying a Ca^{2+}-free extracellular solution (82). These observations suggest that Ca^{2+} may be required for minis, and that Ca^{2+} influx and RYR-mediated Ca^{2+} release are the only sources of Ca^{2+} for triggering synaptic exocytosis at the *C. elegans* NMJ.

If Ca^{2+} is indeed required for the occurrence of minis, application of the fast Ca^{2+} chelators BAPTA-AM (BAPTA-tetraacetoxymethyl ester) might be able to eliminate all minis. However, BAPTA-AM showed no effect on the frequency of minis in rat dorsolateral periaqueductal gray neurons (127), at glycinergic inhibitory synapses of rat auditory brainstem nuclei (90), and at glutamatergic excitatory synapses in cultured rat CA3-CA1 hippocampal neurons (128). Application of a Ca^{2+}-free extracellular solution containing BAPTA-AM (100 µM) reduced the frequency of minis recorded from the mouse calyx of Held synapse and NMJ, and from rat barrel cortex layer II pyramidal neurons by ~90% and ~50%, respectively (93,109). These observations suggest that either Ca^{2+} is not essential to minis at these synapses or a very tight functional coupling exists between Ca^{2+} channels or RYRs and the Ca^{2+} sensor of synaptic exocytosis. Thus, it may be helpful to analyze the combined effects of a Ca^{2+}-free extracellular solution and RYR mutation on the frequency of minis in other systems to determine whether the findings from *C. elegans* are of general importance.

Acknowledgment   This work is supported by National Science Foundation grant 0619427 to the first author.

References

1. Locke FS. Notiz uber den Einfluss physiologischer Kochsalz-losung auf die elektrische Erregbarkeit von Muskel und Nerv. Zbl Physiol 1894;8:166–167.
2. Harvey AM, Macintosh FC. Calcium and synaptic transmission in a sympathetic ganglion. J Physiol 1940;97(3):408–416.
3. Del Castillo J, Stark L. The effect of calcium ions on the motor end-plate potentials. J Physiol 1952;116(4):507–515.

4. Dodge FA Jr, Rahamimoff R. Co-operative action a calcium ions in transmitter release at the neuromuscular junction. J Physiol 1967;193(2):419–432.
5. Katz B, Miledi R. The effect of calcium on acetylcholine release from motor nerve terminals. Proc R Soc Lond B Biol Sci 1965;161:496–503.
6. Verkhratsky A. The endoplasmic reticulum and neuronal calcium signalling. Cell Calcium 2002;32(5–6):393–404.
7. Berridge MJ. Neuronal calcium signaling. Neuron 1998;21(1):13–26.
8. Schneggenburger R, Neher E. Intracellular calcium dependence of transmitter release rates at a fast central synapse. Nature 2000;406(6798):889–893.
9. Heidelberger R, Heinemann C, Neher E, Matthews G. Calcium dependence of the rate of exocytosis in a synaptic terminal. Nature 1994;371(6497):513–515.
10. Lando L, Zucker RS. Ca2+ cooperativity in neurosecretion measured using photolabile Ca2+ chelators. J Neurophysiol 1994;72(2):825–830.
11. Bollmann JH, Sakmann B, Borst JG. Calcium sensitivity of glutamate release in a calyx-type terminal. Science 2000;289(5481):953–957.
12. Goda Y, Stevens CF. Two components of transmitter release at a central synapse. Proc Natl Acad Sci U S A 1994;91(26):12942–12946.
13. Fernandez-Chacon R, Konigstorfer A, Gerber SH, et al. Synaptotagmin I functions as a calcium regulator of release probability. Nature 2001;410(6824):41–49.
14. Yoshihara M, Littleton JT. Synaptotagmin I functions as a calcium sensor to synchronize neurotransmitter release. Neuron 2002;36(5):897–908.
15. Broadie K, Bellen HJ, DiAntonio A, Littleton JT, Schwarz TL. Absence of synaptotagmin disrupts excitation-secretion coupling during synaptic transmission. Proc Natl Acad Sci U S A 1994;91(22):10727–10731.
16. Stewart BA, Mohtashami M, Trimble WS, Boulianne GL. SNARE proteins contribute to calcium cooperativity of synaptic transmission. Proc Natl Acad Sci U S A 2000;97 (25):13955–13960.
17. Augustine GJ, Adler EM, Charlton MP. The calcium signal for transmitter secretion from presynaptic nerve terminals. Ann N Y Acad Sci 1991;635:365–381.
18. Felmy F, Neher E, Schneggenburger R. Probing the intracellular calcium sensitivity of transmitter release during synaptic facilitation. Neuron 2003;37(5):801–811.
19. Rickman C, Hu K, Carroll J, Davletov B. Self-assembly of SNARE fusion proteins into star-shaped oligomers. Biochem J 2005;388(pt 1):75–79.
20. Liu Q, Chen B, Ge Q, Wang ZW. Presynaptic Ca2+/calmodulin-dependent protein kinase II modulates neurotransmitter release by activating BK channels at Caenorhabditis elegans neuromuscular junction. J Neurosci 2007;27(39):10404–10413.
21. Gentile L, Stanley EF. A unified model of presynaptic release site gating by calcium channel domains. Eur J Neurosci 2005;21(1):278–282.
22. Kuno M, Takahashi T. Effects of calcium and magnesium on transmitter release at Ia synapses of rat spinal motoneurones in vitro. J Physiol 1986;376:543–553.
23. Hubbard JI, Jones SF, Landau EM. On the mechanism by which calcium and magnesium affect the release of transmitter by nerve impulses. J Physiol 1968;196(1):75–86.
24. Shimosawa T, Takano K, Ando K, Fujita T. Magnesium inhibits norepinephrine release by blocking N-type calcium channels at peripheral sympathetic nerve endings. Hypertension 2004;44(6):897–902.
25. Zhang A, Fan SH, Cheng TP, Altura BT, Wong RK, Altura BM. Extracellular Mg2+ modulates intracellular Ca2+ in acutely isolated hippocampal CA1 pyramidal cells of the guinea-pig. Brain Res 1996;728(2):204–208.
26. Shi J, Krishnamoorthy G, Yang Y, et al. Mechanism of magnesium activation of calcium-activated potassium channels. Nature 2002;418(6900):876–880.
27. Robitaille R, Garcia ML, Kaczorowski GJ, Charlton MP. Functional colocalization of calcium and calcium-gated potassium channels in control of transmitter release. Neuron 1993;11 (4):645–655.
28. Wang ZW, Saifee O, Nonet ML, Salkoff L. SLO-1 potassium channels control quantal content of neurotransmitter release at the C. elegans neuromuscular junction. Neuron 2001;32 (5):867–881.

29. Adler EM, Augustine GJ, Duffy SN, Charlton MP. Alien intracellular calcium chelators attenuate neurotransmitter release at the squid giant synapse. J Neurosci 1991;11(6):1496–1507.
30. Tandon A, Bannykh S, Kowalchyk JA, Banerjee A, Martin TF, Balch WE. Differential regulation of exocytosis by calcium and CAPS in semi-intact synaptosomes. Neuron 1998;21 (1):147–154.
31. Wolfel M, Schneggenburger R. Presynaptic capacitance measurements and Ca2+ uncaging reveal submillisecond exocytosis kinetics and characterize the Ca2+ sensitivity of vesicle pool depletion at a fast CNS synapse. J Neurosci 2003;23(18):7059–7068.
32. Augustine GJ, Santamaria F, Tanaka K. Local calcium signaling in neurons. Neuron 2003;40(2):331–346.
33. Fogelson AL, Zucker RS. Presynaptic calcium diffusion from various arrays of single channels. Implications for transmitter release and synaptic facilitation. Biophys J 1985;48(6): 1003–1017.
34. Simon SM, Llinas RR. Compartmentalization of the submembrane calcium activity during calcium influx and its significance in transmitter release. Biophys J 1985;48(3):485–498.
35. Zucker RS, Fogelson AL. Relationship between transmitter release and presynaptic calcium influx when calcium enters through discrete channels. Proc Natl Acad Sci U S A 1986;83(9):3032–3036.
36. Llinas R, Sugimori M, Silver RB. Microdomains of high calcium concentration in a presynaptic terminal. Science 1992;256(5057):677–679.
37. Beaumont V, Llobet A, Lagnado L. Expansion of calcium microdomains regulates fast exocytosis at a ribbon synapse. Proc Natl Acad Sci U S A 2005;102(30):10700–10705.
38. Yazejian B, Sun XP, Grinnell AD. Tracking presynaptic Ca2+ dynamics during neurotransmitter release with Ca2+-activated K+ channels. Nat Neurosci 2000;3(6):566–571.
39. DiGregorio DA, Peskoff A, Vergara JL. Measurement of action potential-induced presynaptic calcium domains at a cultured neuromuscular junction. J Neurosci 1999;19(18):7846–7859.
40. Demuro A, Parker I. Imaging single-channel calcium microdomains. Cell Calcium 2006;40(5–6):413–422.
41. Zenisek D, Davila V, Wan L, Almers W. Imaging calcium entry sites and ribbon structures in two presynaptic cells. J Neurosci 2003;23(7):2538–2548.
42. Heidelberger R, Matthews G. Calcium influx and calcium current in single synaptic terminals of goldfish retinal bipolar neurons. J Physiol 1992;447:235–256.
43. Neves G, Lagnado L. The kinetics of exocytosis and endocytosis in the synaptic terminal of goldfish retinal bipolar cells. J Physiol 1999;515(pt 1):181–202.
44. Zenisek D, Matthews G. The role of mitochondria in presynaptic calcium handling at a ribbon synapse. Neuron 2000;25(1):229–237.
45. von Gersdorff H, Matthews G. Dynamics of synaptic vesicle fusion and membrane retrieval in synaptic terminals. Nature 1994;367(6465):735–739.
46. Borst JG, Sakmann B. Calcium influx and transmitter release in a fast CNS synapse. Nature 1996;383(6599):431–434.
47. Meinrenken CJ, Borst JG, Sakmann B. Calcium secretion coupling at calyx of held governed by nonuniform channel-vesicle topography. J Neurosci 2002;22(5):1648–1667.
48. Schneggenburger R, Neher E. Presynaptic calcium and control of vesicle fusion. Curr Opin Neurobiol 2005;15(3):266–274.
49. Lacinova L. Voltage-dependent calcium channels. Gen Physiol Biophys 2005;24(suppl 1): 1–78.
50. Catterall WA, Perez-Reyes E, Snutch TP, Striessnig J. International Union of Pharmacology. XLVIII. Nomenclature and structure-function relationships of voltage-gated calcium channels. Pharmacol Rev 2005;57(4):411–425.
51. Randall A, Tsien RW. Pharmacological dissection of multiple types of Ca2+ channel currents in rat cerebellar granule neurons. J Neurosci 1995;15(4):2995–3012.
52. Birnbaumer L, Campbell KP, Catterall WA, et al. The naming of voltage-gated calcium channels. Neuron 1994;13(3):505–506.
53. Ertel EA, Campbell KP, Harpold MM, et al. Nomenclature of voltage-gated calcium channels. Neuron 2000;25(3):533–535.

54. Wheeler DB, Randall A, Tsien RW. Roles of N-type and Q-type Ca2+ channels in supporting hippocampal synaptic transmission. Science 1994;264(5155):107–111.
55. Wu LG, Saggau P. Pharmacological identification of two types of presynaptic voltage-dependent calcium channels at CA3–CA1 synapses of the hippocampus. J Neurosci 1994;14(9):5613–5622.
56. Takahashi T, Momiyama A. Different types of calcium channels mediate central synaptic transmission. Nature 1993;366(6451):156–158.
57. Luebke JI, Dunlap K, Turner TJ. Multiple calcium channel types control glutamatergic synaptic transmission in the hippocampus. Neuron 1993;11(5):895–902.
58. Turner TJ, Adams ME, Dunlap K. Multiple Ca2+ channel types coexist to regulate synaptosomal neurotransmitter release. Proc Natl Acad Sci U S A 1993;90(20):9518–9522.
59. Uchitel OD, Protti DA, Sanchez V, Cherksey BD, Sugimori M, Llinas R. P-type voltage-dependent calcium channel mediates presynaptic calcium influx and transmitter release in mammalian synapses. Proc Natl Acad Sci U S A 1992;89(8):3330–3333.
60. Protti DA, Reisin R, Mackinley TA, Uchitel OD. Calcium channel blockers and transmitter release at the normal human neuromuscular junction. Neurology 1996;46(5):1391–1396.
61. Protti DA, Sanchez VA, Cherksey BD, Sugimori M, Llinas R, Uchitel OD. Mammalian neuromuscular transmission blocked by funnel web toxin. Ann N Y Acad Sci 1993; 681:405–407.
62. Bowersox SS, Miljanich GP, Sugiura Y, et al. Differential blockade of voltage-sensitive calcium channels at the mouse neuromuscular junction by novel omega-conopeptides and omega-agatoxin-IVA. J Pharmacol Exp Ther 1995;273(1):248–256.
63. Araque A, Clarac F, Buno W. P-type Ca2+ channels mediate excitatory and inhibitory synaptic transmitter release in crayfish muscle. Proc Natl Acad Sci U S A 1994;91(10):4224–4228.
64. Wu LG, Westenbroek RE, Borst JG, Catterall WA, Sakmann B. Calcium channel types with distinct presynaptic localization couple differentially to transmitter release in single calyx-type synapses. J Neurosci 1999;19(2):726–736.
65. Pan ZH, Hu HJ, Perring P, Andrade R. T-type Ca(2+) channels mediate neurotransmitter release in retinal bipolar cells. Neuron 2001;32(1):89–98.
66. Tachibana M, Okada T, Arimura T, Kobayashi K, Piccolino M. Dihydropyridine-sensitive calcium current mediates neurotransmitter release from bipolar cells of the goldfish retina. J Neurosci 1993;13(7):2898–2909.
67. Mochida S, Westenbroek RE, Yokoyama CT, Itoh K, Catterall WA. Subtype-selective reconstitution of synaptic transmission in sympathetic ganglion neurons by expression of exogenous calcium channels. Proc Natl Acad Sci U S A 2003;100(5):2813–2818.
68. Iwasaki S, Momiyama A, Uchitel OD, Takahashi T. Developmental changes in calcium channel types mediating central synaptic transmission. J Neurosci 2000;20(1):59–65.
69. Iwasaki S, Takahashi T. Developmental changes in calcium channel types mediating synaptic transmission in rat auditory brainstem. J Physiol 1998;509(pt 2):419–423.
70. Urbano FJ, Piedras-Renteria ES, Jun K, Shin HS, Uchitel OD, Tsien RW. Altered properties of quantal neurotransmitter release at endplates of mice lacking P/Q-type Ca2+ channels. Proc Natl Acad Sci U S A 2003;100(6):3491–3496.
71. Pardo NE, Hajela RK, Atchison WD. Acetylcholine release at neuromuscular junctions of adult tottering mice is controlled by N-(cav2.2) and R-type (cav2.3) but not L-type (cav1.2) Ca2+ channels. J Pharmacol Exp Ther 2006;319(3):1009–1020.
72. Kaja S, Van de Ven RC, Ferrari MD, Frants RR, Van den Maagdenberg AM, Plomp JJ. Compensatory contribution of Cav2.3 channels to acetylcholine release at the neuromuscular junction of tottering mice. J Neurophysiol 2006;95(4):2698–2704.
73. Inchauspe CG, Martini FJ, Forsythe ID, Uchitel OD. Functional compensation of P/Q by N-type channels blocks short-term plasticity at the calyx of held presynaptic terminal. J Neurosci 2004;24(46):10379–10383.
74. Ishikawa T, Kaneko M, Shin HS, Takahashi T. Presynaptic N-type and P/Q-type Ca2+ channels mediating synaptic transmission at the calyx of Held of mice. J Physiol 2005;568(pt 1): 199–209.
75. Bouchard R, Pattarini R, Geiger JD. Presence and functional significance of presynaptic ryanodine receptors. Prog Neurobiol 2003;69(6):391–418.

76. De Crescenzo V, Fogarty KE, Zhuge R, et al. Dihydropyridine receptors and type 1 ryanodine receptors constitute the molecular machinery for voltage-induced Ca2+ release in nerve terminals. J Neurosci 2006;26(29):7565–7574.
77. Berridge MJ. The endoplasmic reticulum: a multifunctional signaling organelle. Cell Calcium 2002;32(5–6):235–249.
78. Zalk R, Lehnart SE, Marks AR. Modulation of the ryanodine receptor and intracellular calcium. Annu Rev Biochem 2007;76:367–385.
79. Llano I, Gonzalez J, Caputo C, et al. Presynaptic calcium stores underlie large-amplitude miniature IPSCs and spontaneous calcium transients. Nat Neurosci 2000;3(12):1256–1265.
80. Sutko JL, Airey JA, Welch W, Ruest L. The pharmacology of ryanodine and related compounds. Pharmacol Rev 1997;49(1):53–98.
81. Sharma G, Vijayaraghavan S. Modulation of presynaptic store calcium induces release of glutamate and postsynaptic firing. Neuron 2003;38(6):929–939.
82. Liu Q, Chen B, Yankova M, et al. Ryanodine receptors are required for normal quantal size at the C. elegans neuromuscular junction. J Neurosci 2005;25:6745–6754.
83. Galante M, Marty A. Presynaptic ryanodine-sensitive calcium stores contribute to evoked neurotransmitter release at the basket cell-Purkinje cell synapse. J Neurosci 2003;23(35):11229–11234.
84. Emptage NJ, Reid CA, Fine A. Calcium stores in hippocampal synaptic boutons mediate short-term plasticity, store-operated Ca2+ entry, and spontaneous transmitter release. Neuron 2001;29(1):197–208.
85. Unni VK, Zakharenko SS, Zablow L, DeCostanzo AJ, Siegelbaum SA. Calcium release from presynaptic ryanodine-sensitive stores is required for long-term depression at hippocampal CA3–CA3 pyramidal neuron synapses. J Neurosci 2004;24(43):9612–9622.
86. De Crescenzo V, ZhuGe R, Velazquez-Marrero C, et al. Ca2+ syntillas, miniature Ca2+ release events in terminals of hypothalamic neurons, are increased in frequency by depolarization in the absence of Ca2+ influx. J Neurosci 2004;24(5):1226–1235.
87. Nakai J, Dirksen RT, Nguyen HT, Pessah IN, Beam KG, Allen PD. Enhanced dihydropyridine receptor channel activity in the presence of ryanodine receptor. Nature 1996;380(6569):72–75.
88. Bardo S, Robertson B, Stephens GJ. Presynaptic internal Ca2+ stores contribute to inhibitory neurotransmitter release onto mouse cerebellar Purkinje cells. Br J Pharmacol 2002;137(4):529–537.
89. Carter AG, Vogt KE, Foster KA, Regehr WG. Assessing the role of calcium-induced calcium release in short-term presynaptic plasticity at excitatory central synapses. J Neurosci 2002;22(1):21–28.
90. Lim R, Oleskevich S, Few AP, Leao RN, Walmsley B. Glycinergic mIPSCs in mouse and rat brainstem auditory nuclei: modulation by ruthenium red and the role of calcium stores. J Physiol 2003;546(pt 3):691–699.
91. Savic N, Sciancalepore M. Intracellular calcium stores modulate miniature GABA-mediated synaptic currents in neonatal rat hippocampal neurons. Eur J Neurosci 1998;10(11):3379–3386.
92. Narita K, Akita T, Hachisuka J, Huang S, Ochi K, Kuba K. Functional coupling of Ca(2+) channels to ryanodine receptors at presynaptic terminals. Amplification of exocytosis and plasticity. J Gen Physiol 2000;115(4):519–532.
93. Simkus CR, Stricker C. The contribution of intracellular calcium stores to mEPSCs recorded in layer II neurones of rat barrel cortex. J Physiol 2002;545(pt 2):521–535.
94. Laughlin SB. Energy as a constraint on the coding and processing of sensory information. Curr Opin Neurobiol 2001;11(4):475–480.
95. Rizzuto R, Duchen MR, Pozzan T. Flirting in little space: the ER/mitochondria Ca2+ liaison. Sci STKE 2004;2004(215):re1.
96. Colegrove SL, Albrecht MA, Friel DD. Dissection of mitochondrial Ca2+ uptake and release fluxes in situ after depolarization-evoked [Ca2+](i) elevations in sympathetic neurons. J Gen Physiol 2000;115(3):351–370.
97. David G, Barrett JN, Barrett EF. Evidence that mitochondria buffer physiological Ca2+ loads in lizard motor nerve terminals. J Physiol 1998;509(pt 1):59–65.
98. Billups B, Forsythe ID. Presynaptic mitochondrial calcium sequestration influences transmission at mammalian central synapses. J Neurosci 2002;22(14):5840–5807.

99. Talbot JD, David G, Barrett EF. Inhibition of mitochondrial Ca2+ uptake affects phasic release from motor terminals differently depending on external [Ca2+]. J Neurophysiol 2003;90(1):491–502.

100. Tang Y, Zucker RS. Mitochondrial involvement in post-tetanic potentiation of synaptic transmission. Neuron 1997;18(3):483–491.

101. Saitoe M, Schwarz TL, Umbach JA, Gundersen CB, Kidokoro Y. Absence of junctional glutamate receptor clusters in Drosophila mutants lacking spontaneous transmitter release. Science 2001;293(5529):514–517.

102. Barria A, Malinow R. Subunit-specific NMDA receptor trafficking to synapses. Neuron 2002;35(2):345–353.

103. Sutton MA, Wall NR, Aakalu GN, Schuman EM. Regulation of dendritic protein synthesis by miniature synaptic events. Science 2004;304(5679):1979–1983.

104. Sutton MA, Ito HT, Cressy P, Kempf C, Woo JC, Schuman EM. Miniature neurotransmission stabilizes synaptic function via tonic suppression of local dendritic protein synthesis. Cell 2006;125(4):785–799.

105. McKinney RA, Capogna M, Durr R, Gahwiler BH, Thompson SM. Miniature synaptic events maintain dendritic spines via AMPA receptor activation. Nat Neurosci 1999;2(1):44–49.

106. Carter AG, Regehr WG. Quantal events shape cerebellar interneuron firing. Nat Neurosci 2002;5(12):1309–1318.

107. Sara Y, Virmani T, Deak F, Liu X, Kavalali ET. An isolated pool of vesicles recycles at rest and drives spontaneous neurotransmission. Neuron 2005;45(4):563–573.

108. Geppert M, Goda Y, Hammer RE, et al. Synaptotagmin I: a major Ca2+ sensor for transmitter release at a central synapse. Cell 1994;79(4):717–727.

109. Pang ZP, Sun J, Rizo J, Maximov A, Sudhof TC. Genetic analysis of synaptotagmin 2 in spontaneous and Ca2+-triggered neurotransmitter release. EMBO J 2006;25(10):2039–2050.

110. Maximov A, Shin OH, Liu X, Sudhof TC. Synaptotagmin-12, a synaptic vesicle phosphoprotein that modulates spontaneous neurotransmitter release. J Cell Biol 2007;176(1):113–124.

111. Katz E, Ferro PA, Cherksey BD, Sugimori M, Llinas R, Uchitel OD. Effects of Ca2+ channel blockers on transmitter release and presynaptic currents at the frog neuromuscular junction. J Physiol 1995;486(pt 3):695–706.

112. Bao J, Li JJ, Perl ER. Differences in Ca2+ channels governing generation of miniature and evoked excitatory synaptic currents in spinal laminae I and II. J Neurosci 1998;18(21):8740–8750.

113. Losavio A, Muchnik S. Spontaneous acetylcholine release in mammalian neuromuscular junctions. Am J Physiol 1997;273(6 Pt 1):C1835–1841.

114. Schoch S, Deak F, Konigstorfer A, et al. SNARE function analyzed in synaptobrevin/VAMP knockout mice. Science 2001;294(5544):1117–1122.

115. Washbourne P, Thompson PM, Carta M, et al. Genetic ablation of the t-SNARE SNAP-25 distinguishes mechanisms of neuroexocytosis. Nat Neurosci 2002;5(1):19–26.

116. Littleton JT, Stern M, Schulze K, Perin M, Bellen HJ. Mutational analysis of Drosophila synaptotagmin demonstrates its essential role in Ca(2+)-activated neurotransmitter release. Cell 1993;74(6):1125–1134.

117. Rosenmund C, Stevens CF. Definition of the readily releasable pool of vesicles at hippocampal synapses. Neuron 1996;16(6):1197–1207.

118. Sudhof TC. The synaptic vesicle cycle: a cascade of protein-protein interactions. Nature 1995;375(6533):645–653.

119. Capogna M, Gahwiler BH, Thompson SM. Presynaptic inhibition of calcium-dependent and -independent release elicited with ionomycin, gadolinium, and alpha-latrotoxin in the hippocampus. J Neurophysiol 1996;75(5):2017–2028.

120. Richmond JE, Davis WS, Jorgensen EM. UNC-13 is required for synaptic vesicle fusion in C. elegans. Nat Neurosci 1999;2(11):959–964.

121. Han MH, Kawasaki A, Wei JY, Barnstable CJ. Miniature postsynaptic currents depend on Ca2+ released from internal stores via PLC/IP3 pathway. Neuroreport 2001;12(10):2203–2207.

122. Hajos N, Katona I, Naiem SS, et al. Cannabinoids inhibit hippocampal GABAergic transmission and network oscillations. Eur J Neurosci 2000;12(9):3239–3249.

123. Silinsky EM. On the mechanism by which adenosine receptor activation inhibits the release of acetylcholine from motor nerve endings. J Physiol 1984;346:243–256.
124. Scanziani M, Capogna M, Gahwiler BH, Thompson SM. Presynaptic inhibition of miniature excitatory synaptic currents by baclofen and adenosine in the hippocampus. Neuron 1992;9(5):919–927.
125. Scholz KP, Miller RJ. Inhibition of quantal transmitter release in the absence of calcium influx by a G protein-linked adenosine receptor at hippocampal synapses. Neuron 1992;8(6):1139–1150.
126. Fatt P, Katz B. Spontaneous subthreshold activity at motor nerve endings. J Physiol 1952;117:109–128.
127. Yang YM, Chung JM, Rhim H. Cellular action of cholecystokinin-8S-mediated excitatory effects in the rat periaqueductal gray. Life Sci 2006;79(18):1702–1711.
128. Abenavoli A, Forti L, Bossi M, Bergamaschi A, Villa A, Malgaroli A. Multimodal quantal release at individual hippocampal synapses: evidence for no lateral inhibition. J Neurosci 2002;22(15):6336–6346.
129. Meinrenken CJ, Borst JG, Sakmann B. Local routes revisited: the space and time dependence of the Ca2+ signal for phasic transmitter release at the rat calyx of Held. J Physiol 2003;547(pt 3):665–689.
130. Xu J, Wu LG. The decrease in the presynaptic calcium current is a major cause of short-term depression at a calyx-type synapse. Neuron 2005;46(4):633–645.
131. Augustine GJ. How does calcium trigger neurotransmitter release? Curr Opin Neurobiol 2001;11(3):320–326.

Chapter 5
Regulation of Presynaptic Calcium Channels

Allen W. Chan and Elise F. Stanley

Contents

Abstract Calcium ion influx through voltage-gated calcium channels is an essential step in action potential–triggered release of neurotransmitters from presynaptic terminals and, hence, in the transfer of information in the nervous system. In addition to their role as calcium ion entry points, these ion channels are subject to both positive and negative modulation via a number of molecular signaling pathways. These regulatory mechanisms are important to the control of synaptic strength and plasticity and as potential pharmaceutical targets. This chapter reviews the principal mechanisms of presynaptic calcium channel regulation via pathways that include G-protein–coupled receptors, phosphorylation by protein kinase C, and their interaction with companion elements of the transmitter release site.

Elise F. Stanley Ph.D.
MP14-320, Toronto Western Research Institute, Toronto Ontario M5T 2S8, Canada
e-mail: estanley@uhnres.utoronto.ca

Allen W. Chan
MP14-320, Toronto Western Research Institute, Toronto Ontario M5T 2S8, Canada
e-mail: alchan@uhnres.utoronto.ca

Z.-W. Wang (ed.) *Molecular Mechanisms of Neurotransmitter Release,*
© Humana Press 2008 a part of Springer Science+Business Media, LLC

Keywords Voltage-gated calcium channel (VGCC), G-protein, syntaxin, Munc18, PKC.

In a classic experiment, Katz and Miledi (1) demonstrated at the frog neuromuscular junction that transmitter release from presynaptic terminals required both membrane depolarization and the presence of calcium ions. Subsequent work has shown that the combined application of these elements was necessary both to open voltage-gated calcium channels and to allow Ca^{2+} to enter the terminal and bind to a calcium sensor. Binding of the ion to the calcium sensor initiates a sequence of events that culminates in the fusion of the synaptic vesicle (SV) with the plasma membrane, discharging its contents. Thus, in this role the channels act as a key element of an electromechanical transducer (2).

The advent of the squid giant synapse experimental preparation opened up the presynaptic terminal for direct, real-time analysis using intracellular recording (3) and analysis of the ion channels by voltage clamp. Unequivocal evidence was presented both for inward Ca^{2+} currents (4,5) and for the entry of Ca^{2+} ions into the cytoplasm (6). The finding of a ~200 μs minimum latency between Ca^{2+} influx and transmitter release (7) combined with theoretical diffusion rates suggested that the channels are located within a few hundred nanometers of the calcium sensor. Subsequent experiments demonstrating that calcium sensor activation could be triggered by Ca^{2+} influx through a *single* calcium channel, admitting as few as ~200 Ca^{2+} ions, restricted this diffusion distance to ~25 nm and favored the conclusion that the channel(s) is (are) actually tethered to the synaptic vesicle fusion machinery (8). Recent detailed studies on release site gating favor a highly localized organizational model and a bridging protein tether (9–12).

The calcium dependence of neurotransmitter release has been investigated in numerous studies. Dodge and Rahamimoff's (13) seminal work demonstrated that the amount of evoked neurotransmitter release is steeply dependent on calcium concentration with release rates proportional to calcium concentration raised to the power of ~4 (see Chapter 4 for further discussion). This steep power dependence most likely evolved to minimize the likelihood of random activation of the release mechanism by small fluctuations in cytoplasmic Ca^{2+} levels. Mutant analyses, and *in vitro* and molecular studies suggest that synaptotagmin-1 serves, or at least contributes to, the calcium sensing mechanism (reviewed extensively in refs. 14 to 17). However, the full biology of presynaptic calcium channels cannot be fully comprehended without placing the channel within the context of an organized, multifunctional presynaptic transmitter release site organelle (13,18). The apposition to, and interaction with, the release site provides numerous opportunities for molecular conversations between the channel and its release site neighbors and reveal additional modulation pathways. In summary, the fundamental role of calcium signaling in triggering neurotransmitter release, the steep dependence of release on cytoplasmic Ca^{2+}, and its interaction with numerous membrane-associated and cytoplasmic proteins combine to make the calcium channels a powerful effecter for the regulation of synaptic strength.

Molecular Structure of Voltage-Gated Calcium Channels

Calcium Channel α_1 Subunit

Voltage-gated calcium channels are heteromultimeric proteins composed of four or five subunits (reviewed extensively in refs. 19 to 24). They consist of a large (190 to 250 kDa), pore forming, α_1 subunit containing four homologous domains (I, II, III, and IV) that are connected via intracellular loops (I–II, II–III, III–IV). Each homologous domain is composed of six membrane-spanning segments (S1 to S6) and a "P" (pore) loop between S5 and S6. In addition, the positively charged S4 segments have been implicated as the voltage sensor that allows the channel to open and close in response to changes in membrane potential (Fig. 5.1A).

Calcium channels have been classified according to pharmacologic/physiologic properties, α_1 subunit composition, and genetic family type, resulting in a sometimes confusing array of names. The current naming system is mainly based on the primary sequence of the α_1 subunits (20,25). Under this system, voltage-gated calcium channel α_1 subunits are grouped into three families (Ca_V1, Ca_V2, and Ca_V3) (26) and are encoded for by at least 10 genes in mammals (Fig. 5.1B).

Ca^{2+} channels of the Ca_V1 family, including $Ca_V1.1$, 1.2, 1.3, and 1.4, are also called L-type calcium channels because the currents that they conduct are often long-lasting (27–31). They are susceptible to blockade by dihydropyridines and are primarily known for their roles in excitation-contraction coupling of muscles, although they are also expressed in neurons (32,33). Ca^{2+} channels of the Ca_V2 family include $Ca_V2.1$, $Ca_V2.2$, and $Ca_V2.3$, which conduct the P/Q-, N-, and R-type calcium currents, respectively, and are widely expressed in neurons. $Ca_V2.1$ (P/Q-type) currents were initially described in Purkinje cells (34,35) and can be blocked by the funnel web spider venom ω-agatoxin-IVA (36). $Ca_V2.2$ currents were originally designated N-type and were first identified in chick dorsal root ganglion (DRG) neurons (37). They are blocked with high specificity by low concentrations of the cone snail toxin ω-conotoxin GVIA (38). $Ca_V2.3$ is responsible for the R-type currents, so named because of their resistance to all the known calcium channel antagonists at the time of their initial description (39–41). Lastly, Ca^{2+} channels of the Ca_V3 family include $Ca_V3.1$, 3.2, and 3.3, and were originally grouped as T-type calcium channels. Ca_V3 currents, as opposed to Ca_V1 and Ca_V2 currents, are low voltage–activated and inactivate rapidly (42,43). This family is expressed in many tissues and is blocked by the scorpion toxin kurotoxin and nickel but with varying efficacy (44–46).

Typically only the Ca_V2 family of calcium channels is expressed at presynaptic terminals and often in various combinations so that neurotransmitter release is controlled by calcium influx from more than one type of calcium channels (47,48). At some synapses, such as the much-studied calyx of Held synapse of the medial nucleus of the trapezoid body (MNTB), the identities of presynaptic calcium channels are developmentally regulated. Here, calcium influx from all members of the Ca_V2 family contributes to neurotransmitter release in neonatal rats, but during

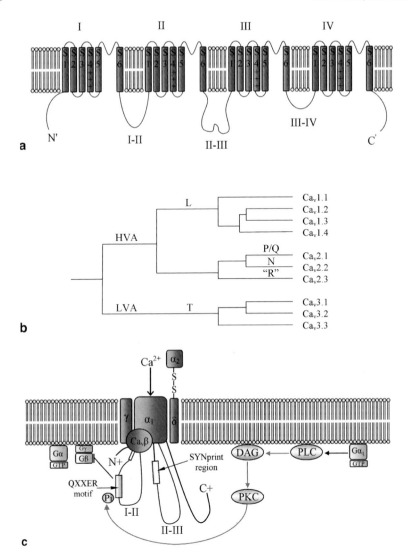

Fig. 5.1 Calcium channel structure, phylogeny, and interaction with key regulatory molecules. (A) A schematic diagram of the structure and membrane topology of the calcium channel α_1 subunit. Depicted are the four homologous domains (I–IV) each containing six membrane-spanning helices (S1 to S6). Connecting the four domains are intracellular linker regions (I–II, II–III, and III–IV). The positively charged nature of the S4 segments contributes to the voltage sensitivity of the channel and is denoted by "+" symbols. Also depicted between S5 and S6 segments are the "P"-loop that forms the channel pore. (B) A dendrogram illustrating the phylogenetic relationship between the three families of voltage-gated calcium channel α_1 subunits (Ca_V1, Ca_V2, and Ca_V3), their division into high- and low-voltage activated populations (HVA and LVA), and their corresponding identities under previous nomenclature. (C) A schematic diagram illustrating interaction sites of Ca_V2 with key regulatory molecules. G-protein $\beta\gamma$ subunits can inhibit the calcium channel via interaction sites on the I–II linker as well as less well defined sites in the N- and C-terminals. G$\beta\gamma$-induced channel inhibition can be antagonized by phosphorylation of consensus sites in the I–II linker region by protein kinase C (PKC) leading to channel upregulation. This pathway is activated by $G\alpha_q$ activation of phospholipase C via diacylglycerol (DAG) synthesis

postnatal development the expression of $Ca_V2.2$ and $Ca_V2.3$ is eventually lost, leaving $Ca_V2.1$ as the only presynaptic calcium channel (49,50).

Calcium Channel Auxiliary Subunits

Voltage-gated calcium channels exist as multisubunit complexes. In addition to the pore-forming α_1 subunit, there are auxiliary β, α_2-δ, and γ subunits. In the case of the Ca_V1 and Ca_V2 family of calcium channels, the α_1 subunit interacts with an intracellular β subunit ($Ca_V\beta$ In mammals, four genes encode various subtypes of $Ca_V\beta$ (β_1, β_2, β_3, and β_4) (22). β subunits contain two conserved domains, an N-terminal *src* homology-3 (SH3) domain and a C-terminal guanylate kinase (GK)-like domain, and hence belong to a family of proteins commonly associated with scaffolding functions called membrane-associated GK (MAGUK) proteins (51–53). β subunits interact with the pore-forming α_1 subunit at an 18 amino acid sequence in the I–II cytoplasmic linker region called the α_1-interaction domain (AID) (54) not found in low-voltage activated channels. One of the primary functional consequences of $Ca_V\beta$ subunit interaction with the α_1 subunit is an increase in calcium current density. β subunits accomplish this by increasing the number of channels located at the plasma membrane (55,56). The mechanism by which this occurs involves the masking of an endoplasmic reticulum retention signal within the I–II linker region of the α_1 subunit that occurs when it is bound to the β subunit, thereby allowing the trafficking of the channel to the plasma membrane (57,58). In addition, β subunits have been shown to profoundly affect biophysical properties of the calcium channel including shifting the current-voltage relationship toward more hyperpolarized membrane potentials, increasing the channel open probability, altering the sensitivity to steady-state inactivation, and altering the kinetics of activation and inactivation (59–63).

The $\alpha_2\delta$ subunit (reviewed in ref. 23) is encoded by a single transcriptional product that is posttranslationally cleaved into α_2 and δ peptides and linked together via disulfide bridges (64–66). To date, four genes encoding different $\alpha_2\delta$ subunit have been identified ($\alpha_2\delta$-1, $\alpha_2\delta$-2, $\alpha_2\delta$-3, and $\alpha_2\delta$-4) (64,67–69). The $\alpha_2\delta$ subunits exhibit a wide tissue distribution with the $\alpha_2\delta$-1, $\alpha_2\delta$-2, and $\alpha_2\delta$-3 isoforms being expressed in the brain (70). Additionally, all $\alpha_2\delta$ subunits exhibit further heterogeneity via alternative splicing (71). Structurally, the α_2 subunit is predicted to exist entirely extracellularly with the δ subunit containing a single membrane-spanning region with a short intracellular region (72). In addition, the α_2 subunit is heavily glycosylated, a posttranslational modification that is critical to its ability of interacting with the channel α_1 subunit (72). Studies have shown that $\alpha_2\delta$-2 subunits, like the β subunit, play an important role in trafficking the calcium channel to the plasma membrane resulting in an increase in calcium current amplitude (73–75) without altering the single channel conductance (67,76). Recent work identified the presence of a von Willebrand factor type A (VWA) domain in the extracellular sequence of all $\alpha_2\delta$ subunits, which contains a metal ion-dependent adhesion site (MIDAS) necessary for the abilities of $\alpha_2\delta$ subunits to facilitate trafficking and currents (75).

The γ subunit was initially found to be a component of voltage-gated calcium channels in skeletal muscle (77) (reviewed in ref. 78). Subsequent studies have revealed the presence of a neuronal isoform. At least eight genes encoding the γ subunit (γ_1 to γ_8) have been identified in mammals with a broad tissue distribution (79–83). The predicted conserved structure for the γ subunit consists of four transmembrane-spanning segments and intracellular N- and C-termini (77). The amino terminal half of the γ subunit that includes the first two transmembrane segments interacts with the α_1 subunit, as shown by analyses of interactions between $\alpha_1 1.1$ and γ_1 in a heterologous expression system (84). While β subunits appear to be able to interact with various α_1 subunits, γ subunits are restricted in their ability to interact with different α_1 subunits. Additionally, γ subunits, unlike the β and $\alpha_{2\delta}$ subunits, do not increase the number of calcium channels in the plasma membrane by facilitating trafficking (84). Instead, the γ_1 and γ_2 subunits appear to have inhibitory effects on calcium currents (85,86). Interestingly, the γ_7 subunit nearly abolished all $Ca_V2.2$ current when coexpressed with $Ca_V2.2$ in *Xenopus* oocytes or COS-7 cells but did not affect the calcium current mediated by preexisting endogenous $Ca_V2.2$ channels when it was transiently overexpressed in sympathetic neurons from the rat superior cervical ganglion, suggesting that the γ_7 subunit regulates the expression rather than trafficking or function of $Ca_V2.2$ channels (87).

In summary, there is considerable diversity in voltage-gated calcium channels. This diversity manifests itself in distinct channel biophysical properties, tissue distribution, and pharmacology. Much of this can be attributed to differences in the intrinsic molecular composition of the calcium channel pore-forming subunit with further functional modulation achieved by coupling with different auxiliary subunits. Thus, even in the absence of outside modulating factors, the diversity resulting from the plurality of voltage-gated calcium channel subtypes makes them exquisitely flexible for various tissue-specific demands.

G-Protein Modulation of Calcium Channels

G-Protein–Coupled Receptor Signaling

G-protein–coupled receptors (GPCRs) are responsible for mediating the signal transduction of a diverse array of extracellular stimuli including sensory stimuli, hormones, and neurotransmitters (extensively reviewed in refs. 88 and 89). The GPCRs are a superfamily of receptor proteins characterized by a seven membrane-spanning domain topology with an extracellular N-terminus and an intracellular C-terminus. Specific GPCRs exist for various types of neuromodulators, including, but not limited to, amines, amino acid transmitters, and peptides. Over 400 different types of non–sensory-activated GPCRs have been identified, but physiologic ligands are known for only about half of them.

The GPCRs are coupled to an intracellular heterotrimeric complex of G-protein subunits. Heterotrimeric G-proteins are ubiquitous signal transduction mediators between the receptor and various intracellular signaling pathways, and in some instances, further discussed below, they can themselves act as the effecter molecule. Heterotrimeric G-proteins consist of a Gα subunit containing a guanosine nucleotide binding site as well as Gβ and Gγ subunits. The Gβ and Gγ subunits are tightly associated forming a structural and functional complex, typically referred to as the Gβγ dimer. In the absence of a GPCR agonist, the heterotrimeric G-protein generally remains in an inactive Gα–guanosine diphosphate (GDP) bound state. Upon GPCR activation, nucleotide exchange is facilitated on the Gα subunit such that GDP is exchanged for guanosine triphosphate (GTP). Upon GTP binding to the Gα subunit, a conformational change is induced in the heterotrimeric G-protein promoting both the dissociation of the G-protein from the receptor and the dissociation of the Gα and Gβ subunits from one another. Once liberated, the mobile Gα and Gβγ are now free to modulate the activities of various effecter molecules such as enzymes and ion channels. Termination of G-protein signaling occurs by the hydrolysis of the bound GTP by the intrinsic guanosine triphosphatase (GTPase) activity of the Gα subunit. The resultant GDP-bound Gα can reassociate with the Gβγ and enter a new cycle of activation depending on the state of GPCR activation.

There are 16 isoforms of Gα subunits, which are divided into four families based on structural and functional similarities, including $G\alpha_s$, $G\alpha_i/G\alpha_o$, $G\alpha_q/G\alpha_{11}$, and $G\alpha_{12}/G\alpha_{13}$. Additionally, there are five isoforms of the Gβ subunit and 12 isoforms of the Gγ subunits. Although a single isoform of the Gβ subunit may associate with several isoforms of the Gγ subunit and vice versa, their associations are not entirely promiscuous. G-protein subunits are highly subject to reversible covalent lipid modifications that are critical to their ability to localize to the plasma membrane.

Voltage-Dependent G-Protein Modulation

The G-protein–mediated direct modulation of voltage-gated calcium channels (extensively reviewed in ref. 90) was first indicated by Dunlap and Fischbach (91,92), who observed a significant reduction in the calcium component of somatic action potentials upon application of neurotransmitters γ–aminobutyric acid (GABA), noradrenaline, and 5-hydroxytryptamine (5-HT) to chick dorsal root ganglion (DRG) neurons (91). Subsequent voltage-clamp experiments with chick DRG neurons confirmed that the neurotransmitters directly attenuated high-voltage–activated calcium currents (92) now known to be mainly mediated by $Ca_V2.2$ channels (93,94). Later studies confirmed the presence of this mode of calcium channel inhibition in a variety of native cells mediated by diverse GPCRs (95–105). Central to these studies was the use of pertussis toxin as a specific inhibitor of the G_i/G_o G-protein signaling. Pertussis toxin inhibits the G_i/G_o G-protein signaling by catalyzing the permanent adenosine diphosphate (ADP) ribosylation of the Gα subunit, rendering it unable to couple with GPCRs (106). However, the molecular mechanisms underpinning this regulatory pathway would not be clear until 15 years after the initial observation of Dunlap and Fischbach (91). A key observation on the underlying mechanism of action was made when it was determined that G-protein inhibition was membrane delimited, such that the second messenger effecter molecule remained associated with the plasma membrane and did not require diffusible, cytosolic signaling cascades (107,108). This observation supported the idea that the Gβγ subunits, which are constrained to the inner leaflet of the plasma membrane, could be candidates for the effecter molecule despite the prevailing idea at the time that the Gα subunit was the predominant signaling component of the heterotrimeric G-protein. This direct role for the Gβγ subunit was eventually confirmed in experiments where G-protein inhibition of calcium currents could be replicated either by direct injection or transient overexpression of Gβγ but not Gα subunits, into neurons (109,110).

Many important structural determinants of interaction between the calcium channel $α_1$ subunit and the Gβγ subunit have been identified. However, the manner in which they function together is complex and has been difficult to resolve. *In vitro* binding assays using recombinant Gβγ revealed two sites of interaction along the I–II linker region of the calcium channel $α_1$ subunit (111,112). One of these two sites contained a QXXER motif, a known Gβγ interacting domain found on adenylyl cyclase. The C-terminal of the $α_1$ subunit enhances the binding affinity of the channel with the Gβγ subunit (112,113). The N-terminal of the $α_1$ subunit is also essential to modulation of the channel by G-protein (111,114,115) through an intramolecular interaction with the I–II linker region of the $α_1$ subunit (116) (Fig. 5.1C).

The inhibition of whole-cell currents by G-protein is characterized by a reduction in current amplitude and a depolarizing shift in the voltage-dependence of current activation. Additionally, this can be accompanied by slowed activation and inactivation kinetics. However, the key defining characteristic of this direct, membrane-delimited G-protein inhibition is its voltage-dependence. Early studies noted that the magnitude of inhibition was greatest at more hyperpolarized membrane potentials and less at more depolarized potentials. Furthermore, it was determined that the effects of inhibition could be temporarily relieved following a strong (for example, +80 mV) membrane depolarization (117–120). This finding led to a useful method to assay the presence, magnitude, and kinetics of G-protein inhibition by comparing current amplitudes with, or without, a depolarizing prepulse, an effect often referred to as "prepulse facilitation."

Single-channel analyses showed that the first latency to opening of Ca_V2 channels during a depolarizing pulse was prolonged by G-protein–mediated inhibition, which explains several of the observed characteristics of macroscopic current inhibition, including slowed activation kinetics and reduced current amplitude (121,122). The observations were consistent with a "reluctant"–"willing" model of action for G-protein inhibition of the calcium channel, whereby a Gβγ-bound channel exhibits "reluctant" gating properties, such that longer and or stronger depolarizations are necessary for the channel to open. It is hypothesized that with strong membrane depolarization the Gβγ subunit is displaced from the channel, shifting the channel gating behavior to an uninhibited "willing" mode (119,120,123,124), rebinding with a time constant of about 5 ms. Analysis of the kinetics of G-protein re-inhibition following strongly depolarizing prepulses has provided experimental evidence to support this model and further elucidate the stoichiometry of the G-protein-channel interaction. In HEK293 cells expressing $Ca_V2.2$ channels, G-protein inhibition was induced by the application of purified G-protein $\beta\gamma$ subunits. $Ca_V2.2$ currents evoked by test pulses were facilitated when preceded by strongly depolarizing prepulses followed by rapid re-inhibition. When the interpulse duration between the prepulse and the test pulse was increased, the decrease in the magnitude of facilitation could be described by a monoexponential function. Additionally, the inverse of the time constant for the decay of prepulse facilitation was related linearly on $G\beta\gamma$ concentration. These observations support the idea that G-protein inhibition is mediated by the interaction of a single $G\beta\gamma$ molecule and the calcium channel(125).

In contrast to the activation of inhibited channels via a gating mode transition from an inhibited reluctant state to an uninhibited willing state with strong depolarizing membrane potentials, a direct reluctant channel gating state was identified. This reluctant form of channel activity was characterized by sparse gating behaviors and reduced open probability. A Ca^{2+} channel in the reluctant state may be activated by strongly depolarizing stimuli in the membrane potential range seen by the peaks of action potentials with implications on altering the kinetics of calcium influx. Such a direct transition from the reluctant closed state to open state was only observed for $Ca_V2.2$, and not $Ca_V2.1$, suggesting further heterogeneity in the modulation of presynaptic calcium channels (121,122,126).

G-protein–mediated inhibition of presynaptic calcium channels is a fundamental mechanism by which presynaptic calcium influx is modulated. However, few studies have systematically investigated the spectrum of G-protein subtypes found at synapses. At the giant, calyx-type, presynaptic terminal of the chick ciliary ganglion, immunocytochemistry and deconvolution microscopy have indicated that all four $G\alpha$ families are present (127). However, only members of the $G\alpha_i/G\alpha_o$ and $G\alpha_q/G\alpha_{11}$ families appear to be closely associated with the neurotransmitter release face membrane. Consistent with the presence of the $G\alpha_i/G\alpha_o$ family, the chick ciliary ganglion calyx shows robust, pertussis toxin-sensitive, voltage-dependent G-protein inhibition that is activated via application of adenosine (127,128). Adenosine has been demonstrated to inhibit synaptic transmission in a variety of synapses and is endogenously produced from the rapid conversion of adenosine triphosphate (ATP) released from nerve terminals under stimulation. The adenosine A1 receptor is believed to reside on the presynaptic membrane and to act as a negative autoreceptor at many synapses (128–135) and may contribute to short-term synaptic plasticity. In autapses of cultured hippocampal neurons, relief of tonic G-protein inhibition of presynaptic calcium channels by trains of action potentials underlies a form of short-term facilitation (136) unrelated to a previously described Ca^{2+} entry-associated facilitation (137,138). Synapses exhibiting this type of plasticity act as a high-pass filter such that low-frequency stimulation, unable to promote relief of G-protein inhibition, will remain unfacilitated (118,139,140). It is likely that this mechanism of short-term plasticity may be present in many synapses (127,128,141–144)

G-Protein Interaction with Syntaxin

Syntaxin-1A is a release site-associated protein (24,145,146). It has been implicated as an essential component of the vesicle fusion machinery and has been shown to be a potent modulator of presynaptic calcium channels as will be discussed below. Interestingly, at the site of the chick ciliary ganglion calyx-type presynaptic terminal, cleavage of syntaxin-1 with botulinum neurotoxin C1 eliminated the ability of intracellular GTPγS to induce G-protein inhibition of presynaptic calcium channels (147). Heterologous expression systems have shown that coexpression of syntaxin-1A and $Ca_V2.2$ results in a tonic and voltage-dependent inhibition of G-protein that is independent of GPCR activation (148–150). Furthermore, *in vitro* binding assays illustrate an interaction between syntaxin-1A and Gβ and may suggest a chaperone role for syntaxin-1A in localizing Gβ subunits to the calcium channel.

Voltage-Independent G-Protein Modulation

The activation of GPCRs can result in a plurality of other signaling events besides liberating the G$\beta\gamma$ subunit to inhibit Ca_V2 channels. Indeed, both the Gα and G$\beta\gamma$ subunits have numerous potential cytoplasmic signaling interacting partners that can in turn impact calcium channel activity. In some systems, GPCR activation can result in the concurrent activation of such pathways. G-protein–dependent calcium channel inhibition that cannot be relieved by a strong depolarizing prepulse is termed voltage-independent inhibition. The mechanism by which voltage-independent inhibition occurs is not entirely understood and may reflect distinct signaling pathways that have been adapted to specific GPCRs.

Studies from chick sensory neurons have identified a voltage-independent form of Ca^{2+} channel inhibition by G-protein that is activated by $GABA_B$ receptors. This inhibition is mediated by the $G\alpha_o$ family of G-proteins and requires the activation of Src kinase, which phosphorylates tyrosine sites in the II–III linker region as well as the C-terminus of the α_1 subunit (151).

In addition, another form of voltage-independent inhibition is observed in superior cervical ganglion neurons triggered by muscarinic M_1 and neurokinin 1 receptors. This signaling pathway is coupled to the $G\alpha_{q/11}$ family of G-proteins and will be discussed further below (see Regulation by Phosphatidylinositol-4,5-Bisphosphate).

Protein Kinase C Phosphorylation

The modulation of voltage-gated calcium channels by phosphorylation is another key mechanism by which channel activity can be regulated (101,152–154). Activation of protein kinase C (PKC), a serine/threonine kinase, with diacylglycerol analogues or phorbol esters has profound effects on whole-cell $Ca_V2.2$ calcium currents, including enhancement of current amplitude and changes in activation and steady-state inactivation kinetics (155,156). Phosphorylation of the calcium channel occurs at two adjacent serine/threonine kinase (or PKC) consensus phosphorylation sites (Thr422, Ser425) in the cytoplasmic linker between domains I and II (113,155). Interestingly, PKC modulates $Ca_V2.2$ strongly but has little effect on $Ca_V2.1$.

Crosstalk Between PKC and G-Protein Signaling Pathways

Intriguingly, PKC- and G-protein–dependent modulations generally have opposite effects on calcium channel activity. The fact that both regulatory pathways target consensus sequences in the I–II linker region of the calcium channel suggests that the two signaling pathways may crosstalk (157–159). Indeed, in neurons where the PKC pathways have been activated using the phorbol ester phorbol 12-myristate 13-acetate (PMA), the magnitude of G-protein–mediated inhibition is greatly attenuated. This led to the hypothesis that PKC regulates calcium channel activity by antagonizing a tonic G-protein–mediated inhibition (152,160,161). Consistent with this notion, the inhibition of calcium channels by GTPγS could be relieved by treatment with PMA and strong depolarizing prepulses in rat superior cervical ganglion neurons. Once inhibition was relieved, PKC activation precluded re-inhibition of the channels, indicating that phosphorylation of the channel may occur only after dissociation of the G-protein (162). In heterologous expression systems, pretreatment with PMA or amino acid substitution that mimics phosphorylation (T422E) antagonized somatostatin and opiate-induced inhibition of $Ca_V2.2$ (158). It was subsequently determined that the ability of PKC to modulate G-protein inhibition of the channel depends on the particular isoform of the Gβ subunit such that the Gβ₁γ subunit-mediated inhibition is antagonized by PKC but not other Gβγ subunit combinations (159,163).

There are, however, reports of a PKC-mediated upregulation of calcium currents that is independent of the removal of tonic G-protein inhibition. This has been shown with *Xenopus* oocytes expressing $Ca_V2.2$ where calcium currents were still potentiated by PMA treatment despite pretreatment of oocytes with pertussis toxin (PTX) (155). Additionally, in rat superior cervical ganglion neurons (156) as well as frog sympathetic neurons (154), the removal of any underlying tonic G-protein inhibition via intracellular application of GDPβS did not preclude the potentiation of calcium currents with PMA. The differential phosphorylation of the PKC consensus sites Thr422 and Ser425 in the I–II linker region of the channel α subunit has been implicated as serving as an integration center by which these opposing outcomes may be controlled (158).

Regulation by Phosphatidylinositol-4,5-Bisphosphate

Calcium currents recorded in the whole-cell or excised patch configuration often decrease spontaneously, a phenomenon called "rundown." Rundown has been attributed to the washout of a calcium channel cofactor. Phosphatidylinositol-4,5-bisphosphate (PtdIns(4,5)P2), a major phosphoinositide of the plasma membrane and critical precursor of the second messengers inositol-1,4,5-triphosphate (IP_3) and diacylglycerol (DAG), appears to contribute to maintenance of channel activity. Thus, in *Xenopus* oocytes increasing PtdIns(4,5)P2 concentration in the membrane after patch excision could greatly slow the rate of expressed $Ca_V2.1$ current rundown (116). Further, if PtdIns(4,5)P2 was sequestered by applying a specific antibody, rundown was accelerated. Surprisingly, however, PtdIns(4,5)P2 application has been reported to induce G-protein–like voltage-dependent inhibition of $Ca_V2.1$ currents that could be antagonized by activation of PKA (164).

Phosphatidylinositol-4,5-bisphosphate depletion-mediated rundown was also observed for $Ca_V2.2$ currents. PtdIns(4,5)P2-treated patches containing $Ca_V2.2$ channels also showed a depolarizing shift in current activation similar to that observed with $Ca_V2.1$ channels (165); however, PKA activation was only partially able to occlude this effect. In addition, PtdIns(4,5)P2 appeared to be essential to voltage-independent inhibition caused by M1 muscarinic receptor activation in superior cervical ganglion (SCG) neurons. This inhibitory pathway is mediated by the $G_q/_{11}$ family of G-proteins and is pertussis toxin insensitive. It was demonstrated that M1 receptor activation activates phospholipase C (PLC), which in turn depletes the membrane of PtdIns(4,5)P2, resulting in an inhibition of calcium currents. Interestingly, not all $G_q/_{11}$-coupled receptors mediate suppression of calcium channels in this manner despite being able to deplete PtdIns(4,5)P2 (165). This has been attributed to specific GPCRs that concomitantly facilitate PtdIns(4,5)P2 synthesis by raising intracellular Ca^{2+} concentration. An alternative pathway for slow and voltage-independent inhibition of calcium channels is via arachidonic acid liberated from M1 receptor-mediated stimulation of phospholipase activity (164,166–168). Few studies have explored the role of PtdIns(4,5)P2 in the maintenance of calcium channel currents at intact presynaptic nerve terminals (169,170).

Calcium Channel Regulation by Synaptic Proteins

Syntaxin-1/Munc-18

Syntaxin-1 is an integral membrane protein that interacts with numerous proteins at the presynaptic site and is a critical member of the exocytotic machinery (145,146). Syntaxin-1 (HPC-1) was originally identified as a $Ca_V2.2$-coprecipitating protein (171) and interacts with the calcium channel via a conserved region in the II–III linker called the SYNaptic PRotein INTeraction (synprint) site (172,173). Discovery of this interaction led to investigations of whether syntaxin could modulate calcium channel function (174,175). Indeed, when syntaxin was coexpressed with calcium channels in tsA-201 cells and in *Xenopus* oocytes, a hyperpolarizing shift in steady-state inactivation was observed (148,176–178). Thus, it was suggested that syntaxin could regulate neurotransmitter release by downregulating the activity of presynaptic calcium channels, irrespective of its role in the exocytotic fusion machinery (179–182). Indeed, at the chick ciliary ganglion calyx-type presynaptic terminal, cleavage of endogenous syntaxin-1 by botulinum C1 toxin induced a moderate but significant depolarizing shift in steady-state inactivation of a population of presynaptic calcium channels, suggesting that syntaxin-1 accelerates channel inactivation. However, it is unclear if this effect plays a biologic role since it requires a sustained depolarization that is not normally experienced by presynaptic terminals (183). In heterologous expression systems, coexpression of synaptic proteins SNAP-25 and Munc18 blocked the facilitatory effect of syntaxin-1 on calcium channel inactivation (148,184). In chick DRG neurons, siRNA knockdown of the endogenous chick homologue of Munc18 enhanced channel inactivation (185) consistent with the idea that Munc18 serves as a molecular "buffer" for the effect of syntaxin-1 on calcium channel inactivation. Similarly, phosphorylation of the channel by PKC inhibited the effect of syntaxin-1 on channel inactivation (148).

14-3-3

14-3-3 proteins interact with a variety of other proteins implicated in diverse cellular processes including cell cycle and transcriptional control, signal transduction, protein trafficking, and the regulation of ion channels (reviewed in ref. 186). There are seven isoforms of 14-3-3 in mammals (β, γ, ϵ, η, δ, σ, and τ/θ). The expression of 14-3-3 proteins is ubiquitous in all eukaryotic organisms and is highly expressed within the brain. Although the function of these proteins is not fully understood, they have aroused particular interest because their levels in the cerebrospinal fluid are increased in patients of several neurologic disorders, which, perhaps, hints at a role of 14-3-3 in the neuropathophysiology of these diseases.

A recent study showed that 14-3-3 proteins are novel modulator of $Ca_V2.2$ channels (187). In this study, immunohistochemistry with specific antibodies showed that 14-3-3 proteins colocalized with the presynaptic terminal marker protein synapsin I in cultured rat hippocampal neurons. In addition, 14-3-3 coimmunoprecipitated with the $Ca_V2.2$ α_1 subunit from rat brain lysates. Using fusion protein pull-down assays, two putative 14-3-3 interaction sites were identified in the C-terminal of the $Ca_V2.2$ α_1 subunit. Voltage-clamp analysis of currents obtained from tsA-201 cells expressing $Ca_V2.2$ and 14-3-3 revealed vastly slowed open- and closed-state inactivation kinetics. Furthermore, in cultured rat hippocampal neurons, which contain endogenous $Ca_V2.2$ and 14-3-3, open-state inactivation could be accelerated by transfection with the 14-3-3–binding antagonist pSCM138, suggesting a role for endogenous 14-3-3 in neurons (187,188).

References

1. Katz B, Miledi R. The timing of calcium action during neuromuscular transmission. J Physiol 1967;189(3):535–544.
2. Stanley EF. The calcium channel and the organization of the presynaptic transmitter release face. Trends Neurosci 1997;20(9):404–409.

3. Bullock TH. Properties of a single synapse in the stellate ganglion of squid. J Neurophysiol 1948;11(4):343–364.
4. Katz B, Miledi R. Tetrodotoxin-resistant electric activity in presynaptic terminals. J Physiol 1969;203(2):459–487.
5. Llinas R, Steinberg IZ, Walton K. Presynaptic calcium currents in squid giant synapse. Biophys J 1981;33(3):289–321.
6. Llinas R, Steinberg IZ, Walton K. Presynaptic calcium currents and their relation to synaptic transmission: voltage clamp study in squid giant synapse and theoretical model for the calcium gate. Proc Natl Acad Sci U S A 1976;73(8):2918–2922.
7. Llinas R, Steinberg IZ, Walton K. Relationship between presynaptic calcium current and postsynaptic potential in squid giant synapse. Biophys J 1981;33(3):323–351.
8. Stanley EF. Single calcium channels and acetylcholine release at a presynaptic nerve terminal. Neuron 1993;11(6):1007–1011.
9. Shahrezaei V, Cao A, Delaney KR. Ca2+ from one or two channels controls fusion of a single vesicle at the frog neuromuscular junction. J Neurosci 2006;26(51):13240–13249.
10. Fedchyshyn MJ, Wang LY. Developmental transformation of the release modality at the calyx of Held synapse. J Neurosci 2005;25(16):4131–4140.
11. Wachman ES, Poage RE, Stiles JR, Farkas DL, Meriney SD. Spatial distribution of calcium entry evoked by single action potentials within the presynaptic active zone. J Neurosci 2004;24(12):2877–2885.
12. Gentile L, Stanley EF. A unified model of presynaptic release site gating by calcium channel domains. Eur J Neurosci 2005;21(1):278–282.
13. Dodge FA Jr, Rahamimoff R. Co-operative action of calcium ions in transmitter release at the neuromuscular junction. J Physiol 1967;193(2):419–432.
14. Koh TW, Bellen HJ. Synaptotagmin I, a Ca2+ sensor for neurotransmitter release. Trends Neurosci 2003;26(8):413–422.
15. Yoshihara M, Adolfsen B, Littleton JT. Is synaptotagmin the calcium sensor? Curr Opin Neurobiol 2003;13(3):315–323.
16. Rizo J, Chen X, Arac D. Unraveling the mechanisms of synaptotagmin and SNARE function in neurotransmitter release. Trends Cell Biol 2006;16(7):339–350.
17. Sudhof TC. The synaptic vesicle cycle. Annu Rev Neurosci 2004;27(1):509–547.
18. Khanna R, Li Q, Schlichter LC, Stanley EF. The transmitter release-site CaV2.2 channel cluster is linked to an endocytosis coat protein complex. Eur J Neurosci 2007;26(3): 560–574.
19. Catterall WA. Structure and regulation of voltage-gated Ca2+ channels. Annu Rev Cell Dev Biol 2000;16(1):521–555.
20. Catterall WA, Perez-Reyes E, Snutch TP, Striessnig J. International Union of Pharmacology. XLVIII. Nomenclature and structure-function relationships of voltage-gated calcium channels. Pharmacol Rev 2005;57(4):411–425.
21. Catterall WA, Perez-Reyes E, Snutch TP, Striessnig J. International Union of Pharmacology. XLVIII. Nomenclature and structure-function relationships of voltage-gated calcium channels. Pharmacol Rev 2005;57(4):411–425.
22. Richards MW, Butcher AJ, Dolphin AC. Ca2+ channel beta-subunits: structural insights AID our understanding. Trends Pharmacol Sci 2004;25(12):626–632.
23. Davies A, Hendrich J, Van Minh AT, Wratten J, Douglas L, Dolphin AC. Functional biology of the [alpha]2[delta] subunits of voltage-gated calcium channels. Trends Pharmacol Sci 2007;28(5):220–228.
24. Evans RM, Zamponi GW. Presynaptic Ca2+ channels—integration centers for neuronal signaling pathways. Trends Neurosci 2006;29(11):617–624.
25. Ertel EA, Campbell KP, Harpold MM, et al. Nomenclature of voltage-gated calcium channels. Neuron 2000;25(3):533–535.
26. Birnbaumer L, Campbell KP, Catterall WA, et al. The naming of voltage-gated calcium channels. Neuron 1994;13(3):505–506.
27. Bean BP. Two kinds of calcium channels in canine atrial cells. Differences in kinetics, selectivity, and pharmacology. J Gen Physiol 1985;86(1):1–30.

28. Nilius B, Hess P, Lansman JB, Tsien RW. A novel type of cardiac calcium channel in ventricular cells. Nature 1985;316(6027):443–446.

29. Nowycky MC, Fox AP, Tsien RW. Long-opening mode of gating of neuronal calcium channels and its promotion by the dihydropyridine calcium agonist Bay K 8644. Proc Natl Acad Sci 1985;82(7):2178–2182.

30. Fox AP, Nowycky MC, Tsien RW. Single-channel recordings of three types of calcium channels in chick sensory neurones. J Physiol 1987;394(1):173–200.

31. Fox AP, Nowycky MC, Tsien RW. Kinetic and pharmacological properties distinguishing three types of calcium currents in chick sensory neurones. J Physiol 1987;394(1):149–172.

32. Mori Y, Friedrich T, Kim MS, et al. Primary structure and functional expression from complementary DNA of a brain calcium channel. Nature 1991;350(6317):398–402.

33. Tanabe T, Takeshima H, Mikami A, et al. Primary structure of the receptor for calcium channel blockers from skeletal muscle. Nature 1987;328(6128):313–318.

34. Llinas RR, Sugimori M, Cherksey B. Voltage-dependent calcium conductances in mammalian neurons. The P channel. Ann N Y Acad Sci 1989;560:103–111.

35. Wheeler DB, Randall A, Tsien RW. Roles of N-type and Q-type Ca2+ channels in supporting hippocampal synaptic transmission. Science 1994;264(5155):107–111.

36. Mintz IM, Venema VJ, Swiderek KM, Lee TD, Bean BP, Adams ME. P-type calcium channels blocked by the spider toxin [omega]-Aga-IVA. Nature 1992;355(6363):827–829.

37. Nowycky MC, Fox AP, Tsien RW. Three types of neuronal calcium channel with different calcium agonist sensitivity. Nature 1985;316(6027):440–443.

38. Kerr LM, Yoshikami D. A venom peptide with a novel presynaptic blocking action. Nature 1984;308(5956):282–284.

39. Soong TW, Stea A, Hodson CD, Dubel SJ, Vincent S, Snutch TP. Structure and functional expression of a member of the low voltage-activated calcium channel family. Science 1993;260(5111):1133–1136.

40. Niidome T, Kim MS, Friedrich T, Mori Y. Molecular cloning and characterization of a novel calcium channel from rabbit brain. FEBS Lett 1992;308(1):7–13.

41. Bourinet E, Zamponi GW, Stea A, et al. The alpha 1E calcium channel exhibits permeation properties similar to low-voltage-activated calcium channels. J Neurosci 1996;16(16):4983–4993.

42. Perez-Reyes E, Cribbs LL, Daud A, et al. Molecular characterization of a neuronal low-voltage-activated T-type calcium channel. Nature 1998;391(6670):896–900.

43. Nilius B, Hess P, Lansman JB, Tsien RW. A novel type of cardiac calcium channel in ventricular cells. Nature 1985;316(6027):443–446.

44. Chuang RSI, Jaffe H, Cribbs L, Perez-Reyes E, Swartz KJ. Inhibition of T-type voltage-gated calcium channels by a new scorpion toxin. Nat Neurosci 1998;1(8):668–674.

45. Lee JH, Gomora JC, Cribbs LL, Perez-Reyes E. Nickel block of three cloned t-type calcium channels: low concentrations selectively block alpha 1H. Biophys J 1999;77(6):3034–3042.

46. Perez-Reyes E. Molecular physiology of low-voltage-activated t-type calcium channels. Physiol Rev 2003;83(1):117–161.

47. Wu LG, Saggau P. Presynaptic inhibition of elicited neurotransmitter release. Trends Neurosci 1997;20(5):204–212.

48. Atlas D. Functional and physical coupling of voltage-sensitive calcium channels with exocytotic proteins: ramifications for the secretion mechanism. J Neurochem 2001;77(4):972–985.

49. Iwasaki S, Takahashi T. Developmental changes in calcium channel types mediating synaptic transmission in rat auditory brainstem. J Physiol 1998;509(2):419–423.

50. Iwasaki S, Momiyama A, Uchitel OD, Takahashi T. Developmental changes in calcium channel types mediating central synaptic transmission. J Neurosci 2000;20(1):59–65.

51. Takahashi SX, Miriyala J, Colecraft HM. Membrane-associated guanylate kinase-like properties of {beta}-subunits required for modulation of voltage-dependent Ca2+ channels. Proc Natl Acad Sci 2004;101(18):7193–7198.

52. Takahashi SX, Miriyala J, Tay LH, Yue DT, Colecraft HM. A CaV{beta} SH3/guanylate kinase domain interaction regulates multiple properties of voltage-gated Ca2+ channels. J Gen Physiol 2005;126(4):365–377.

53. Opatowsky Y, Chen CC, Campbell KP, Hirsch JA. Structural analysis of the voltage-dependent calcium channel [beta] subunit functional core and its complex with the [alpha]1 interaction domain. Neuron 2004;42(3):387–399.

54. Pragnell M, De WM, Mori Y, Tanabe T, Snutch TP, Campbell KP. Calcium channel beta-subunit binds to a conserved motif in the I–II cytoplasmic linker of the alpha 1–subunit. Nature 1994;368(6466):67–70.

55. Chien AJ, Zhao X, Shirokov RE, et al. Roles of a membrane-localized beta subunit in the formation and targeting of functional L-type Ca[image] Channels. J Biol Chem 1995;270(50): 30036–30044.

56. Gao T, Chien AJ, Hosey MM. Complexes of the alpha 1C and beta subunits generate the necessary signal for membrane targeting of class C L-type calcium channels. J Biol Chem 1999;274(4):2137–2144.

57. Bichet D, Cornet V, Geib S, et al. The I–II loop of the Ca2+ channel alpha1 subunit contains an endoplasmic reticulum retention signal antagonized by the beta subunit. Neuron 2000;25(1):177–190.

58. Brice NL, Berrow NS, Campbell V, et al. Importance of the different beta subunits in the membrane expression of the alpha1A and alpha2 calcium channel subunits: studies using a depolarization-sensitive alpha1A antibody. Eur J Neurosci 1997;9(4):749–759.

59. Perez-Reyes E, Castellano A, Kim HS, et al. Cloning and expression of a cardiac/brain beta subunit of the L-type calcium channel. J Biol Chem 1992;267(3):1792–1797.

60. De WM, Pragnell M, Campbell KP. Ca2+ channel regulation by a conserved beta subunit domain. Neuron 1994;13(2):495–503.

61. Gerster U, Neuhuber B, Groschner K, Striessnig J, Flucher BE. Current modulation and membrane targeting of the calcium channel alpha1C subunit are independent functions of the beta subunit. J Physiol 1999;517(2):353–368.

62. Hullin R, Khan IFY, Wirtz S, et al. Cardiac L-type calcium channel {beta}-subunits expressed in human heart have differential effects on single channel characteristics. J Biol Chem 2003;278(24):21623–21630.

63. Kanevsky N, Dascal N. Regulation of maximal open probability is a separable function of cav{beta} subunit in L-type Ca2+ channel, dependent on NH2 terminus of {alpha}1C (Cav1.2{alpha}). J Gen Physiol 2006;128(1):15–36.

64. Ellis SB, Williams ME, Ways NR, et al. Sequence and expression of mRNAs encoding the α_1 and α_2 subunits of a DHP-sensitive calcium channel. Science 1988;241(4873): 1661–1664.

65. De Jongh KS, Warner C, Catterall WA. Subunits of purified calcium channels ?2 and ? are encoded by the same gene. J Biol Chem 1990;265(25):14738–14741.

66. Jay SD, Sharp AH, Kahl SD, Vedvick TS, Harpold MM, Campbell KP. Structural characterization of the dihydropyridine-sensitive calcium channel α_2–subunit and the associated δ peptides. J Biol Chem 1991;266(5):3287–3293.

67. Barclay J, Balaguero N, Mione M, et al. Ducky mouse phenotype of epilepsy and ataxia is associated with mutations in the Cacna2d2 gene and decreased calcium channel current in cerebellar Purkinje cells. J Neurosci 2001;21(16):6095–6104.

68. Klugbauer N, Lacinova L, Marais E, Hobom M, Hofmann F. Molecular diversity of the calcium channel $\alpha_2\delta$ subunit. J Neurosci 1999;19(2):684–691.

69. Qin N, Yagel S, Momplaisir ML, Codd EE, D'Andrea MR. Molecular cloning and characterization of the human voltage-gated calcium channel alpha 2 delta 4 subunit. Mol Pharmacol 2002;62(3):485–496.

70. Klugbauer N, Marais E, Hofmann F. Calcium channel alpha2delta subunits: differential expression, function, and drug binding. J Bioenerg Biomembr 2003;35(6):639–647.

71. Klugbauer N, Lacinova L, Marais E, Hobom M, Hofmann F. Molecular diversity of the calcium channel $\alpha_2\delta$ subunit. J Neurosci 1999;19(2):684–691.

72. Gurnett CA, De WM, Campbell KP. Dual function of the voltage-dependent Ca2+ channel alpha 2 delta subunit in current stimulation and subunit interaction. Neuron 1996;16(2): 431–440.
73. Gao B, Sekido Y, Maximov A, et al. Functional properties of a new voltage-dependent calcium channel alpha 2delta auxiliary subunit gene (CACNA2D2). J Biol Chem 2000;275 (16):12237–12242.
74. Canti C, Dolphin AC. CaVbeta subunit-mediated up-regulation of CaV2.2 currents triggered by D2 dopamine receptor activation. Neuropharmacology 2003;45(6):814–827.
75. Canti C, Nieto-Rostro M, Foucault I, et al. The metal-ion-dependent adhesion site in the Von Willebrand factor-A domain of {alpha}2{delta} subunits is key to trafficking voltage-gated Ca2+ channels. Proc Natl Acad Sci 2005;102(32):11230–11235.
76. Brodbeck J, Davies A, Courtney JM, et al. The Ducky mutation in Cacna2d2 results in altered Purkinje cell morphology and is associated with the expression of a truncated alpha 2delta -2 protein with abnormal function. J Biol Chem 2002;277(10):7684–7693.
77. Jay SD, Ellis SB, McCue AF, et al. Primary structure of the δ subunit of the DHP-sensitive calcium channel from skeletal muscle. Science 1990;248(4954):490–492.
78. Kang MG, Campbell KP. {gamma} Subunit of voltage-activated calcium channels. J Biol Chem 2003;278(24):21315–21318.
79. Chu PJ, Robertson HM, Best PM. Calcium channel [gamma] subunits provide insights into the evolution of this gene family. Gene 2001;280(1–2):37–48.
80. Burgess DL, Gefrides LA, Foreman PJ, Noebels JL. A cluster of three novel Ca2+ channel [gamma] subunit genes on chromosome 19q13.4: evolution and expression profile of the [gamma] subunit gene family. Genomics 2001;71(3):339–350.
81. Klugbauer N, Dai S, Specht V, et al. A family of [gamma]-like calcium channel subunits. FEBS Lett 2000;470(2):189–197.
82. Sharp AH, Black JL, Dubel SJ, et al. Biochemical and anatomical evidence for specialized voltage-dependent calcium channel [gamma] isoform expression in the epileptic and ataxic mouse, stargazer. Neuroscience 2001;105(3):599–617.
83. Black JL, III. The voltage-gated calcium channel gamma subunits: a review of the literature. J Bioenerg Biomembr 2003;35(6):649–660.
84. Arikkath J, Chen CC, Ahern C, et al. gamma 1 Subunit interactions within the skeletal muscle L-type voltage-gated calcium channels. J Biol Chem 2003;278(2):1212–1219.
85. Kang MG, Chen CC, Felix R, et al. Biochemical and biophysical evidence for gamma 2 subunit association with neuronal voltage-activated Ca2+ channels. J Biol Chem 2001;276(35):32917–32924.
86. Rousset M, Cens T, Restituito S, et al. Functional roles of {gamma}2, {gamma}3 and {gamma}4, three new Ca2+ channel subunits, in P/Q-type Ca2+ channel expressed in Xenopus oocytes. J Physiol 2001;532(3):583–593.
87. Moss FJ, Viard P, Davies A, et al. The novel product of a five-exon stargazin-related gene abolishes Ca(V)2.2 calcium channel expression. EMBO J 2002;21(7):1514–1523.
88. Wettschureck N, Offermanns S. Mammalian G proteins and their cell type specific functions. Physiol Rev 2005;85(4):1159–1204.
89. Gudermann T, Schoneberg T, Schultz G. Functional and structural complexity of signal transduction via G-protein-coupled receptors. Annu Rev Neurosci 1997;20(1):399–427.
90. Tedford HW, Zamponi GW. Direct G protein modulation of Cav2 calcium channels. Pharmacol Rev 2006;58(4):837–862.
91. Dunlap K, Fischbach GD. Neurotransmitters decrease the calcium component of sensory neurone action potentials. Nature 1978;276(5690):837–839.
92. Dunlap K, Fischbach GD. Neurotransmitters decrease the calcium conductance activated by depolarization of embryonic chick sensory neurones. J Physiol 1981;317:519–535.
93. Cox DH, Dunlap K. Pharmacological discrimination of N-type from L-type calcium current and its selective modulation by transmitters. J Neurosci 1992;12(3):906–914.
94. Chan AW, Stanley EF. Slow inhibition of N-type calcium channels with GTP gamma S reflects the basal G protein-GDP turnover rate. Pflugers Arch 2003;446(2):183–188.

95. Forscher P, Oxford GS, Schulz D. Noradrenaline modulates calcium channels in avian dorsal root ganglion cells through tight receptor-channel coupling. J Physiol 1986; 379(1):131–144.

96. Holz GG, Shefner SA, Anderson EG. Serotonin decreases the duration of action potentials recorded from tetraethylammonium-treated bullfrog dorsal root ganglion cells. J Neurosci 1986;6(3):620–626.

97. Ikeda SR, Schofield GG. Somatostatin blocks a calcium current in rat sympathetic ganglion neurones. J Physiol 1989;409(1):221–240.

98. Bernheim L, Mathie A, Hille B. Characterization of muscarinic receptor subtypes inhibiting Ca2+ current and M current in rat sympathetic neurons. Proc Natl Acad Sci 1992;89(20):9544–9548.

99. Zhu Y, Ikeda SR. Adenosine modulates voltage-gated Ca2+ channels in adult rat sympathetic neurons. J Neurophysiol 1993;70(2):610–620.

100. Lipscombe D, Kongsamut S, Tsien RW. [alpha]-Adrenergic inhibition of sympathetic neurotransmitter release mediated by modulation of N-type calcium-channel gating. Nature 1989;340(6235):639–642.

101. Golard A, Role LW, Siegelbaum SA. Protein kinase C blocks somatostatin-induced modulation of calcium current in chick sympathetic neurons. J Neurophysiol 1993;70(4):1639–1643.

102. Bean BP. Neurotransmitter inhibition of neuronal calcium currents by changes in channel voltage dependence. Nature 1989;340(6229):153–156.

103. Caulfield MP, Jones S, Vallis Y, et al. Muscarinic M-current inhibition via G alpha q/11 and alpha-adrenoceptor inhibition of Ca2+ current via G alpha o in rat sympathetic neurones. J Physiol 1994;477(pt_3):415–422.

104. Beech DJ, Bernheim L, Hille B. Pertussis toxin and voltage dependence distinguish multiple pathways modulating calcium channels of rat sympathetic neurons. Neuron 1992;8(1):97–106.

105. Shapiro MS, Hille B. Substance P and somatostatin inhibit calcium channels in rat sympathetic neurons via different G protein pathways. Neuron 1993;10(1):11–20.

106. Fields TA, Casey PJ. Signalling functions and biochemical properties of pertussis toxin-resistant G-proteins. Biochem J 1997;321(3):561–571.

107. Forscher P, Oxford GS, Schulz D. Noradrenaline modulates calcium channels in avian dorsal root ganglion cells through tight receptor-channel coupling. J Physiol 1986;379(1): 131–144.

108. Hille B. Modulation of ion-channel function by G-protein-coupled receptors. Trends Neurosci 1994;17(12):531–536.

109. Herlitze S, Garcia DE, Mackie K, Hille B, Scheuer T, Catterall WA. Modulation of Ca2+ channels by G-protein beta gamma subunits. Nature 1996;380(6571):258–262.

110. Ikeda SR. Voltage-dependent modulation of N-type calcium channels by G-protein beta gamma subunits. Nature 1996;380(6571):255–258.

111. Page KM, Canti C, Stephens GJ, Berrow NS, Dolphin AC. Identification of the amino terminus of neuronal Ca2+ channel alpha 1 subunits alpha 1B and alpha 1E as an essential determinant of G-protein modulation. J Neurosci 1998;18(13):4815–4824.

112. Li B, Zhong H, Scheuer T, Catterall WA. Functional role of a C-terminal Gbetagamma-binding domain of Ca(v)2.2 channels. Mol Pharmacol 2004;66(3):761–769.

113. Hamid J, Nelson D, Spaetgens R, Dubel SJ, Snutch TP, Zamponi GW. Identification of an integration center for cross-talk between protein kinase C and G protein modulation of N-type calcium channels. J Biol Chem 1999;274(10):6195–6202.

114. Canti C, Page KM, Stephens GJ, Dolphin AC. Identification of residues in the N terminus of alpha 1B critical for inhibition of the voltage-dependent calcium channel by Gbeta gamma. J Neurosci 1999;19(16):6855–6864.

115. Simen AA, Miller RJ. Structural features determining differential receptor regulation of neuronal Ca channels. J Neurosci 1998;18(10):3689–3698.

116. Agler HL, Evans J, Tay LH, Anderson MJ, Colecraft HM, Yue DT. G protein-gated inhibitory module of N-type (ca(v)2.2) Ca2+ channels. Neuron 2005;46(6):891–904.

117. Boland LM, Bean BP. Modulation of N-type calcium channels in bullfrog sympathetic neurons by luteinizing hormone-releasing hormone: kinetics and voltage dependence. J Neurosci 1993;13(2):516–533.
118. Elmslie KS, Zhou W, Jones SW. LHRH and GTP-gamma-S modify calcium current activation in bullfrog sympathetic neurons. Neuron 1990;5(1):75–80.
119. Bean BP. Neurotransmitter inhibition of neuronal calcium currents by changes in channel voltage dependence. Nature 1989;340(6229):153–156.
120. Hille B. Modulation of ion-channel function by G-protein-coupled receptors. Trends Neurosci 1994;17(12):531–536.
121. Colecraft HM, Patil PG, Yue DT. Differential occurrence of reluctant openings in G-protein-inhibited N- and P/Q-type calcium channels. J Gen Physiol 2000;115(2):175–192.
122. Lee HK, Elmslie KS. Reluctant gating of single N-type calcium channels during neurotransmitter-induced inhibition in bullfrog sympathetic neurons. J Neurosci 2000;20(9):3115–3128.
123. Kasai H, Aosaki T. Modulation of Ca-channel current by an adenosine analog mediated by a GTP-binding protein in chick sensory neurons. Pflugers Arch 1989;414(2):145–149.
124. Elmslie KS. Calcium current modulation in frog sympathetic neurones: multiple neurotransmitters and G proteins. J Physiol 1992;451(1):229–246.
125. Zamponi GW, Snutch TP. Decay of prepulse facilitation of N type calcium channels during G protein inhibition is consistent with binding of a single Gbeta subunit. Proc Natl Acad Sci U S A 1998;95(7):4035–4039.
126. Colecraft HM, Brody DL, Yue DT. G-protein inhibition of N- and P/Q-type calcium channels: distinctive elementary mechanisms and their functional impact. J Neurosci 2001;21(4):1137–1147.
127. Mirotznik RR, Zheng X, Stanley EF. G-protein types involved in calcium channel inhibition at a presynaptic nerve terminal. J Neurosci 2000;20(20):7614–7621.
128. Yawo H, Chuhma N. Preferential inhibition of o[omega]-conotoxin-sensitive presynaptic Ca2+ channels by adenosine autoreceptors. Nature 1993;365(6443):256–258.
129. Wu LG, Saggau P. Adenosine inhibits evoked synaptic transmission primarily by reducing presynaptic calcium influx in area CA1 of hippocampus. Neuron 1994;12(5):1139–1148.
130. Ginsborg BL, Hirst GDS. The effect of adenosine on the release of the transmitter from the phrenic nerve of the rat. J Physiol 1972;224(3):629–645.
131. Umemiya M, Berger AJ. Activation of adenosine A1 and A2 receptors differentially modulates calcium channels and glycinergic synaptic transmission in rat brainstem. Neuron 1994;13(6):1439–1446.
132. Barnes-Davies M, Forsythe ID. Pre- and postsynaptic glutamate receptors at a giant excitatory synapse in rat auditory brainstem slices. J Physiol 1995;488(pt_2):387–406.
133. Bagley EE, Vaughan CW, Christie MJ. Inhibition by adenosine receptor agonists of synaptic transmission in rat periaqueductal grey neurons. J Physiol 1999;516(1):219–225.
134. Arrigoni E, Rainnie DG, McCarley RW, Greene RW. Adenosine-mediated presynaptic modulation of glutamatergic transmission in the laterodorsal tegmentum. J Neurosci 2001;21(3):1076–1085.
135. Kimura M, Saitoh N, Takahashi T. Adenosine A1 receptor-mediated presynaptic inhibition at the calyx of Held of immature rats. J Physiol 2003;553(2):415–426.
136. Brody DL, Yue DT. Relief of G-protein inhibition of calcium channels and short-term synaptic facilitation in cultured hippocampal neurons. J Neurosci 2000;20(3):889–898.
137. Borst JGG, Sakmann B. Facilitation of presynaptic calcium currents in the rat brainstem. J Physiol 1998;513(1):149–155.
138. Cuttle MF, Tsujimoto T, Forsythe ID, Takahashi T. Facilitation of the presynaptic calcium current at an auditory synapse in rat brainstem. J Physiol 1998;512(3):723–729.
139. Bertram R. Differential filtering of two presynaptic depression mechanisms. Neural Comp 2001;13(1):69–85.

140. Bertram R, Swanson J, Yousef M, Feng ZP, Zamponi GW. A minimal model for G protein-mediated synaptic facilitation and depression. J Neurophysiol 2003;90(3):1643–1653.
141. Takahashi T, Forsythe ID, Tsujimoto T, Barnes-Davies M, Onodera K. Presynaptic calcium current modulation by a metabotropic glutamate receptor. Science 1996;274(5287):594–597.
142. Dittman JS, Regehr WG. Contributions of calcium-dependent and calcium-independent mechanisms to presynaptic inhibition at a cerebellar synapse. J Neurosci 1996;16(5): 1623–1633.
143. Shen WX, Horn JP. Presynaptic muscarinic inhibition in bullfrog sympathetic ganglia. J Physiol 1996;491(pt_2):413–421.
144. Matsushima T, Tegner J, Hill RH, Grillner S. GABAB receptor activation causes a depression of low- and high-voltage-activated Ca2+ currents, postinhibitory rebound, and postspike afterhyperpolarization in lamprey neurons. J Neurophysiol 1993;70(6):2606–2619.
145. O'Connor VM, Shamotienko O, Grishin E, Betz H. On the structure of the "synaptosecretosome." Evidence for a neurexin/synaptotagmin/syntaxin/Ca2+ channel complex. FEBS Lett 1993;326(1–3):255–260.
146. Leveque C, el Far O, Martin-Moutot N, et al. Purification of the N-type calcium channel associated with syntaxin and synaptotagmin. A complex implicated in synaptic vesicle exocytosis. J Biol Chem 1994;269(9):6306–6312.
147. Stanley EF, Mirotznik RR. Cleavage of syntaxin prevents G-protein regulation of presynaptic calcium channels. Nature 1997;385(6614):340–343.
148. Jarvis SE, Zamponi GW. Distinct molecular determinants govern syntaxin 1A-mediated inactivation and G-protein inhibition of N-type calcium channels. J Neurosci 2001;21(9):2939–2948.
149. Jarvis SE, Barr W, Feng ZP, Hamid J, Zamponi GW. Molecular determinants of syntaxin 1 modulation of N-type calcium channels. J Biol Chem 2002;277(46):44399–44407.
150. Lu Q, Atkisson MS, Jarvis SE, Feng ZP, Zamponi GW, Dunlap K. Syntaxin 1A supports voltage-dependent inhibition of alpha1B Ca2+ channels by Gbetagamma in chick sensory neurons. J Neurosci 2001;21(9):2949–2957.
151. Richman RW, Tombler E, Lau KK, et al. N-type Ca2+ channels as scaffold proteins in the assembly of signaling molecules for GABAB receptor effects. J Biol Chem 2004;279(23):24649–24658.
152. Swartz KJ. Modulation of Ca2+ channels by protein kinase C in rat central and peripheral neurons: disruption of G protein-mediated inhibition. Neuron 1993;11(2):305–320.
153. Swartz KJ, Merritt A, Bean BP, Lovinger DM. Protein kinase C modulates glutamate receptor inhibition of Ca2+ channels and synaptic transmission. Nature 1993;361(6408):165–168.
154. Yang J, Tsien RW. Enhancement of N- and L-type calcium channel currents by protein kinase C in frog sympathetic neurons. Neuron 1993;10(2):127–136.
155. Stea A, Soong TW, Snutch TP. Determinants of PKC-dependent modulation of a family of neuronal calcium channels. Neuron 1995;15(4):929–940.
156. Garcia-Ferreiro RE, Hernandez-Ochoa EO, Garcia DE. Modulation of N-type Ca2+ channel current kinetics by PMA in rat sympathetic neurons. Pflugers Arch 2001;442(6):848–858.
157. Zamponi GW, Bourinet E, Nelson D, Nargeot J, Snutch TP. Crosstalk between G proteins and protein kinase C mediated by the calcium channel [alpha]1 subunit. Nature 1997;385(6615):442–446.
158. Hamid J, Nelson D, Spaetgens R, Dubel SJ, Snutch TP, Zamponi GW. Identification of an integration center for cross-talk between protein kinase C and G protein modulation of N-type calcium channels. J Biol Chem 1999;274(10):6195–6202.
159. Cooper CB, Arnot MI, Feng ZP, Jarvis SE, Hamid J, Zamponi GW. Cross-talk between G-protein and protein kinase C modulation of N-type calcium channels is dependent on the G-protein beta subunit isoform. J Biol Chem 2000;275(52):40777–40781.
160. Zhu Y, Ikeda SR. Modulation of Ca(2+)-channel currents by protein kinase C in adult rat sympathetic neurons. J Neurophysiol 1994;72(4):1549–1560.

161. Shapiro MS, Zhou J, Hille B. Selective disruption by protein kinases of G-protein-mediated Ca2+ channel modulation. J Neurophysiol 1996;76(1):311–320.
162. Barrett CF, Rittenhouse AR. Modulation of N-type calcium channel activity by G-proteins and protein kinase C. J Gen Physiol 2000;115(3):277–286.
163. Doering CJ, Kisilevsky AE, Feng ZP, et al. A single G{beta} subunit locus controls crosstalk between protein kinase C and G protein regulation of N-type calcium channels. J Biol Chem 2004;279(28):29709–29717.
164. Michailidis IE, Zhang Y, Yang J. The lipid connection-regulation of voltage-gated Ca(2+) channels by phosphoinositides. Pflugers Arch 2007;455(1):147–155.
165. Gamper N, Reznikov V, Yamada Y, Yang J, Shapiro MS. Phosphatidylinositol [correction] 4,5–bisphosphate signals underlie receptor-specific Gq/11–mediated modulation of N-type Ca2+ channels. J Neurosci 2004;24(48):10980–10992.
166. Liu L, Barrett CF, Rittenhouse AR. Arachidonic acid both inhibits and enhances whole cell calcium currents in rat sympathetic neurons. Am J Physiol Cell Physiol 2001;280(5): C1293–C1305.
167. Liu L, Rittenhouse AR. Arachidonic acid mediates muscarinic inhibition and enhancement of N-type Ca2+ current in sympathetic neurons. Proc Natl Acad Sci 2003;100(1): 295–300.
168. Liu L, Zhao R, Bai Y, et al. M1 muscarinic receptors inhibit L-type Ca2+ current and M-current by divergent signal transduction cascades. J Neurosci 2006;26(45):11588–11598.
169. Lechner SG, Hussl S, Schicker KW, Drobny H, Boehm S. Presynaptic inhibition via a phospholipase C- and phosphatidylinositol bisphosphate-dependent regulation of neuronal Ca2+ channels. Mol Pharmacol 2005;68(5):1387–1396.
170. Zamponi GW, Snutch TP. Modulating modulation: crosstalk between regulatory pathways of presynaptic calcium channels. Mol Intervent 2002;2(8):476–478.
171. Saisu H, Ibaraki K, Yamaguchi T, Sekine Y, Abe T. Monoclonal antibodies immunoprecipitating [omega]-conotoxin-sensitive calcium channel molecules recognize two novel proteins localized in the nervous system. Biochem Biophys Res Commun 1991;181(1):59–66.
172. Sheng ZH, Rettig J, Takahashi M, Catterall WA. Identification of a syntaxin-binding site on N-type calcium channels. Neuron 1994;13(6):1303–1313.
173. Rettig J, Sheng ZH, Kim DK, Hodson CD, Snutch TP, Catterall WA. Isoform-specific interaction of the alpha1A subunits of brain Ca2+ channels with the presynaptic proteins syntaxin and SNAP-25. Proc Natl Acad Sci U S A 1996;93(14):7363–7368.
174. Sheng ZH, Rettig J, Takahashi M, Catterall WA. Identification of a syntaxin-binding site on N-type calcium channels. Neuron 1994;13(6):1303–1313.
175. Rettig J, Sheng ZH, Kim DK, Hodson CD, Snutch TP, Catterall WA. Isoform-specific interaction of the alpha1A subunits of brain Ca2+ channels with the presynaptic proteins syntaxin and SNAP-25. Proc Natl Acad Sci U S A 1996;93(14):7363–7368.
176. Bezprozvanny I, Scheller RH, Tsien RW. Functional impact of syntaxin on gating of N-type and Q-type calcium channels. Nature 1995;378(6557):623–626.
177. Wiser O, Bennett MK, Atlas D. Functional interaction of syntaxin and SNAP-25 with voltage-sensitive L- and N-type Ca2+ channels. EMBO J 1996;15(16):4100–4110.
178. Degtiar VE, Scheller RH, Tsien RW. Syntaxin modulation of slow inactivation of N-type calcium channels. J Neurosci 2000;20(12):4355–4367.
179. Marsal J, Ruiz-Montasell B, Blasi J, et al. Block of transmitter release by botulinum C1 action on syntaxin at the squid giant synapse. Proc Natl Acad Sci 1997;94(26): 14871–14876.
180. Sugimori M, Tong CK, Fukuda M, et al. Presynaptic injection of syntaxin-specific antibodies blocks transmission in the squid giant synapse. Neuroscience 1998;86(1):39–51.
181. Sakaba T, Stein A, Jahn R, Neher E. Distinct kinetic changes in neurotransmitter release after SNARE protein cleavage. Science 2005;309(5733):491–494.
182. Bergsman JB, Tsien RW. Syntaxin modulation of calcium channels in cortical synaptosomes as revealed by botulinum toxin C1. J Neurosci 2000;20(12):4368–4378.

183. Stanley EF. Syntaxin I modulation of presynaptic calcium channel inactivation revealed by botulinum toxin C1. Eur J Neurosci 2003;17(6):1303–1305.

184. Gladycheva SE, Ho CS, Lee YY, Stuenkel EL. Regulation of syntaxin1A-munc18 complex for SNARE pairing in HEK293 cells. J Physiol 2004;558(Pt 3):857–871.

185. Chan AW, Khanna R, Li Q, Stanley EF. A presynaptic transmitter release site N type (CaV2.2) calcium channel interacting protein. Channels 2007;1(1):11–20.

186. Berg D, Holzmann C, Riess O. 14-3-3 proteins in the nervous system. Nat Rev Neurosci 2003;4(9):752–762.

187. Li Y, Wu Y, Zhou Y. Modulation of inactivation properties of CaV2.2 channels by 14-3-3 proteins. Neuron 2006;51(6):755–771.

188. Li Y, Wu Y, Li R, Zhou Y. The role of 14-3-3 dimerization in its modulation of the CaV2.2 channel. Channels 2007;1(1):1–2.

Chapter 6
Synaptotagmin: Transducing Ca²⁺-Binding to Vesicle Fusion

Carin Loewen and Noreen Reist

Contents

Abstract Synaptotagmins are a large family of transmembrane proteins consisting of at least 15 isoforms in mammals (1), and seven in *Drosophila* (2). Synaptotagmin 1 is the most conserved of the synaptotagmin isoforms (3) and is known to play a role in the synaptic vesicle cycle. Genetic studies in mice (4–10), *Caenorhabditis elegans* (11), and *Drosophila* (12–22) have shown that synaptotagmin 1 is required for efficient synaptic transmission. Although synaptic transmission persists in synaptotagmin knockouts (4,11,12), it is severely disrupted. Biochemical and genetic studies have implicated synaptotagmin function during several stages in the synaptic vesicle cycle, including (1) docking synaptic vesicles at release sites, (2) priming synaptic vesicles for quick release, (3) binding the Ca²⁺ required to trigger

Noreen Reist
Colorado State University, BMS Dept., Fort Collins, CO 80523, USA
e-mail: Noreen.Reist@Colostate.edu

Z.-W. Wang (ed.) *Molecular Mechanisms of Neurotransmitter Release*,
© Humana Press 2008 a part of Springer Science+Business Media, LLC

fusion, and (4) endocytosis of synaptic vesicles after fusion. This chapter reviews the evidence supporting each of these hypotheses, and discusses the molecular interactions that may underlie these abilities.

Keywords Synaptotagmin, asynchronous fusion, synchronous fusion, docking, priming.

The primary way that neurons communicate with their targets is Ca^{2+}-triggered release of a chemical neurotransmitter contained within synaptic vesicles in the presynaptic terminal (23). As described in previous chapters, much has been learned about the synaptic vesicle cycle, including the role of Ca^{2+} and soluble *N*-ethylmaleimide–sensitive factor attachment receptor (SNARE) proteins in synaptic vesicle fusion. We now know that the synaptic vesicle protein, synaptotagmin 1 (24–26), is also a critical regulator of the synaptic vesicle cycle.

The Structure of Synaptotagmin

Clues to synaptotagmin's function may be found in its molecular structure. Synaptotagmin 1 contains several domains (27): an amino terminal, intravesicular domain that is glycosylated; a single transmembrane region that spans the synaptic vesicle membrane; and a large cytoplasmic region that is composed primarily of two C_2 domains, C_2A and C_2B (Fig. 6.1, top), each of which is homologous to the regulatory C_2 region of protein kinase C. The structure of synaptotagmin was solved by x-ray crystallography and nuclear magnetic resonance (NMR) (28–31). These studies show that both C_2 domains form a stable, eight-stranded, β-sandwich with flexible loops emerging from the top and bottom (Fig. 6.1, top). The β-sandwich is formed by two, four-stranded, antiparallel, β-sheets. Both C_2 domains of synaptotagmin 1 bind Ca^{2+} ions (Fig. 6.1 top, spheres; bottom, black circles) exclusively at the tip of the β-sandwich in a cuplike cavity formed by the loops connecting β2 with β3 (loop 1) and β6 with β7 (loop 3). In each domain, the bound Ca^{2+} ions are partially coordinated by five highly conserved acidic residues that reside in these two flexible loops (Fig. 6.1 and 6.2. bottom, D_1, D_2, D_3, D_4, D_5; and Fig. 6.1, top, black stick residues) (28–32).

To refer to specific residues, we indicate the C_2 domain by letter and the residue by its label in Figure 6.2. For example, the second conserved acidic residue in the C_2B domain is indicated as B-D_2. The C_2A domain binds three Ca^{2+} ions, while the C_2B domain binds two. These highly conserved, Ca^{2+}-binding pockets support the hypothesis that synaptotagmin 1 is the Ca^{2+} sensor for evoked transmitter release (i.e., the molecule that binds Ca^{2+} upon influx into the presynaptic terminal and consequently triggers fusion of synaptic vesicles with the presynaptic membrane).

In addition to the Ca^{2+}-binding motif in the C_2A and C_2B domains, synaptotagmin 1 also contains a polylysine motif in the fourth strand of the C_2B β-sandwich (Fig. 6.1 top, space-filled residues marked by asterisks; Fig. 6.2, asterisks). This motif supplies a patch of positively charged residues on the side of the C_2B domain,

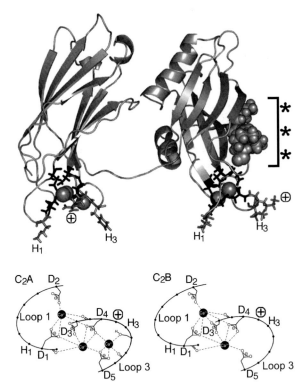

Fig. 6.1 Synaptotagmin structure. Top: Structure of the C_2A and C_2B domains of synaptotagmin 1 [PDB files 1BYN and K5W visualized using the PyMOL molecular graphics system (154)]. The connection between the C_2A and C_2B domains was drawn by hand. The spheres represent Ca^{2+} ions. The space-filled residues in the C_2B domain marked with asterisks are the polylysine motif. The black stick residues represent the Ca^{2+}-binding residues (D_{1-5}). Two hydrophobic residues (H_1 and H_3) and the acidic residue $\oplus$ found at the tip of each Ca^{2+}-binding pocket are indicated. Bottom: Schematic of the Ca^{2+}-binding loops of each C_2 domain showing the coordination of Ca^{2+} ions by D_{1-5}. $\oplus$, acidic residue. H_1 and H_3, hydrophobic residues. (Modified from Fernandez et al [31]. The original figure was published in *Neuron,* copyright Elsevier.)

near the Ca^{2+}-binding pocket. Despite the fact that the entire synaptotagmin sequence is only approximately 50% to 65% conserved, the C_2B, polylysine motif is virtually identical in all synaptotagmin isoforms among various species (Fig. 6.2, asterisks) (33). Such a high level of conservation suggests that this motif plays an important role in synaptotagmin function.

Synaptotagmin and Neurotransmitter Release

At least two kinetically distinct components of neurotransmitter release have been identified at both neuromuscular junctions and central synapses (6,20,34–39). In the first component, the rate of neurotransmitter release is fast, and release occurs

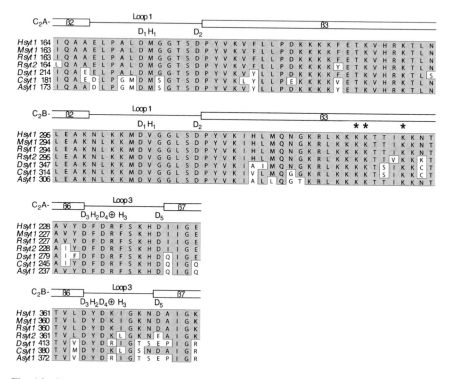

Fig. 6.2 ClustalW sequence alignment of the highly conserved Ca²⁺-binding loops and adjacent ß-sheets in the C₂A and C₂B domains of synaptotagmin. Bars, ß-sheets; D₁₋₅, Ca²⁺-binding residues; H₁₋₃, hydrophobic residues; ⊕, acidic residues; *, polybasic motif

nearly synchronously with the stimulus. This fast, synchronous release component comprises the majority of evoked release. In the second component, the rate of neurotransmitter release is slower and occurs asynchronously with the stimulus. Both components are dependent on Ca²⁺ influx into the presynaptic terminal.

Synaptotagmin and Synchronous Release

Strong evidence supports the hypothesis that synaptotagmin 1 is the Ca²⁺ sensor for the fast, synchronous release of neurotransmitter. Knocking out synaptotagmin selectively abolishes, or at least severely decreases, the fast, synchronous component of neurotransmitter release (4,6,9,10,16–18,20,39). For example, at the *Drosophila* neuromuscular junction the synchronous response is decreased ~95% in synaptotagmin knockouts (*syt*^null^) (Fig. 6.3). However, slow, asynchronous release persists in synaptotagmin knockouts, as exhibited by the increased number

Fig. 6.3 The amplitude of synchronous evoked neurotransmitter release is decreased in synaptotagmin
knockouts (*syt^null*). Representative evoked junctional
potentials recorded from *wild-type* and *syt^null*
Drosophila larvae. (Modified from Loewen et al [17].)

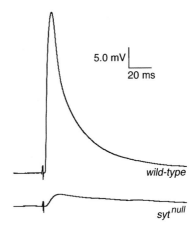

of longer latency events in Figure 6.4, indicating that another Ca^{2+} sensor mediates
this release (4,6,9,10,16–18,20,39). Most studies examining release after a single
stimulus show that the slow, asynchronous component of release increases in synaptotagmin knockouts by approximately the same extent as the synchronous component decreases (6,9,20). In other words, the total amount of Ca^{2+}-triggered release
measured over a relatively long period after the stimulus (20 to 50 times the duration of the synchronous event) is similar between synaptotagmin knockouts and
wild-type controls. The majority of release at wild-type synapses is synchronous
(Fig. 6.4, *wild-type*, occurring within tens to hundreds of milliseconds after the
stimulus, depending on the synapse), while the release remaining at synaptotagmin
knockout synapses is asynchronous (Fig. 6.4, *syt^null*, spread out over a 20 to 50 times
longer time period). These findings indicate that if synaptotagmin is present, it catalyzes fast, synchronous release. If synaptotagmin is absent, vesicles are triggered to
fuse asynchronously by an unknown, slow sensor.

Synaptotagmin and Asynchronous Release

The relationship between synaptotagmin and the asynchronous sensor remains
unclear. The finding that approximately the same number of vesicles fuse after a
single stimulus in wild-type and synaptotagmin knockouts suggests that the reason
asynchronous release is low in the presence of synaptotagmin is because the population of releasable vesicles is depleted by synchronous fusion and few vesicles are
left for the asynchronous sensor to trigger to fuse. However, other data suggest that
asynchronous release is low in the presence of synaptotagmin because synaptotagmin inhibits the asynchronous sensor when synaptotagmin is in its Ca^{2+}-free state
(i.e., as soon as intracellular Ca^{2+} levels begin to drop after stimulation).

During high-frequency stimulation, asynchronous release in wild-type neurons
is a more prominent mode of release than it is following a single stimulus, and

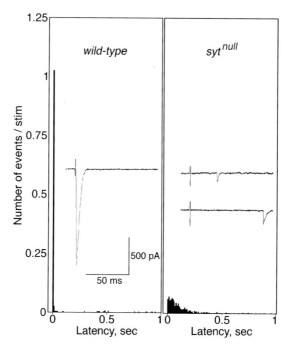

Fig. 6.4 Latency analysis of evoked neurotransmitter release in synaptotagmin knockouts (*syt^null*). In *Drosophila* embryos, the latencies of synaptic currents within 1 second following nerve stimulation in 4 mM extracellular Ca^{2+} were measured and plotted (100 stimuli for each cell). Results from each animal were averaged and presented as the number of events per stimulation in 10-ms bins. The value is slightly greater than 1 in *wild-type* as two release events from a single stimulus were occasionally observed. (The small number of random asynchronous events in *wild-type* are due to spontaneous neural firing originating from the intact central nervous system [CNS] as they are large-amplitude events. Traces containing spontaneous bursting activity originating from the CNS were excluded from the analysis. Spontaneous CNS activity is abolished in synaptotagmin knockouts (*syt^null*) due to the dramatic reduction in neurotransmission.) The small number of release events in the first 10-ms bin in *syt^null* reflects asynchronous events, as most occurred after the first 6 ms; normal release in the first few milliseconds was rarely observed. (Modified from Yoshihara and Littleton [20]. The original figure was published in *Neuron,* copyright Elsevier.)

appears unaffected in synaptotagmin knockouts (Fig. 6.5) (39,40). When synaptotagmin is present, release drops rapidly when the high-frequency stimulation ceases; however, release continues longer in synaptotagmin knockouts (Fig. 6.5, arrow) (39). This delayed release in synaptotagmin knockouts is triggered by the buildup of residual Ca^{2+} in the nerve terminals as a result of the high-frequency stimulus train. Since synaptotagmin is a low-affinity Ca^{2+}-sensor (8,30,41), it should release Ca^{2+} very shortly after the cessation of stimulation, before Ca^{2+} levels are back down to resting levels. In wild-type terminals, this Ca^{2+}-free synaptotagmin inhibits the asynchronous sensor. While in synaptotagmin knockouts terminals, the asynchronous sensor can continue to trigger fusion, resulting in delayed release.

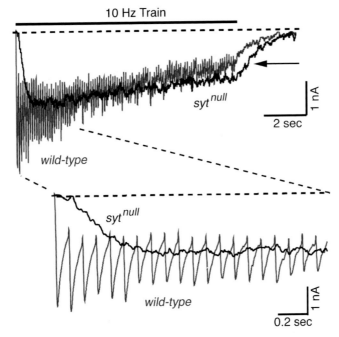

Fig. 6.5 Ca²⁺-free synaptotagmin inhibits asynchronous release. Representative inhibitory post-synaptic currents during a 10-second stimulus train at 10 Hz from cultured cortical neurons of *wild-type* or synaptotagmin knockout (*syt^null^*) mice; a similar plateau level of release mediated by the asynchronous sensor is present in both. Arrow points to the asynchronous release that persists in the synaptotagmin knockouts after stimulation ceases and intracellular Ca²⁺ levels drop. (Modified from Tang et al [40]. The original figure was published in *Cell,* copyright Elsevier.)

The finding that the asynchronous sensor can trigger release for a longer period of time than synaptotagmin can (Fig. 6.5, arrow) demonstrates that this sensor has a higher affinity for Ca²⁺ than synaptotagmin (i.e., it can still trigger release at Ca²⁺ levels insufficient to activate synaptotagmin's fusogenic activity). These findings show that synaptotagmin is a low-affinity, fast Ca²⁺ sensor, while the asynchronous sensor is a high-affinity, slow sensor. They further suggest that synaptotagmin competes with the asynchronous Ca²⁺ sensor and, when synaptotagmin is not Ca²⁺-bound, it inhibits release mediated by the asynchronous sensor (Fig. 6.6).

In summary, release resulting from a single action potential is mainly synchronous, and is triggered by synaptotagmin. It may be that release triggered by a single action potential is mainly synchronous because synchronous release depletes the population of releasable vesicles, leaving few for the asynchronous sensor to trigger to fuse. In addition, asynchronous release may be a minor component because Ca²⁺-free synaptotagmin impedes release by the slow, asynchronous sensor. In this scenario, upon Ca²⁺ influx, synaptotagmin binds Ca²⁺ and triggers fast fusion. As soon as Ca²⁺ levels begin to drop, synaptotagmin (the low-affinity sensor) releases Ca²⁺ and inhibits the asynchronous sensor (Fig. 6.6). The asynchronous sensor, being slow, has not yet triggered

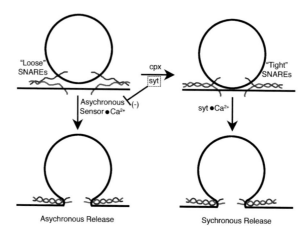

Fig. 6.6 Model of asynchronous release versus synchronous release. Prior to Ca^{2+} entry, SNAREs may exist in either a partially coiled, "loose" conformation (top left) or a fully assembled, "tight" conformation (top right). Complexin (cpx) and synaptotagmin (syt) may participate in vesicle priming by stabilizing the "tight" conformation. Ca^{2+} can trigger fusion from either conformation. Ca^{2+}-triggered fusion from the "loose" state of SNARE assembly is mediated by the asynchronous sensor•Ca^{2+} (left), while fusion from the "tight" state of SNARE assembly is mediate by synaptotagmin•Ca^{2+} (right). When synaptotagmin is not bound to Ca^{2+}, it inhibits the asynchronous sensor (-) and, thus, asynchronous release

the fusion of many vesicles. During prolonged periods of elevated intracellular Ca^{2+}, like that which occurs during high-frequency stimulation, synaptotagmin is predominantly in its Ca^{2+}-bound state (synaptotagmin•Ca^{2+}). Thus, it ceases to inhibit the asynchronous sensor, and release quickly becomes primarily asynchronous (Fig. 6.5). After high-frequency stimulation stops, synaptotagmin returns to its Ca^{2+} free state and inhibits any further release that might be triggered by residual intracellular Ca^{2+} via the high-affinity asynchronous sensor (Fig. 6.5, arrow).

Consistent with the hypothesis that synaptotagmin must bind Ca^{2+} to relieve its inhibition of the asynchronous sensor, mutations of synaptotagmin's C_2B Ca^{2+}-binding residues that severely disrupt Ca^{2+}-binding by the C_2B domain disrupt *both* synchronous and asynchronous release (5). Indeed, similar inhibition of both synchronous and asynchronous release are seen when the entire C_2B domain of synaptotagmin is deleted (20). Thus, the C_2A domain alone appears to be able to inhibit the asynchronous sensor, and Ca^{2+} must bind to the C_2B domain to release this inhibition.

Synaptotagmin and Spontaneous Release

Finally, spontaneous release is increased in *Drosophila* knockouts of synaptotagmin 1 (16,17; however, see refs. 20 and 42) and mouse knockouts of synaptotagmin II (43). The increased rate of spontaneous fusion seen in some preparations has led to the hypothesis that in addition to facilitating fast, synchronous release and inhibiting asynchronous release, synaptotagmin may also inhibit spontaneous release (44). Alternatively, an increase in spontaneous release may be a compensatory response to the severe decrease in Ca^{2+}-triggered, synchronous releases that occurs in synaptotagmin knockouts.

Mechanism of Ca^{2+}-Sensing

Genetic studies indicate that binding of Ca^{2+} to synaptotagmin's C_2B domain is critical for synaptotagmin's Ca^{2+}-sensing role. In *Drosophila*, mutation of two acidic, Ca^{2+}-binding residues in synaptotagmin's C_2B domain to asparagines (N) decreases evoked release by >99% (Fig. 6.2, B-D$_3$ and B-D$_4$ to N = B-D$_{3,4}$N), or results in lethality (B-D$_{1,2}$N) (18). The second and third aspartates in the C_2B Ca^{2+}-binding pocket (Figs. 6.1 and 6.2, B-D$_2$ and B-D$_3$) are the most critical residues for synaptotagmin function; mutation of either nearly abolishes all release (5). These experiments demonstrate that synaptotagmin's ability to bind Ca^{2+} by the C_2B domain is required for synchronous synaptic transmission.

Curiously, unlike the C_2B domain, the C_2A domain is not required for synaptotagmin's Ca^{2+}-sensing role. Mutation of the second Ca^{2+}-binding aspartate residue in synaptotagmin's C_2A domain to asparagine (A-D$_2$N) has no effect on the Ca^{2+}-dependent properties of synaptic transmission (22). Similarly, mutation of either the fourth or fifth Ca^{2+}-binding residues of C_2A (A-D$_4$N or A-D$_5$N) (45,46) or even mutation of all five Ca^{2+}-binding residues (A-D$_{1-5}$N) (7) causes little to no change in synaptic transmission. Thus, unlike the C_2B domain, Ca^{2+}-binding to the C_2A domain is not critical for synaptotagmin's Ca^{2+}-sensing role.

Transducing Ca^{2+}-Binding to Neurotransmitter Release

As the main Ca^{2+} sensor for synchronous neurotransmitter release, synaptotagmin must link Ca^{2+} influx to synaptic vesicle fusion. Ca^{2+}-binding to synaptotagmin does not cause a major conformational change, but instead changes synaptotagmin's electrostatic potential (47). Therefore, it is likely that Ca^{2+}-binding to synaptotagmin acts as an "electrostatic switch" for neurotransmitter release by regulating synaptotagmin's interactions with presynaptic molecules (29,30,47–49). Indeed, *in vitro* studies have demonstrated that synaptotagmin undergoes Ca^{2+}-stimulated interactions with numerous presynaptic molecules. Thus, it is important to identify the molecules that interact with synaptotagmin, understand how Ca^{2+} affects these interactions, and map the interaction sites in both synaptotagmin and its partners. The next section reviews what is currently known regarding the Ca^{2+}-dependent binding partners of synaptotagmin in the context of how these interactions may mediate synaptic vesicle fusion.

The Ca²⁺-Dependent Binding Partners of Synaptotagmin

Phospholipids

Synaptotagmin was first proposed to function as a Ca^{2+} sensor for neurotransmitter release when it was found to bind Ca^{2+} at physiological levels in a complex with negatively charged phospholipids (50). Indeed, Ca^{2+}-dependent phospholipid binding is a highly conserved property of C_2 domains (51), and numerous biochemical studies have confirmed the Ca^{2+}-dependent interaction between synaptotagmin and negatively charged phospholipids (18,25,31,49,52–59), including phosphatidylinositol-4,5-bisphosphate (PtdIns(4,5)P2)-containing membranes (49,60,61), such as the presynaptic membrane.

The intrinsic affinity of synaptotagmin for Ca^{2+} is quite low (8,30,41) because the negatively charged, Ca^{2+}-binding residues found in the C_2A and C_2B Ca^{2+}-binding pockets of synaptotagmin only partially coordinate the Ca^{2+} ions. However, synaptotagmin's affinity for Ca^{2+} increases in the presence of negatively charged phospholipid membranes (8,30,49,50) because the negatively charged phospholipid headgroups complete the coordination sphere for the Ca^{2+} ions. Thus, a major component of synaptotagmin's interaction with phospholipids is electrostatic.

An additional component of this electrostatic interaction is a positively charged amino acid (indicated by $\oplus$ in Figs. 6.1 and 6.2) at the tip of each C_2 domain, immediately adjacent to the fourth, Ca^{2+}-binding residue. In the C_2A domain, this basic amino acid is an arginine, and in the C_2B domain it is a lysine or an arginine. This positively charged residue likely mediates a Ca^{2+}-dependent interaction with negatively-charged phospholipids in both the C_2A (8,56) and C_2B (62,63) (see, however, ref. 64) domains. Thus, upon Ca^{2+} influx, the positive charge of the bound Ca^{2+} in combination with these C_2A and C_2B basic residues (Figs. 6.1 and 6.2, A-$\oplus$, and B-$\oplus$) produces an electrostatic attraction between synaptotagmin on the synaptic vesicle and the negatively charged presynaptic membrane. This electrostatic interaction would draw the synaptic vesicle membrane closer to the presynaptic membrane.

Although the interaction between synaptotagmin and the presynaptic plasma membrane is triggered by the change in synaptotagmin's electrostatic potential upon Ca^{2+} binding (49,55,63), this interaction may be mostly mediated by hydrophobic interactions (65). Three highly conserved hydrophobic residues are exposed on the tips of the Ca^{2+} binding pocket in each C_2 domain of synaptotagmin (Fig. 6.2, H_1, H_2, H_3). *In vitro* studies have demonstrated that one or more of these hydrophobic residues in each C_2 domain penetrate the plasma membrane in the presence of Ca^{2+} (55–57,59,66–68). When these hydrophobic residues are made more hydrophobic by mutation to tryptophan, there is an increase in the apparent Ca^{2+} affinity of synaptotagmin for negatively charged phospholipids (69).

Role of Phospholipids

Inclusion of SNARE proteins in synthetic lipid vesicles results in SNARE-mediated fusion of the vesicles (70–72) and led to the hypothesis that SNARE proteins constitute the minimal machinery for fusion (see Chapter 3). When soluble synaptotagmin and Ca^{2+} are added to the fusion reaction, the rate of fusion increases (73). Although the presence of negatively charged phospholipids in the synthetic vesicles is not necessary for SNARE-mediated fusion, negatively charged lipids are required for the stimulation of fusion by soluble synaptotagmin that has bound Ca^{2+} (synaptotagmin•Ca^{2+}) (74). This *in vitro* study suggests that synaptotagmin's interaction with negatively charged phospholipids is important for Ca^{2+}-stimulated fusion. [It must be noted, however, that the physiological relevance of the stimulation of SNARE-mediated fusion by soluble synaptotagmin•Ca^{2+} is currently controversial. Two pieces of data argue against its physiological relevance. First, *in vivo*, synaptotagmin is not soluble but tethered to synaptic vesicles. Indeed, when synaptotagmin is incorporated into the vesicle-associated membrane protein (VAMP)/synaptobrevin containing vesicles, it still stimulates SNARE-mediated fusion, but the stimulation is Ca^{2+}-independent (75,76). Second, Ca^{2+}-dependent stimulation of SNARE-mediated fusion by soluble synaptotagmin•Ca^{2+} is more severely disrupted by mutations in synaptotagmin's C_2A Ca^{2+}-binding motif than in its C_2B Ca^{2+}-binding motif (74), while the opposite is true *in vivo*.]

Role of the Basic Residue in C_2A

In vivo experiments support the hypothesis that the electrostatic interaction between synaptotagmin and negatively charged phospholipids plays a role in triggering neurotransmitter release. Mutation of the C_2A, Ca^{2+}-binding pocket, basic residue (Fig. 6.2, A-⊕) to a glutamine decreases Ca^{2+}-dependent phospholipid binding and neurotransmitter release (8,49,63). The decrease in Ca^{2+}-dependent neurotransmitter release caused by this mutation is somewhat surprising in light of the findings discussed above, which demonstrate that mutations of Ca^{2+}-binding residues in C_2A have little to no effect on neurotransmitter release (7,45,46). How can it be that a mutation that disrupts Ca^{2+}-dependent phospholipid binding by the C_2A domain decreases release when mutations that disrupt Ca^{2+} binding by C_2A have little effect on neurotransmitter release? The answer to this conundrum may lie in the nature of the amino acids used to substitute for the Ca^{2+}-binding residues of the C_2A domain; the negatively charged aspartates in C_2A were replaced by neutral asparagines. It may be that neutralization of the negatively charged amino acids in the C_2A, Ca^{2+}-binding pocket (which would normally repel the negatively charged plasma membrane) permit the C_2A basic residue to interact with the plasma membrane and facilitate fusion upon Ca^{2+} binding to the intact C_2B domain. In this scenario, Ca^{2+}-binding to the C_2A domain is important for neurotransmitter release because it neutralizes the negatively charged Ca^{2+}-binding pocket, thereby permitting the basic residue to interact with the plasma membrane. Consistent with this hypothesis, neutralization of this positively charged residue by mutation to an asparagine (N) increased the intrinsic affinity of synaptotagmin for Ca^{2+} even though it decreased neurotransmitter release (8). Interestingly, neutralization of the fourth Ca^{2+}-binding residue in C_2A (A-D_4N), which is located immediately adjacent to the conserved basic residue (Figs. 6.1 and 6.2, A-⊕), actually increases the apparent Ca^{2+}-affinity of release (7,46). Thus, the A-D_4N mutation may partially mimic Ca^{2+} binding and permit the arginine to interact with the plasma membrane.

Role of the Basic Residue in C_2B

The role of the conserved basic residue in the C_2B, Ca^{2+}-binding pocket (Figs. 6.1 and 6.2, B-⊕) during neurotransmitter release is likely similar to that of the corresponding residue in C_2A. Although one study found that mutation of the C_2B basic residue does not effect phospholipid binding *in vitro* or neurotransmitter release from cultured cells (64), others demonstrate that the mutation decreases the ability of synaptotagmin to bind negatively charged phospholipids and decreases neurotransmitter release (62,63). Indeed, at an intact synapse, mutation of this basic residue in the C_2B domain results in a more severe decrease in neurotransmitter release than mutation of the corresponding basic residue in the C_2A domain (62). These results support the hypothesis that the Ca^{2+}-dependent interaction between the negatively charged presynaptic membrane and these positively charged residues in both the C_2A and C_2B domains is important for synaptic vesicle fusion.

Role of the Hydrophobic Residues

The hydrophobic interaction between synaptotagmin and the membrane plays a key role in triggering neurotransmitter release. The ability of soluble synaptotagmin•Ca^{2+} to stimulate SNARE-mediated fusion of synthetic vesicles depends on the presence of the hydrophobic residues found around the rim of synaptotagmin's two Ca^{2+}-binding pockets (Figs. 6.1 and 6.2, H_1 and H_3). Indeed, soluble synaptotagmin•Ca^{2+} stimulates SNARE-mediated fusion of synthetic vesicles to an even greater extent when these two hydrophobic residues in each C_2 domain are made more hydrophobic (77). Furthermore, increasing the hydrophobicity of these residues also increases Ca^{2+}-triggered release at cultured synapses (69). Insertion of these hydrophobic residues should force the plasma membrane to bend to relieve the tension created by the insertion (77). If synaptotagmin 1 does induce membrane curvature, it should preferentially bind to membranes with curvatures similar to those produced when synaptotagmin 1 inserts. Indeed, *in vitro* studies demonstrate that synaptotagmin 1 shows a strong preference for binding small diameter vesicles, and is actually able to induce positive membrane curvature. Both the preference for binding smaller diameter membranes and the ability to induce positive membrane curvature are dependent on the presence of Ca^{2+} (77). Thus, insertion of these hydrophobic residues triggered by synaptotagmin•Ca^{2+} may lower the fusion activation barrier by inducing high, positive curvature in the presynaptic membrane and thereby stimulate SNARE-mediate fusion.

Indeed, the hydrophobic interaction between the C_2B domain of synaptotagmin and the plasma membrane is more critical for exocytosis than its electrostatic interaction with the plasma membrane. While mutation of a key hydrophobic residue in the C_2A domain (A-H_3E or A-H_3Y) disrupts synaptic transmission to approximately the same extent as mutation of the C_2A basic residue (~50% decrease), mutation of the homologous hydrophobic residue on the tip of the C_2B Ca^{2+}-binding pocket (B-H_3E) results in such a severe deficit that it is lethal (78). Yet disruption of the C_2B electrostatic interaction with the plasma membrane is viable, although evoked release is decreased by 80% (62). To date, the only *Drosophila* synaptotagmin point mutations to results in embryonic lethality are those of the C_2B, Ca^{2+}-binding residues and the C_2B, hydrophobic residues (78,79). Thus, the hydrophobic interaction mediated by synaptotagmin's C_2B domain appears to be the most critical of synaptotagmin's Ca^{2+}-triggered interactions.

Summary of Ca^{2+}-Dependent Phospholipid Binding by Synaptotagmin

Ca^{2+}-dependent synaptic vesicle fusion depends on both electrostatic and hydrophobic interactions between synaptotagmin•Ca^{2+} and the presynaptic plasma membrane. These interactions, which include the direct penetration of phospholipid membranes by hydrophobic residues of synaptotagmin, may directly influence the lipid transition states during fusion. Consistent with this hypothesis, it has recently been demonstrated that soluble synaptotagmin•Ca^{2+} induces positive membrane curvature due to the Ca^{2+}-dependent penetration of two, Ca^{2+}-binding pocket, hydrophobic residues in each C_2 domain (Figs. 6.1 and 6.2, A-H_1, A-H_3, B-H_1 and B-H_3) into the phospholipid membrane (77). As this ability is correlated with its ability to stimulate SNARE-mediated fusion of synthetic vesicles (77), the induction of high, positive membrane curvature by synaptotagmin•Ca^{2+} may be sufficient to directly trigger fusion pore opening (80). Alternatively, Ca^{2+}-triggered phospholipid binding by synaptotagmin, including insertion of its hydrophobic residues, may destabilize a fusion intermediate (see discussion of "loose" vs. "tight" SNARE complexes, below) to trigger fusion pore opening (81). Finally, consistent with the preeminent role of the C_2B Ca^{2+}-binding motif in triggering vesicle fusion, the electrostatic and hydrophobic interactions between the plasma membrane and the tip of the C_2B domain's Ca^{2+}-binding pocket are more critical for neurotransmitter release than those of the C_2A domain.

SNARE Proteins

Biochemical experiments have shown that synaptotagmin does not bind VAMP/synaptobrevin directly (82). However, many *in vitro* studies demonstrate that synaptotagmin is able to interact directly with syntaxin (9,22,48,52,57,82–87; see however, 88), SNAP-25 (9,52,82,85,88,89), a syntaxin/SNAP-25 complex (the t-SNARE complex) (9,33,82,85,88,90,91), and the fully assembled SNARE complex (52,57,82,85,89,92–94).

Whether the interaction between synaptotagmin and isolated or complexed SNARE proteins is dependent on Ca^{2+} is somewhat unclear because *in vitro* reaction conditions greatly affect the results (22,57,86), and both synaptotagmin and SNAREs are "sticky" proteins in biochemical experiments. However, most studies show that Ca^{2+} greatly promotes the interaction between synaptotagmin and isolated syntaxin and isolated SNAP-25. Thus, any interaction between synaptotagmin and these proteins *in vivo* is likely to be Ca^{2+} dependent. Although Ca^{2+} promotes the interaction between synaptotagmin and t-SNARE complexes (85,88,91) as well as full SNARE complexes (52,57,82,85,89,92–94), these molecules exhibit a Ca^{2+}-independent interaction with synaptotagmin as well (9,33,82,90–93). The physiological relevance of the Ca^{2+}-independent binding of synaptotagmin to SNAREs is currently under debate. Although one study suggests that in physiological conditions the levels of Ca^{2+}-independent binding is low (40), another study argues that the Ca^{2+}-independent interaction of synaptotagmin with t-SNARE complexes is synaptotagmin's most conserved activity, even more conserved than Ca^{2+}-dependent phospholipid binding, and that many synaptotagmin isoforms that do not bind Ca^{2+} still bind t-SNARE complexes (33).

Role of SNAREs

Numerous studies have demonstrated that SNARE function is intimately linked to Ca^{2+}-triggered fusion. For example: (1) Botulinum and tetanus neurotoxins (BoTx and TeTx) cleave SNARE proteins and completely inhibit Ca^{2+}-triggered neurotransmitter release (95). Ca^{2+} can, at least partly, rescue the inhibition of neurotransmitter release caused by BoTx A cleavage of SNAP-25 (96–98). (2) Genetic knockouts of SNAP-25 and VAMP/synaptobrevin show greater disruption in Ca^{2+}-triggered release than in spontaneous release (99–103). (3) A mutation in SNAP-25 that impairs SNARE complex assembly decreases the Ca^{2+}-cooperativity of exocytosis (104,105). (4) Adding the 65 amino acid C-terminal fragment of SNAP-25 that is cleaved off by BoTx E rescues the inhibition of neurotransmitter released caused by this toxin, but only in the presence of Ca^{2+} (106).

Consistent with the tight coupling between Ca^{2+} and SNARE function, numerous studies indicate that interactions between synaptotagmin and SNARES are likely important for neurotransmitter release. For example: (1) Synaptotagmin fragments can inhibit neurotransmitter release from cracked PC12 cells (52,91,107) and chromaffin cells (33). The inhibitory activity of the fragments in cracked PC12 cells is correlated with their Ca^{2+}-dependent ability to bind SNAP-25, syntaxin (52) and t-SNARE complexes (91), whereas the inhibitory activity in chromaffin cells is correlated with their Ca^{2+}-independent ability to bind t-SNARE complexes (33). Likewise, the ability of SNAP-25 to bind synaptotagmin is correlated with its ability to mediate release from cracked PC12 cells (89). (2) Lengthening the linker region between synaptotagmin's two C_2 domains does not have an affect on synaptotagmin's Ca^{2+}-dependent membrane binding. But it does disrupt synaptotagmin's Ca^{2+}-dependent interaction with t-SNARE complexes, the inhibitory activity of synaptotagmin fragments in PC12 cell secretion assays, and the stability of fusion pores (85). (3) Membrane fusion mediated by SNAREs in synthetic vesicles can be accelerated by soluble synaptotagmin only in the presence of Ca^{2+} (73). This activity is specific for neuronal SNAREs and is correlated with synaptotagmin's Ca^{2+}-dependent binding of t-SNARE heterodimers; synaptotagmin does not undergo

Ca^{2+}-stimulated binding to yeast t-SNARE heterodimers, and synaptotagmin•Ca^{2+} cannot stimulate fusion of synthetic vesicles mediated by yeast SNAREs (108). Together these data demonstrate that the interaction between synaptotagmin and SNAREs is a critical component of Ca^{2+}-triggered vesicle fusion.

The mechanism by which synaptotagmin interacts with SNAREs to mediate Ca^{2+}-dependent fusion, however, is still unclear. Ca^{2+}-binding to synaptotagmin could initiate an interaction with SNAREs, release already bound SNAREs, or strengthen/rearrange existing Ca^{2+}-independent interactions with SNAREs. Synaptotagmin's interaction with SNAP-25, which is likely to be predominantly Ca^{2+}-dependent, has been proposed to participate in synaptic vesicle docking at active zones (82,109,110). In support of this theory, Ca^{2+} induces the formation of SNAP-25–synaptotagmin complexes and stimulates granule cell docking in neuroendocrine cells (110). This docking was dependent on SNAP-25 in that it was decreased when SNAP-25 was cleaved by BoTx E. Granule cell docking was also disrupted by addition of either antisynaptotagmin antibodies or C$_2$AB peptides, but not by addition of C$_2$B peptides (110).

Another hypothesis regarding how synaptotagmin interacts with SNAREs to mediate Ca^{2+}-dependent fusion is that synaptotagmin•Ca^{2+} may facilitate SNARE complex formation. In support of this hypothesis, synaptotagmin is able to promote the recruitment of SNAP-25 into t-SNARE heterodimers only in the presence of Ca^{2+} (108). Interestingly, this ability, as well as its ability to facilitate SNARE-mediated fusion of synthetic vesicles, is dependent on the presence of negatively charged phospholipids (108). Thus, synaptotagmin, Ca^{2+}, and negatively charged phospholipids may work together to facilitate t-SNARE heterodimer formation. Consistent with this hypothesis, synaptotagmin•Ca^{2+} binds simultaneously to SNARE complexes and negatively charged phospholipid membranes (93).

Alternatively, synaptotagmin•Ca^{2+} may interact with SNARE complexes after they've already, at least partially, assembled. Synaptotagmin•Ca^{2+} has been shown to displace the protein complexin from SNARE complexes (40,93). Complexins are small, soluble molecules (111,112) that do not bind to the individual SNARE proteins, but only to assembled SNARE complexes (112–114). These studies demonstrate that synaptotagmin•Ca^{2+} interacts with preformed SNARE complexes, and thus indicate that binding of synaptotagmin•Ca^{2+} is not required for formation of the SNARE complex.

Complexins are thought to stabilize the C-terminal, membrane-proximal portion of assembled SNARE complexes (115) and hold the SNARE complex in a state where the transmembrane regions of syntaxin and VAMP/synaptobrevin can interact (116). The interaction between complexin and SNARE complexes likely serves as a fusion clamp, as overexpression of complexin in chromaffin cells, PC12 cells, and primary cortical neurons inhibits neurotransmitter release (40,117,118). Complexins also inhibit SNARE-mediated fusion of synthetic vesicles and cells expressing surface exposed SNAREs on their plasma membranes. Importantly, synaptotagmin•Ca^{2+} relieves this inhibition (119,120). Thus, an attractive hypothesis is that, in the absence of Ca^{2+}, complexins bind to and stabilize assembled SNARE complexes. Although this binding inhibits fusion (a "clamping" function), it also acts to prime vesicles by holding SNARE complexes in a more assembled conformation (a function that facilitates fusion) (40). According to this hypothesis, when Ca^{2+} enters the cell, it not only triggers synaptotagmin's penetration into the plasma membrane, it also triggers a synaptotagmin/SNARE interaction that displaces complexin. Together these three phenomena—membrane penetration by synaptotagmin, displacement of complexin, and full assembly of the SNARE complex—work together to trigger Ca^{2+}-dependent fusion. Consistent with complexin and synaptotagmin functioning together to mediate fusion, the phenotype of complexin knockouts is very similar to that of synaptotagmin knockouts, namely that Ca^{2+}-dependent synchronous release is specifically disrupted (121).

Why Two C_2 Domains?

Why does synaptotagmin contain two C_2 domains? The C_2B domain seems to play a more critical role in synaptotagmin function than the C_2A domain. Mutations in the Ca^{2+}-binding residues, phospholipid-interacting residues, and polylysine motif in the C_2B domain of synaptotagmin disrupt exocytosis more severely than analogous mutations in the C_2A domain (5,7,8,18,22,45,46,62,64,76,78,122,123). Furthermore, two *in vitro* abilities of synaptotagmin thought to be important for fusion *in vivo*, namely, the ability to induce membrane curvature and the ability to displace complexin from SNARE complexes, are more severely disrupted by mutations in the C_2B domain than by mutations in the C_2A domain (77,93).

What, then, is the role of the C_2A domain? One possibility is to assist the C_2B domain in its critical function(s). Several observations support this: (1) The Ca^{2+}-dependent, electrostatic interactions between isolated C_2B domains and membranes are disrupted by increasing ionic strength, but these interactions become more resistant to changes in ionic strength when C_2B is tethered to a C_2A domain (66). (2) The C_2B domain must be tethered to a C_2A domain to induce positive membrane curvature (77). (3) Both C_2 domains penetrate deeper into phospholipid membranes when they are tethered together than either in isolation (67). Thus, although the C_2B domain is more critical for synaptotagmin function, the presence of the C_2A domain is required for full function. Interestingly, although the two C_2 domains are homologous to each other, they are not able to substitute for one another; stimulation of SNARE-mediated fusion of synthetic vesicles by soluble synaptotagmin• Ca^{2+} is abolished if synaptotagmin consists of two C_2A domains tethered to each other (77).

Other Roles of Synaptotagmin

Synaptotagmin 1 is critical for Ca^{2+}-dependent, synchronous neurotransmitter release. The Ca^{2+}-sensing role of synaptotagmin is predominantly mediated by Ca^{2+} binding to its C_2B domain rather than to its C_2A domain. Once Ca^{2+} is bound, synaptotagmin likely interacts with the plasma membrane and SNARE complexes, facilitating vesicle fusion and neurotransmitter release. However, the ability of synaptotagmin to catalyze Ca^{2+}-dependent, fast, synchronous release may involve interactions between synaptotagmin and presynaptic molecules before the entry of Ca^{2+} into the nerve terminal. These molecular interactions may dock synaptic vesicles at release sites, or subsequently prime synaptic vesicles thereby increasing the speed with which synaptic vesicles can fuse upon Ca^{2+} influx (61,64,124).

Synaptic Vesicle Docking

Neurotransmitter release occurs preferentially at active zones, where synaptic vesicles are clustered (see Chapter 1). The subset of vesicles within this cluster that are located in direct contact with the presynaptic plasma membrane are referred to as docked vesicles. Although the identities of the molecules that mediate docking are currently under investigation, synaptotagmin 1 is likely to play a role. At rest, there is a severe decrease in the number of morphologically docked vesicles in synaptotagmin 1 knockouts (125,126). While the overall synaptic vesicle population was also decreased (~50% of controls), the docked vesicle population was most severely affected (~25% of controls) (125).

In functional studies, SNARE-mediated fusion of synthetic vesicles is accelerated in the *absence* of Ca^{2+} when synaptotagmin is incorporated into the VAMP/synaptobrevin containing vesicles (75,76). This acceleration of fusion may be due to a Ca^{2+}-independent increase in vesicle docking by synaptotagmin. A Ca^{2+}-independent docking ability of synaptotagmin may be mediated by its C_2B polylysine motif, which interacts with t-SNARE complexes or PtdIns(4,5)P2-containing membranes in a Ca^{2+}-independent manner (33,61). As PtdIns(4,5)P2 is located predominantly in the plasma membrane (127,128), where t-SNAREs are also located, the Ca^{2+}-independent interaction between synaptotagmin and PtdIns(4,5)P2 or t-SNARE complexes has been proposed to mediate synaptic vesicle docking (76,82). Indeed, polylysine motif mutations abolish this ability of synaptotagmin to accelerate Ca^{2+}-independent, SNARE-mediated fusion (76). Polylysine motif mutations also decrease vesicular release probability, slow the repopulation of the readily releasable pool after its depletion by high frequency stimulation, and decrease the rate of Ca^{2+}-dependent penetration of synaptotagmin into lipid membranes (61,64,76,82,122). A docking defect could readily explain these deficits.

In addition, a Ca^{2+}-independent docking ability of synaptotagmin may be mediated by a highly conserved WHXL motif in synaptotagmin's C-terminus (129). The WHXL motif has been shown to mediate an interaction between synaptotagmin's cytosolic domain and the plasma membrane in PC12 cells. Injection of a peptide containing the WHXL sequence into squid giant terminals blocked synaptic transmission and decreased morphologically docked vesicles (129).

Synaptic Vesicle Priming

The defects observed in the C_2B polylysine motif mutants (described above) could also be explained by a disruption in synaptic vesicle priming (rather than synaptic vesicle docking). Synaptic vesicle priming likely consists of multiple molecular interactions that transform vesicles from a docked but not releasable state, through multiple releasable states with differing release properties (130). The Ca^{2+}-independent interaction of the C_2B polylysine motif of synaptotagmin with PtdIns(4,5)P2 or t-SNARE complexes may prime vesicles for Ca^{2+}-triggered fusion by positioning the C_2B Ca^{2+}-binding pocket near the negatively charged phospholipids of the presynaptic membrane (Fig. 6.7). Upon Ca^{2+} influx, these lipids would be immediately at hand to complete the coordination sphere of calcium, thereby effectively increasing the affinity of synapto-

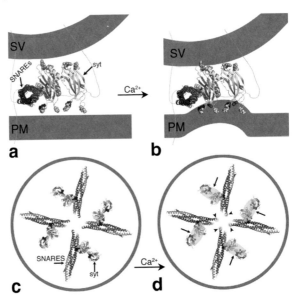

Fig. 6.7 Model of synaptotagmin function. (A,B) Side view of synaptic vesicle (SV) and presynaptic membrane (PM) before (A) and after (B) Ca^{2+} entry into the terminal. (C,D) View from the synaptic cleft toward the presynaptic terminal showing a single synaptic vesicle (large gray circle) before (C) and after (D) Ca^{2+} entry into the terminal. An interaction between the polylysine motif of synaptotagmin's C_2B domain (space-filled residues of synaptotagmin abutting SNAREs) and SNAP-25 within the SNARE complex docks/primes synaptic vesicles at release sites (A). Four such synaptotagmin/SNARE complexes per vesicle (on average) may mediate this docking/priming function (C). Upon Ca^{2+} (spheres in B) binding, synaptotagmin interacts with the plasma membrane via acidic residues (dark gray space-filled residues in the PM in B) and hydrophobic residues (light gray space-filled residues in the PM in B) in each C_2 domain's Ca^{2+}-binding pocket. Insertion of the hydrophobic residues of synaptotagmin into the presynaptic membrane induces positive membrane curvature; synaptotagmin pulls the presynaptic membrane toward the vesicle (B). Thus the presynaptic membrane would be destabilized in multiple places by synaptotagmin (D, gray ovals indicated by arrows) in a ring around syntaxin's penetration of the presynaptic membrane (D, gray circles indicated by arrowheads) and VAMP/synaptobrevin's penetration of the vesicle membrane (not shown.)

tagmin for Ca^{2+} and increasing the probability of vesicle fusion. Consistent with this hypothesis, *in vitro* studies have shown that PtdIns(4,5)P2 increases the rate of synaptotagmin's Ca^{2+}-dependent penetration into lipid membranes (61), a step thought to be important for fusion.

Another possible way in which the interaction of synaptotagmin's C_2B polylysine motif with PtdIns(4,5)P2 or t-SNARE complexes could prime synaptic vesicles is by facilitating the formation of *trans*-SNARE complexes. By positioning syntaxin and SNAP-25 in the plasma membrane in close proximity to VAMP/synaptobrevin on the synaptic vesicle, synaptotagmin may increase the probability of *trans*-SNARE complex formation (33,116). Supporting this hypothesis, the fastest component of dense core granule fusion is selectively abolished in synaptotagmin knockouts (10). This fast component is hypothesized to represent fusion of vesicles whose *trans*-SNARE complexes exist in a "tight" conformation (see Chapter 3). These "tight" *trans*-SNARE complexes are postulated to form a semi-stable, hemifusion intermediate (81) from which full fusion would proceed most rapidly. Accordingly, synaptotagmin may facilitate the formation of "tight" *trans*-SNARE complexes, thereby speeding up membrane fusion.

Synaptic Vesicle Endocytosis

Synaptotagmin was first proposed to function in endocytosis when synaptotagmin 1 knockouts in *C. elegans* mutants showed impaired, but not eliminated, synaptic function (11). Consistent with an endocytic deficit, the nerve terminals in *C. elegans* and *Drosophila* synaptotagmin knockouts are severely depleted of synaptic vesicles (125,126,131). Furthermore, functional studies now demonstrate that synaptotagmin 1 is required for efficient synaptic vesicle endocytosis (94,132–137), and *in vitro* studies suggest that the C_2B domain of synaptotagmin may mediate this role (94,132–135). Specifically, synaptic vesicle endocytosis was originally thought to be mediated by the polylysine motif in the C_2B domain of synaptotagmin (138) via a Ca^{2+}-independent interaction with either AP-2, an endocytic clathrin adaptor protein (94,139–143), or PtdIns(4,5)P2 (61), which is also important during endocytosis. However, *in vivo* studies demonstrate that C_2B polylysine motif mutations in *Drosophila* do not slow synaptic vesicle endocytosis (76,144). Thus, the endocytic role played by synaptotagmin's C_2B domain is not via the polylysine motif. The conserved C_2B WHXL motif is a possible candidate for this role as this motif mediates internalization of synaptotagmin in PC12 cells (134).

What Determines the Apparent Ca^{2+} Cooperativity of Exocytosis?

During synaptic transmission, the amount of neurotransmitter released by nerve stimulation shows a steep, highly nonlinear dependence on extracellular Ca^{2+} (145,146) (see Chapter 4). If transmitter release is plotted as a function of extracellular Ca^{2+} on a double logarithmic plot, the slope (n) corresponds to the exponent of this power relationship. In 1967, Dodge and Rahamimof (145) showed at frog neuromuscular junctions that n is ~4 and concluded that the dependence of vesicle fusion on extracellular Ca^{2+} can be explained by assuming a cooperative action of ~4 Ca^{2+} ions on average. Subsequently, it was demonstrated that n is ~4 at the calyx of Held (147,148), and that n is ~3.5 at *Drosophila* neuromuscular junctions (15,20,149).

This high cooperativity of Ca^{2+} for triggering neurotransmitter release has led to a popular model of vesicle fusion in which the cooperativity arises from the binding of multiple (i.e., "n") Ca^{2+} ions to a single Ca^{2+} sensor. Indeed, the rate of secretion in goldfish retinal bipolar neurons can be modeled quite well by the cooperative binding of four calcium ions (150). At the calyx of Held, two studies have proposed a kinetic model that require the binding of 5 Ca^{2+} ions to the Ca^{2+} sensor in order to achieve an n of ~4 (147,148). In one of these models Ca^{2+}-binding to the sensor was cooperative (148) and in the other Ca^{2+}-binding to each site was assumed to be independent (147). Thus, it may be that the high cooperativity of Ca^{2+} in triggering neurotransmitter release is a measure of the number of binding sites on the Ca^{2+} sensor (7,146,151).

Alternatively, the high cooperativity of Ca^{2+} in triggering neurotransmitter release may arise from the cooperative action of multiple (i.e., "n") Ca^{2+}-activated molecular complexes in triggering each vesicle to fuse (Fig. 6.7C,D) (105). In this model, synaptotagmin 1 would be an important component of this molecular complex, providing the ability of the complex to be activated by Ca^{2+}. Multiple observations support this hypothesis: (1) Reducing the level of the SNARE proteins (either syntaxin 1A or VAMP/synaptobrevin) at intact synapses reduces the Ca^{2+} cooperativity of neurotransmitter release (149). (2) Knocking out complexin, which should neither bind Ca^{2+} itself nor alter Ca^{2+} binding to synaptotagmin, but instead should affect the SNARE complexes, also alters the Ca^{2+} characteristics of exocytosis (121). (3) A mutation in SNAP-25 that severely impairs SNARE complex assembly, but does not affect synaptotagmin's ability to bind to SNAREs, decreases the apparent Ca^{2+}-cooperativity of release as well (105). These results all demonstrate that the SNARE complex is also a component of the molecular complex that contributes to the apparent Ca^{2+} cooperativity of release. Thus, the apparent Ca^{2+}-cooperativity of release is not simply determined by the number of Ca^{2+} ions that can bind to synaptotagmin or even synaptotagmin's ability to bind to the SNARE complex. It may be that the high cooperativity of Ca^{2+} in triggering exocytosis depends on the mean number of SNARE complexes that mediate a vesicle fusion event when Ca^{2+} influx triggers synaptotagmin to activate the fusion reaction. Also, SNARE proteins have the intrinsic ability to oligomerize. Negative stain electron microscopy demonstrated that the quaternary structure of these oligomers was star-shaped with three to four "legs" emanating from the center; each leg was approximately the same size as an individual SNARE complex (152). As the average number of "legs" emanating from the oligomerized particle corresponds well with the Ca^{2+} cooperativity of neurotransmitter release, these results support the hypothesis that the high cooperativity of Ca^{2+} in triggering neurotransmitter release results from fusion events mediated by the cooperative action of three to four (on average) SNARE complexes, each triggered by an associated Ca^{2+}-bound synaptotagmin molecule (153).

Model of Synaptotagmin Function in the Synaptic Vesicle Cycle

Synaptotagmin appears to play multiple roles in the synaptic vesicle cycle, and the exact nature of these roles is an area of intensive research. We favor the following model of synaptotagmin function, although alternative models also exist: Synaptotagmin docks or primes synaptic vesicles at release sites through a Ca^{2+}-independent interaction with SNARE complexes (Fig. 6.7A,C). This Ca^{2+}-independent interaction, which has been mapped to synaptotagmin's C_2B polylysine motif (Fig. 6.7A,C, space-filled residues of synaptotagmin abutting SNAREs), positions synaptotagmin's Ca^{2+}-binding pockets immediately adjacent to the plasma membrane so that they can more rapidly interact with this membrane when Ca^{2+} binding neutralizes the repulsive force of these negatively charged components. Thus, by increasing the rate of fusion upon Ca^{2+} influx, this Ca^{2+}-independent interaction serves a priming function. An additional priming interaction is mediated by complexin (not shown). By stabilizing tight *trans*-SNARE complexes, complexin both prevents fusion, and ensures that formation of the fully zippered SNARE complex proceeds rapidly when complexin is displaced. Upon Ca^{2+} influx, Ca^{2+} binding to synaptotagmin both strengthens its interaction with the SNARE complex, thereby displacing complexin, and rapidly triggers synaptotagmin's interaction with the negatively charged plasma membrane (Fig. 6.7B,D). Membrane penetration by the hydrophobic residues (Fig. 6.7B) found in synaptotagmin's Ca^{2+}-binding pockets, coupled with the complete assembly of the SNARE complex in response to complexin displacement, results in fusion of the vesicle with the presynaptic membrane.

References

1. Südhof TC. Synaptotagmins: why so many? J Biol Chem 2002;277(10):7629–7632.
2. Adolfsen B, Saraswati S, Yoshihara M, Littleton JT. Synaptotagmins are trafficked to distinct subcellular domains including the postsynaptic compartment. J Cell Biol 2004;166(2):249–260.
3. Dai H, Shin OH, Machius M, Tomchick DR, Südhof TC, Rizo J. Structural basis for the evolutionary inactivation of Ca2+ binding to synaptotagmin 4. Nat Struct Mol Biol 2004;11(9):844–849.
4. Geppert M, Goda Y, Hammer RE, et al. Synaptotagmin I: a major Ca2+ sensor for transmitter release at a central synapse. Cell 1994;79(4):717–727.
5. Nishiki T, Augustine GJ. Dual roles of the C2B domain of synaptotagmin I in synchronizing Ca2+-dependent neurotransmitter release. J Neurosci 2004;24(39):8542–8550.
6. Nishiki T, Augustine GJ. Synaptotagmin I synchronizes transmitter release in mouse hippocampal neurons. J Neurosci 2004;24(27):6127–6132.
7. Stevens CF, Sullivan JM. The synaptotagmin C2A domain is part of the calcium sensor controlling fast synaptic transmission. Neuron 2003;39(2):299–308.
8. Fernández-Chacón R, Königstorfer A, Gerber SH, et al. Synaptotagmin I functions as a calcium regulator of release probability. Nature 2001;410(6824):41–49.
9. Shin OH, Rhee JS, Tang J, Sugita S, Rosenmund C, Südhof TC. Sr2+ binding to the Ca2+ binding site of the synaptotagmin 1 C2B domain triggers fast exocytosis without stimulating SNARE interactions. Neuron 2003;37(1):99–108.

10. Voets T, Moser T, Lund PE, et al. Intracellular calcium dependence of large dense-core vesicle exocytosis in the absence of synaptotagmin I. Proc Natl Acad Sci U S A 2001;98 (20):11680–11685.
11. Nonet ML, Grundahl K, Meyer BJ, Rand JB. Synaptic function is impaired but not eliminated in C. elegans mutants lacking synaptotagmin. Cell 1993;73(7):1291–1305.
12. DiAntonio A, Parfitt KD, Schwarz TL. Synaptic transmission persists in synaptotagmin mutants of Drosophila. Cell 1993;73(7):1281–1290.
13. DiAntonio A, Schwarz TL. The effect on synaptic physiology of synaptotagmin mutations in Drosophila. Neuron 1994;12(4):909–920.
14. Littleton JT, Stern M, Schulze K, Perin M, Bellen HJ. Mutational analysis of Drosophila synaptotagmin demonstrates its essential role in Ca(2+)-activated neurotransmitter release. Cell 1993;74(6):1125–1134.
15. Littleton JT, Stern M, Perin M, Bellen HJ. Calcium dependence of neurotransmitter release and rate of spontaneous vesicle fusions are altered in Drosophila synaptotagmin mutants. Proc Natl Acad Sci U S A 1994;91(23):10888–10892.
16. Broadie K, Bellen HJ, DiAntonio A, Littleton JT, Schwarz TL. Absence of synaptotagmin disrupts excitation-secretion coupling during synaptic transmission. Proc Natl Acad Sci U S A 1994;91(22):10727–10731.
17. Loewen CA, Mackler JM, Reist NE. Drosophila synaptotagmin I null mutants survive to early adulthood. Genesis 2001;31(1):30–36.
18. Mackler JM, Drummond JA, Loewen CA, Robinson IM, Reist NE. The C2B Ca2+-binding motif of synaptotagmin is required for synaptic transmission in vivo. Nature 2002;418(6895):340–344.
19. Mackler JM, Reist NE. Mutations in the second C2 domain of synaptotagmin disrupt synaptic transmission at Drosophila neuromuscular junctions. J Comp Neurol 2001;436(1):4–16.
20. Yoshihara M, Littleton JT. Synaptotagmin I functions as a calcium sensor to synchronize neurotransmitter release. Neuron 2002;36(5):897–908.
21. Littleton JT, Barnard RJ, Titus SA, Slind J, Chapman ER, Ganetzky B. SNARE-complex disassembly by NSF follows synaptic-vesicle fusion. Proc Natl Acad Sci U S A 2001;98 (21):12233–12238.
22. Robinson IM, Ranjan R, Schwarz TL. Synaptotagmins I and IV promote transmitter release independently of Ca(2+) binding in the C(2)A domain. Nature 2002;418(6895):336–340.
23. Del Castillo J, Katz B. Local activity at a depolarized nerve-muscle junction. J Physiol 1954;128:396–411.
24. Matthew WD, Tsavaler L, Reichardt LF. Identification of a synaptic vesicle-specific membrane protein with a wide distribution in neuronal and neurosecretory tissue. J Cell Biol 1981;91(1):257–269.
25. Chapman ER, Jahn R. Calcium-dependent interaction of the cytoplasmic region of synaptotagmin with membranes. Autonomous function of a single C2–homologous domain. J Biol Chem 1994;269(8):5735–5741.
26. Takamori S, Holt M, Stenius K, et al. Molecular anatomy of a trafficking organelle. Cell 2006;127(4):831–846.
27. Perin MS, Brose N, Jahn R, Südhof TC. Domain structure of synaptotagmin (p65). J Biol Chem 1991;266(1):623–629.
28. Sutton RB, Davletov BA, Berghuis AM, Südhof TC, Sprang SR. Structure of the first C2 domain of synaptotagmin I: a novel Ca2+/phospholipid-binding fold. Cell 1995;80 (6):929–938.
29. Sutton RB, Ernst JA, Brunger AT. Crystal structure of the cytosolic C2A-C2B domains of synaptotagmin III. Implications for Ca(+2)-independent snare complex interaction. J Cell Biol 1999;147(3):589–598.
30. Ubach J, Zhang X, Shao X, Südhof TC, Rizo J. Ca2+ binding to synaptotagmin: how many Ca2+ ions bind to the tip of a C2–domain? EMBO J 1998;17(14):3921–3930.
31. Fernandez I, Araç D, Ubach J, et al. Three-dimensional structure of the synaptotagmin 1 C2B-domain: synaptotagmin 1 as a phospholipid binding machine. Neuron 2001;32(6): 1057–1069.

32. Shao X, Davletov BA, Sutton RB, Südhof TC, Rizo J. Bipartite Ca2+-binding motif in C2 domains of synaptotagmin and protein kinase C. Science 1996;273(5272):248–251.

33. Rickman C, Archer DA, Meunier FA, et al. Synaptotagmin interaction with the syntaxin/SNAP-25 dimer is mediated by an evolutionarily conserved motif and is sensitive to inositol hexakisphosphate. J Biol Chem 2004;279(13):12574–12579.

34. Goda Y, Stevens CF. Two components of transmitter release at a central synapse. Proc Natl Acad Sci U S A 1994;91(26):12942–12946.

35. Barrett EF, Stevens CF. The kinetics of transmitter release at the frog neuromuscular junction. J Physiol 1972;227(3):691–708.

36. Meiri U, Rahamimoff R. Activation of transmitter release by strontium and calcium ions at the neuromuscular junction. J Physiol 1971;215(3):709–726.

37. Miledi R, Orkand P. Effect of a "fast" nerve on "slow" muscle fibres in the frog. Nature 1966;209(5024):717–718.

38. Atluri PP, Regehr WG. Delayed release of neurotransmitter from cerebellar granule cells. J Neurosci 1998;18(20):8214–8227.

39. Maximov A, Südhof TC. Autonomous function of synaptotagmin 1 in triggering synchronous release independent of asynchronous release. Neuron 2005;48(4):547–554.

40. Tang J, Maximov A, Shin OH, Dai H, Rizo J, Südhof TC. A complexin/synaptotagmin 1 switch controls fast synaptic vesicle exocytosis. Cell 2006;126(6):1175–1187.

41. Ubach J, Lao Y, Fernandez I, Araç D, Südhof TC, Rizo J. The C2B domain of synaptotagmin I is a Ca2+-binding module. Biochemistry 2001;40(20):5854–5860.

42. Marek KW, Davis GW. Transgenically encoded protein photoinactivation (FlAsH-FALI): acute inactivation of synaptotagmin I. Neuron 2002;36(5):805–813.

43. Pang ZP, Sun J, Rizo J, Maximov A, Südhof TC. Genetic analysis of synaptotagmin 2 in spontaneous and Ca2+-triggered neurotransmitter release. EMBO J 2006;25(10):2039–2050.

44. Popov SV, Poo MM. Synaptotagmin: a calcium-sensitive inhibitor of exocytosis? Cell 1993;73(7):1247–1249.

45. Fernández-Chacón R, Shin OH, Königstorfer A, et al. Structure/function analysis of Ca2+ binding to the C2A domain of synaptotagmin 1. J Neurosci 2002;22(19):8438–8446.

46. Pang ZP, Shin OH, Meyer AC, Rosenmund C, Südhof TC. A gain-of-function mutation in synaptotagmin-1 reveals a critical role of Ca2+-dependent soluble N-ethylmaleimide-sensitive factor attachment protein receptor complex binding in synaptic exocytosis. J Neurosci 2006;26(48):12556–12565.

47. Shao X, Fernandez I, Südhof TC, Rizo J. Solution structures of the Ca2+-free and Ca2+-bound C2A domain of synaptotagmin I: does Ca2+ induce a conformational change? Biochemistry 1998;37(46):16106–16115.

48. Shao X, Li C, Fernandez I, Zhang X, Südhof TC, Rizo J. Synaptotagmin-syntaxin interaction: the C2 domain as a Ca2+-dependent electrostatic switch. Neuron 1997;18(1):133–142.

49. Zhang X, Rizo J, Südhof TC. Mechanism of phospholipid binding by the C2A-domain of synaptotagmin I. Biochemistry 1998;37(36):12395–123403.

50. Brose N, Petrenko AG, Südhof TC, Jahn R. Synaptotagmin: a calcium sensor on the synaptic vesicle surface. Science 1992;256(5059):1021–1025.

51. Rizo J, Südhof TC. C2-domains, structure and function of a universal Ca2+-binding domain. J Biol Chem 1998;273(26):15879–15882.

52. Earles CA, Bai J, Wang P, Chapman ER. The tandem C2 domains of synaptotagmin contain redundant Ca2+ binding sites that cooperate to engage t-SNAREs and trigger exocytosis. J Cell Biol 2001;154(6):1117–1123.

53. Li C, Davletov BA, Südhof TC. Distinct Ca2+ and Sr2+ binding properties of synaptotagmins. Definition of candidate Ca2+ sensors for the fast and slow components of neurotransmitter release. J Biol Chem 1995;270(42):24898–24902.

54. Davletov BA, Südhof TC. A single C2 domain from synaptotagmin I is sufficient for high affinity Ca2+/phospholipid binding. J Biol Chem 1993;268(35):26386–26390.

55. Chapman ER, Davis AF. Direct interaction of a Ca2+-binding loop of synaptotagmin with lipid bilayers. J Biol Chem 1998;273(22):13995–14001.

56. Chae YK, Abildgaard F, Chapman ER, Markley JL. Lipid binding ridge on loops 2 and 3 of the C2A domain of synaptotagmin I as revealed by NMR spectroscopy. J Biol Chem 1998;273 (40):25659–25663.

57. Davis AF, Bai J, Fasshauer D, Wolowick MJ, Lewis JL, Chapman ER. Kinetics of synapto-tagmin responses to Ca2+ and assembly with the core SNARE complex onto membranes. Neuron 1999;24(2):363–376.

58. Bai J, Earles CA, Lewis JL, Chapman ER. Membrane-embedded synaptotagmin penetrates cis or trans target membranes and clusters via a novel mechanism. J Biol Chem 2000;275(33):25427–25435.

59. Bai J, Wang P, Chapman ER. C2A activates a cryptic Ca(2+)-triggered membrane penetration activity within the C2B domain of synaptotagmin I. Proc Natl Acad Sci U S A 2002;99(3): 1665–1670.

60. Schiavo G, Gu QM, Prestwich GD, Söllner TH, Rothman JE. Calcium-dependent switching of the specificity of phosphoinositide binding to synaptotagmin. Proc Natl Acad Sci U S A 1996;93(23):13327–13332.

61. Bai J, Tucker WC, Chapman ER. PIP2 increases the speed of response of synaptotagmin and steers its membrane-penetration activity toward the plasma membrane. Nat Struct Mol Biol 2004;11(1):36–44.

62. Paddock BE, Reist NE. Ca2+-dependent, phospholipid-binding residues of synaptotagmin are critical for excitation-secretion coupling. Submitted.

63. Wang P, Wang CT, Bai J, Jackson MB, Chapman ER. Mutations in the effector binding loops in the C2A and C2B domains of synaptotagmin I disrupt exocytosis in a nonadditive manner. J Biol Chem 2003;278(47):47030–47037.

64. Li L, Shin OH, Rhee JS, et al. Phosphatidylinositol phosphates as co-activators of Ca2+ bind-ing to C2 domains of synaptotagmin 1. J Biol Chem 2006;281(23):15845–15852.

65. Gerber SH, Rizo J, Südhof TC. Role of electrostatic and hydrophobic interactions in Ca(2+)-dependent phospholipid binding by the C(2)A-domain from synaptotagmin I. Diabetes 2002;51:S12–18.

66. Hui E, Bai J, Chapman ER. Ca2+-triggered simultaneous membrane penetration of the tan-dem C2–domains of synaptotagmin I. Biophys J 2006;91(5):1767–1777.

67. Herrick DZ, Sterbling S, Rasch KA, Hinderliter A, Cafiso DS. Position of synaptotagmin I at the membrane interface: cooperative interactions of tandem C2 domains. Biochemistry 2006;45(32):9668–9674.

68. Rufener E, Frazier AA, Wieser CM, Hinderliter A, Cafiso DS. Membrane-bound orientation and position of the synaptotagmin C2B domain determined by site-directed spin labeling. Biochemistry 2005;44(1):18–28.

69. Rhee JS, Li LY, Shin OH, et al. Augmenting neurotransmitter release by enhancing the apparent Ca2+ affinity of synaptotagmin 1. Proc Natl Acad Sci U S A 2005;102(51): 18664–18669.

70. Weber T, Zemelman BV, McNew JA, et al. SNAREpins: minimal machinery for membrane fusion. Cell 1998;92(6):759–772.

71. Melia TJ, You D, Tareste DC, Rothman JE. Lipidic antagonists to SNARE-mediated fusion. J Biol Chem 2006;281(40):29597–29605.

72. Chen Y, Xu Y, Zhang F, Shin YK. Constitutive versus regulated SNARE assembly: a structural basis. EMBO J 2004;23(4):681–689.

73. Tucker WC, Weber T, Chapman ER. Reconstitution of Ca2+-regulated membrane fusion by synaptotagmin and SNAREs. Science 2004;304(5669):435–438.

74. Bhalla A, Tucker WC, Chapman ER. Synaptotagmin isoforms couple distinct ranges of Ca2+, Ba2+, and Sr2+ concentration to SNARE-mediated membrane fusion. Mol Biol Cell 2005;16(10):4755–4764.

75. Mahal LK, Sequeira SM, Gureasko JM, Sèollner TH. Calcium-independent stimulation of membrane fusion and SNAREpin formation by synaptotagmin I. J Cell Biol 2002;158(2):273–282.

76. Loewen CA, Lee SM, Shin YK, Reist NE. C2B polylysine motif of synaptotagmin facilitates a Ca2+-independent stage of synaptic vesicle priming in vivo. Mol Biol Cell 2006;17(12):5211–5226.
77. Martens S, Kozlov MM, McMahon HT. How synaptotagmin promotes membrane fusion. Science (New York, NY) 2007;316(5828):1205–1208.
78. Paddock BE, Reist NE. Unpublished observations.
79. Mackler JM, Reist NE. Unpublished observations.
80. Cevc G, Richardsen H. Lipid vesicles and membrane fusion. Adv Drug Deliv Rev 1999;38:207–232.
81. Jahn R, Lang T, Südhof TC. Membrane fusion. Cell 2003;112(4):519–533.
82. Schiavo G, Stenbeck G, Rothman JE, Sèollner TH. Binding of the synaptic vesicle v-SNARE, synaptotagmin, to the plasma membrane t-SNARE, SNAP-25, can explain docked vesicles at neurotoxin-treated synapses. Proc Natl Acad Sci U S A 1997;94(3):997–1001.
83. Li C, Ullrich B, Zhang JZ, Anderson RG, Brose N, Südhof TC. Ca(2+)-dependent and -independent activities of neural and non-neural synaptotagmins. Nature 1995;375(6532):594–599.
84. Chapman ER, Hanson PI, An S, Jahn R. Ca2+ regulates the interaction between synaptotagmin and syntaxin 1. J Biol Chem 1995;270(40):23667–23671.
85. Bai J, Wang CT, Richards DA, Jackson MB, Chapman ER. Fusion pore dynamics are regulated by synaptotagmin*t-SNARE interactions. Neuron 2004;41(6):929–942.
86. Kee Y, Scheller RH. Localization of synaptotagmin-binding domains on syntaxin. J Neurosci 1996;16(6):1975–1981.
87. Bennett MK, Calakos N, Scheller RH. Syntaxin: a synaptic protein implicated in docking of synaptic vesicles at presynaptic active zones. Science (New York, NY) 1992;257(5067):255–259.
88. Gerona RR, Larsen EC, Kowalchyk JA, Martin TF. The C terminus of SNAP25 is essential for Ca(2+)-dependent binding of synaptotagmin to SNARE complexes. J Biol Chem 2000;275(9):6328–6336.
89. Zhang X, Kim-Miller MJ, Fukuda M, Kowalchyk JA, Martin TF. Ca2+-dependent synaptotagmin binding to SNAP-25 is essential for Ca2+-triggered exocytosis. Neuron 2002;34(4):599–611.
90. Rickman C, Davletov B. Mechanism of calcium-independent synaptotagmin binding to target SNAREs. J Biol Chem 2003;278(8):5501–5504.
91. Tucker WC, Edwardson JM, Bai J, Kim HJ, Martin TF, Chapman ER. Identification of synaptotagmin effectors via acute inhibition of secretion from cracked PC12 cells. J Cell Biol 2003;162(2):199–209.
92. Bowen ME, Weninger K, Ernst J, Chu S, Brunger AT. Single-molecule studies of synaptotagmin and complexin binding to the SNARE complex. Biophys J 2005;89(1):690–702.
93. Dai H, Shen N, Araç D, Rizo J. A quaternary SNARE-synaptotagmin-Ca2+-phospholipid complex in neurotransmitter release. J Mol Biol 2007;367(3):848–863.
94. Littleton JT, Bai J, Vyas B, et al. synaptotagmin mutants reveal essential functions for the C2B domain in Ca2+-triggered fusion and recycling of synaptic vesicles in vivo. J Neurosci 2001;21(5):1421–1433.
95. Breidenbach MA, Brunger AT. New insights into clostridial neurotoxin-SNARE interactions. Trends Mol Med 2005;11(8):377–381.
96. Sakaba T, Stein A, Jahn R, Neher E. Distinct kinetic changes in neurotransmitter release after SNARE protein cleavage. Science (New York, NY) 2005;309(5733):491–494.
97. Capogna M, McKinney RA, O'Connor V, Gähwiler BH, Thompson SM. Ca2+ or Sr2+ partially rescues synaptic transmission in hippocampal cultures treated with botulinum toxin A and C, but not tetanus toxin. J Neurosci 1997;17(19):7190–7202.
98. Lawrence GW, Foran P, Dolly JO. Distinct exocytotic responses of intact and permeabilised chromaffin cells after cleavage of the 25–kDa synaptosomal-associated protein (SNAP-25) or synaptobrevin by botulinum toxin A or B. Eur J Biochem/FEBS 1996;236(3):877–886.
99. Washbourne P, Thompson PM, Carta M, et al. Genetic ablation of the t-SNARE SNAP-25 distinguishes mechanisms of neuroexocytosis. Nature Neurosci 2002;5(1):19–26.

100. Schoch S, Deák F, Königstorfer A, et al. SNARE function analyzed in synaptobrevin/VAMP knockout mice. Science (New York, NY) 2001;294(5544):1117–1122.
101. Deitcher DL, Ueda A, Stewart BA, Burgess RW, Kidokoro Y, Schwarz TL. Distinct requirements for evoked and spontaneous release of neurotransmitter are revealed by mutations in the Drosophila gene neuronal-synaptobrevin. J Neurosci 1998;18(6):2028–2039.
102. Broadie K, Prokop A, Bellen HJ, O'Kane CJ, Schulze KL, Sweeney ST. Syntaxin and synaptobrevin function downstream of vesicle docking in Drosophila. Neuron 1995;15(3):663–673.
103. Yoshihara M, Ueda A, Zhang D, Deitcher DL, Schwarz TL, Kidokoro Y. Selective effects of neuronal-synaptobrevin mutations on transmitter release evoked by sustained versus transient Ca2+ increases and by cAMP. J Neurosci 1999;19(7):2432–2441.
104. Sørensen JB, Matti U, Wei SH, et al. The SNARE protein SNAP-25 is linked to fast calcium triggering of exocytosis. Proc Natl Acad Sci U S A 2002;99(3):1627–1632.
105. Chen X, Tang J, Südhof TC, Rizo J. Are neuronal SNARE proteins Ca2+ sensors? J Mol Biol 2005;347(1):145–158.
106. Chen YA, Scales SJ, Patel SM, Doung YC, Scheller RH. SNARE complex formation is triggered by Ca2+ and drives membrane fusion. Cell 1999;97(2):165–174.
107. Desai RC, Vyas B, Earles CA, et al. The C2B domain of synaptotagmin is a Ca(2+)-sensing module essential for exocytosis. J Cell Biol 2000;150(5):1125–1136.
108. Bhalla A, Chicka MC, Tucker WC, Chapman ER. Ca(2+)-synaptotagmin directly regulates t-SNARE function during reconstituted membrane fusion. Nat Struct Mol Biol 2006;13(4):323–330.
109. Chieregatti E, Chicka MC, Chapman ER, Baldini G. SNAP-23 functions in docking/fusion of granules at low Ca2+. Mol Biol Cell 2004;15(4):1918–1930.
110. Chieregatti E, Witkin JW, Baldini G. SNAP-25 and synaptotagmin 1 function in Ca2+-dependent reversible docking of granules to the plasma membrane. Traffic 2002;3(7):496–511.
111. Ishizuka T, Saisu H, Odani S, Abe T. Synaphin: a protein associated with the docking/fusion complex in presynaptic terminals. Biochem Biophys Res Commun 1995;213(3):1107–1114.
112. McMahon HT, Missler M, Li C, Südhof TC. Complexins: cytosolic proteins that regulate SNAP receptor function. Cell 1995;83(1):111–119.
113. Pabst S, Margittai M, Vainius D, Langen R, Jahn R, Fasshauer D. Rapid and selective binding to the synaptic SNARE complex suggests a modulatory role of complexins in neuroexocytosis. J Biol Chem 2002;277(10):7838–7848.
114. Pabst S, Hazzard JW, Antonin W, et al. Selective interaction of complexin with the neuronal SNARE complex. Determination of the binding regions. J Biol Chem 2000;275(26):19808–19818.
115. Chen X, Tomchick DR, Kovrigin E, et al. Three-dimensional structure of the complexin/SNARE complex. Neuron 2002;33(3):397–409.
116. Hu K, Carroll J, Rickman C, Davletov B. Action of complexin on SNARE complex. J Biol Chem 2002;277(44):41652–41656.
117. Itakura M, Misawa H, Sekiguchi M, Takahashi S, Takahashi M. Transfection analysis of functional roles of complexin I and II in the exocytosis of two different types of secretory vesicles. Biochem Biophys Res Commun 1999;265(3):691–696.
118. Archer DA, Graham ME, Burgoyne RD. Complexin regulates the closure of the fusion pore during regulated vesicle exocytosis. J Biol Chem 2002;277(21):18249–18252.
119. Schaub JR, Lu X, Doneske B, Shin YK, McNew JA. Hemifusion arrest by complexin is relieved by Ca2+-synaptotagmin I. Nat Struct Mol Biol 2006;13(8):748–750.
120. Giraudo CG, Eng WS, Melia TJ, Rothman JE. A clamping mechanism involved in SNARE-dependent exocytosis. Science (New York, NY) 2006;313(5787):676–680.
121. Reim K, Mansour M, Varoqueaux F, et al. Complexins regulate a late step in Ca2+-dependent neurotransmitter release. Cell 2001;104(1):71–81.
122. Borden CR, Stevens CF, Sullivan JM, Zhu Y. Synaptotagmin mutants Y311N and K326/327A alter the calcium dependence of neurotransmission. Mol Cell Neurosci 2005;29(3):462–470.
123. Mace KE, Reist NE. Unpublished observations.

124. Lu X, Xu Y, Zhang F, Shin YK. Synaptotagmin I and Ca(2+) promote half fusion more than full fusion in SNARE-mediated bilayer fusion. FEBS Lett 2006;580(9):2238–2246.

125. Reist NE, Buchanan J, Li J, DiAntonio A, Buxton EM, Schwarz TL. Morphologically docked synaptic vesicles are reduced in synaptotagmin mutants of *Drosophila*. J Neurosci 1998;18(19):7662–7673.

126. Loewen CA, Royer SM, Reist NE. Drosophila synaptotagmin I null mutants show severe alterations in vesicle populations but calcium-binding motif mutants do not. J Comp Neurol 2006;496(1):1–12.

127. Holz RW, Hlubek MD, Sorensen SD, et al. A pleckstrin homology domain specific for phosphatidylinositol 4, 5–bisphosphate (PtdIns-4,5–P2) and fused to green fluorescent protein identifies plasma membrane PtdIns-4,5–P2 as being important in exocytosis. J Biol Chem 2000;275(23):17878–17885.

128. Micheva KD, Holz RW, Smith SJ. Regulation of presynaptic phosphatidylinositol 4,5–biphosphate by neuronal activity. J Cell Biol 2001;154(2):355–368.

129. Fukuda M, Moreira JE, Liu V, Sugimori M, Mikoshiba K, Llinás RR. Role of the conserved WHXL motif in the C terminus of synaptotagmin in synaptic vesicle docking. Proc Natl Acad Sci U S A 2000;97(26):14715–14719.

130. Martin TF. Tuning exocytosis for speed: fast and slow modes. Biochim Biophys Acta 2003;1641(2–3):157–165.

131. Jorgensen EM, Hartwieg E, Schuske K, Nonet ML, Jin Y, Horvitz HR. Defective recycling of synaptic vesicles in synaptotagmin mutants of Caenorhabditis elegans. Nature 1995;378(6553):196–199.

132. von Poser C, Zhang JZ, Mineo C, et al. Synaptotagmin regulation of coated pit assembly. J Biol Chem 2000;275(40):30916–30924.

133. Jarousse N, Kelly RB. The AP2 binding site of synaptotagmin 1 is not an internalization signal but a regulator of endocytosis. J Cell Biol 2001;154(4):857–866.

134. Jarousse N, Wilson JD, Arac D, Rizo J, Kelly RB. Endocytosis of synaptotagmin 1 is mediated by a novel, tryptophan-containing motif. Traffic (Copenhagen, Denmark) 2003;4(7):468–478.

135. Llinás RR, Sugimori M, Moran KA, Moreira JE, Fukuda M. Vesicular reuptake inhibition by a synaptotagmin I C2B domain antibody at the squid giant synapse. Proc Natl Acad Sci U S A 2004;101(51):17855–17860.

136. Poskanzer KE, Marek KW, Sweeney ST, Davis GW. Synaptotagmin I is necessary for compensatory synaptic vesicle endocytosis *in vivo*. Nature 2003;426(6966):559–563.

137. Nicholson-Tomishima K, Ryan TA. Kinetic efficiency of endocytosis at mammalian CNS synapses requires synaptotagmin I. Proc Natl Acad Sci U S A 2004;101(47):16648–16652.

138. Takei K, Haucke V. Clathrin-mediated endocytosis: membrane factors pull the trigger. Trends Cell Biol 2001;11(9):385–391.

139. Zhang JZ, Davletov BA, Südhof TC, Anderson RG. Synaptotagmin I is a high affinity receptor for clathrin AP-2: implications for membrane recycling. Cell 1994;78(5):751–760.

140. Chapman ER, Desai RC, Davis AF, Tornehl CK. Delineation of the oligomerization, AP-2 binding, and synprint binding region of the C2B domain of synaptotagmin. J Biol Chem 1998;273(49):32966–32972.

141. Haucke V, De Camilli P. AP-2 recruitment to synaptotagmin stimulated by tyrosine-based endocytic motifs. Science 1999;285(5431):1268–1271.

142. Haucke V, Wenk MR, Chapman ER, Farsad K, De Camilli P. Dual interaction of synaptotagmin with mu2– and alpha-adaptin facilitates clathrin-coated pit nucleation. EMBO J 2000;19(22):6011–6019.

143. Grass I, Thiel S, Höning S, Haucke V. Recognition of a basic AP-2 binding motif within the C2B domain of synaptotagmin is dependent on multimerization. J Biol Chem 2004;279(52):54872–54880.

144. Poskanzer KE, Fetter RD, Davis GW. Discrete residues in the c(2)b domain of synaptotagmin I independently specify endocytic rate and synaptic vesicle size. Neuron 2006;50(1):49–62.

145. Dodge FA Jr, Rahamimoff R. Co-operative action of calcium ions in transmitter release at the neuromuscular junction. J Physiol 1967;193(2):419–432.
146. Schneggenburger R, Neher E. Presynaptic calcium and control of vesicle fusion. Curr Opin Neurobiol 2005;15(3):266–274.
147. Bollmann JH, Sakmann B, Borst JG. Calcium sensitivity of glutamate release in a calyx-type terminal. Science 2000;289(5481):953–957.
148. Schneggenburger R, Neher E. Intracellular calcium dependence of transmitter release rates at a fast central synapse. Nature 2000;406(6798):889–893.
149. Stewart BA, Mohtashami M, Trimble WS, Boulianne GL. SNARE proteins contribute to calcium cooperativity of synaptic transmission. Proc Natl Acad Sci U S A 2000;97(25):13955–13960.
150. Heidelberger R, Heinemann C, Neher E, Matthews G. Calcium dependence of the rate of exocytosis in a synaptic terminal. Nature 1994;371(6497):513–515.
151. Tamura T, Hou J, Reist NE, Kidokoro Y. Nerve-evoked synchronous release and high K+ -induced quantal events are regulated separately by synaptotagmin I at Drosophila neuromuscular junctions. J Neurophysiol 2007;97(1):540–549.
152. Rickman C, Hu K, Carroll J, Davletov B. Self-assembly of SNARE fusion proteins into star-shaped oligomers. Biochem J 2005;388(Pt):75–79.
153. Hu K, Davletov B. SNAREs and control of synaptic release probabilities. FASEB J 2003;17(2):130–135.
154. DeLano WL. The PyMOL molecular graphics system. http://wwwpymolorg, 2002.

Chapter 7
Functional Interactions Among the SNARE Regulators UNC-13, Tomosyn, and UNC-18

Robby M. Weimer and Janet E. Richmond

Contents

Abstract Neurotransmitters are released from secretory vesicles following calcium-triggered fusion with the plasma membrane. These exocytotic events are driven by assembly of tertiary soluble N-ethylmaleimide–sensitive factor attachment receptor (SNARE) complexes among the vesicle SNARE, synaptobrevin, the plasma membrane-associated SNAREs, syntaxin, and synaptosome-associated protein of 25 kDa (SNAP-25). Proteins that effect SNARE complex assembly are thus important regulators of synaptic strength. This chapter reviews our current understanding of the roles

Janet E. Richmond
Biological Sciences Department, University of Illinois at Chicago, Chicago, IL 60607, USA
e-mail: jer@uic.edu

Z.-W. Wang (ed.) *Molecular Mechanisms of Neurotransmitter Release,*
© Humana Press 2008 a part of Springer Science+Business Media, LLC

played by three SNARE interacting proteins: UNC-13(Munc13), TOM-1(tomosyn) and UNC-18(Munc18). We discuss studies from both invertebrate and vertebrate model systems, highlighting recent advances, the current consensus on molecular mechanisms of action, and unresolved aspects of their function.

Keywords Tomosyn, Munc18, Munc13, exocytosis, priming, docking, SNARE complex, syntaxin, SNAP-25, synaptobrevin, synaptic transmission.

Neurotransmitter release from synaptic terminals is mediated by the fusion of neurotransmitter-filled vesicles with the plasma membrane (1, 2). Synaptic vesicle fusion is triggered by depolarization-induced calcium influx on a microsecond time scale (3). This rapidity suggests that a pool of synaptic vesicles is competent or primed to undergo membrane fusion immediately upon calcium entry. Vesicle priming and fusion require the function of members of the conserved soluble (SNARE) protein families (Fig. 7.1A) (4–8).

a SNAREs

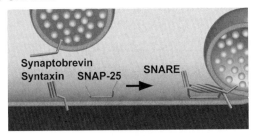

b Membrane-associated/'primed' synaptic vesicles

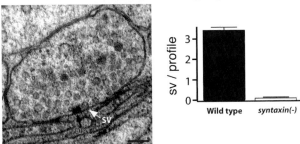

Fig. 7.1 Syntaxin changes its conformation from a "closed" to "open" state to mediate synaptic vesicle priming. (A) In solution, syntaxin adopts a default closed conformation. It must transit to an open conformation in order to from SNARE complexes with synaptobrevin and SNAP-25 to prime vesicles for release. (B) Synaptic vesicles (SV, white arrow) contact the plasma membrane near the dense projection (DP, black arrow) within active zones. Membrane contact requires the Q-SNARE syntaxin; therefore, membrane-contacting vesicles likely represent SNARE-dependent primed vesicles. (Data from Hammarlund et al [12].)

The SNAREs are small membrane-associated proteins that contain a conserved SNARE binding domain (9). Syntaxin and (SNAP-25) are plasma membrane-associated SNAREs (t-SNAREs or Q-SNAREs), whereas synaptobrevin is a vesicle membrane-associated SNARE (v-SNARE or R-SNARE). Single SNARE domains of syntaxin and synaptobrevin interact with two SNARE domains in SNAP-25 to form a parallel four alpha-helical bundle termed the SNARE complex. The SNARE complex assembly in *trans* is predicted to bring the vesicle membrane into close apposition with the plasma membrane (6, 10, 11)—a prerequisite for membrane fusion. In fact, loss of syntaxin function results in a decrease in the number of synaptic vesicles contacting the plasma membrane near presynaptic dense projections (12), suggesting that this population of synaptic vesicles represents the morphologic equivalents of functionally primed vesicles (12, 13).

In solution, syntaxin adopts a default "closed" confirmation in which its N-terminus, containing the Habc alpha-helices, folds over and occludes its C-terminal SNARE domain, also referred to as the H3 domain (14). To prime vesicles for fusion, syntaxin must adopt an "open" configuration to expose its SNARE domain in order for SNARE complex assembly to proceed (Fig. 7.1A). Therefore, proteins that bind syntaxin may regulate vesicle priming by modulating SNARE interactions. UNC-18/Munc18 (15, 16), UNC-13/Munc13 (17, 18) and TOM-1/Tomosyn (19, 20) all bind syntaxin and are implicated in the regulation of synaptic vesicle priming. Here we review the evidence implicating these proteins in vesicle priming, discuss the interaction between these proteins and the SNAREs, and outline current models for how these proteins function in this critical process.

UNC-18/Munc18

Identification

UNC-18 was first implicated in the regulation of synaptic transmission as a result of forward genetic screens conducted by the Nobel Laureate Sydney Brenner (21). Based on the premise that mutations disrupting genes required for synaptic transmission would result in locomotory defects in the soil nematode, *Caenorhabditis elegans*, Brenner identified and named the 18th uncoordinated mutant isolated *unc-18*. Null mutations in the *unc-18* locus result in almost complete paralysis in *C. elegans*. UNC-18 is a ~67-kDa cytosolic protein (22), and is a member of a molecularly and structurally conserved protein family. Most organisms contain between four and seven UNC-18–related protein family members (yeast and *Drosophila* encoding four, *C. elegans* six, and mammals seven), all of which are thought to serve conserved functions in vesicle trafficking and fusion at different intracellular compartments, as reviewed by Toonen and Verhage (23). In yeast, Sec1p most closely resembles UNC-18 (24), whereas the mouse genome encodes for three UNC-18 homologues—Munc18-1/n-sec-1/rbsec1, Munc18-2, and Munc18c (23, 25)—leading to the general classification of this family as SM (Sec/

Munc18) proteins. In *Drosophila*, the homologue is Rop (26). UNC-18, Munc18-1, and Rop are all enriched in neurons, whereas Munc18-2 is largely expressed in epithelial cells and Munc18c is ubiquitous.

Structure

UNC-18/Munc18 proteins contain three domains within the broadly conserved Sec1 homology region, named domains 1 to 3 (Fig. 7.2A). The crystal structure of Munc18-1 reveals a horseshoe-shaped molecule with a central cavity ~15 Å wide (27), domains 1 and 3 providing many of the surface residues within the cavity region. Crystal structures solved for other SM family members, namely, squid Sec-1 (28), yeast Sly1p (29), and Munc18c (30), exhibit a similar horseshoe structure with conserved binding pockets, indicating that SM proteins have universally conserved structural features.

Function

Mutant analyses indicate that SM proteins acting at specific intracellular compartments have a conserved role in membrane fusion at their respective sites of action (23, 31–33). In the case of SM proteins acting at the synapse, disrupting SM function invariably leads to severe release defects as exemplified in *C. elegans unc-18* null mutants (Fig. 7.2B) (34). *Drosophila* Rop null mutants are embryonically lethal and exhibit morphologic defects precluding neuromuscular junction (NMJ) recordings; however, neurotransmission assessed through electroretinograms from temperature-sensitive Rop mutants is blocked at nonpermissive temperatures (26). Similarly, Munc18-1 mouse knockouts that are stillborn are devoid of all synaptic activity despite apparently normal synaptogenesis (35). Chromaffin cells derived from these Munc18-1 nulls also exhibit impaired release (36). In both chromaffin cells and *C. elegans* NMJs (Fig. 7.2C), these evoked release defects are attributed to a reduction in the readily releasable vesicle pool (34, 36, 37). Ultrastructural analysis reveals a corresponding reduction in morphologically docked vesicles at the plasma membrane in NMJs of *unc-18* mutants (34) (Fig. 7.2D) and Munc18-1 heterozygotes (37), as well as in Munc18-1 null chromaffin cells (36).

The SM proteins are one of several protein classes implicated in vesicle docking; however, the molecular events and functional consequences of the docking process are not clearly understood, in part because the definition of docking is based on variable morphologic criteria and differing imaging techniques (12, 13, 38, 39). It is also likely that docking measured by stationary analysis (i.e., fixed tissues) fails to capture the true complexity of vesicle docking events in real time (40). In the case of the Munc18-1–dependent docking defect observed by conventional EM, live cell imaging suggests this represents changes in several kinetically distinct vesicle docking states. Specifically, in wild-type cells vesicle docking can be described by three dwell

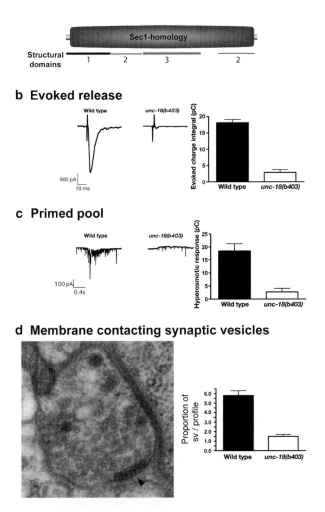

Fig. 7.2 The function of UNC-18/Munc18 in synaptic transmission. (A) UNC-18/Munc18 proteins are members of the larger Sec1/Munc18 (SM) family. The crystal structure predicts that the Sec1 homology region forms a horseshoe-shaped topography with a central cavity lined by domains 1 and 3. (B,C) *unc-18* mutants exhibit reduced evoked and hyperosmolarity-induced neurotransmitter release, suggesting that fewer vesicles are primed (recordings from *C. elegans* neuromuscular junction [NMJ]). (D) Consistent with a decrease in primed vesicles, fewer vesicles contact the plasma membrane at the NMJ in *unc-18* mutants than in wild type. Black arrowhead points to the dense-projection within the presynaptic terminal. (Adapted from Weimer et al [34].)

times: transiently visiting (present for <1 second), short-retained (present for 1 to 10 seconds), and long-retained (present for >10 seconds) based on total internal reflection fluorescence microscopy (TIRFM). The incidence of both visitors and long-retained vesicles is significantly reduced in Munc18-1 mutant chromaffin cells, which together account for the reduced number of docked vesicles observed by conventional EM (41). In the absence of Munc18-1, vesicle docking appears to be hindered by a thickening of the submembrane actin cytomatrix, as actin depolymerization by latrunculin restores morphologic docking in Munc18-1 mutant cells. However, docked vesicles in latrunculin-treated Munc18-1 mutants remain fusion incompetent and exhibit weaker tethering forces than wild-type docked vesicles, measured by autocorrelation analysis (41). This result suggests that strong vesicle tethering correlates with the primed state. Consistent with this notion, enhanced strongly tethered vesicles in chromaffin cells are observed under conditions that promote vesicle priming (40). Since clostridial toxin cleavage of syntaxin in chromaffin cells also reduces strong tethering of vesicles (41) and results in reduced morphologic docking (42), it appears likely that strongly tethered, docked vesicles represent the morphologic correlates of functionally primed vesicles (40, 41). Consistent with this conclusion the synapses of *C. elegans* priming-defective syntaxin and *unc-13* mutants prepared by high-pressure freeze fixation also exhibit a dramatic loss of docked vesicles (12, 13) contrary to previous reports using conventional chemical fixation (5, 43–46).

Together these observations indicate that Munc18-1 is required for at least two distinct processes: the first regulating the submembrane actin cytomatrix permitting vesicle delivery to the plasma membrane, a prerequisite for weak tethering; the second rendering vesicles strongly tethered and fusion-competent. The precise molecular mechanisms by which Munc18 regulates either step have yet to be fully elucidated, but the similarities in phenotypes of Munc18-1 and syntaxin mutants suggest that their ability to promote fusion-competence relies on interactions between these binding partners.

Interaction with Syntaxin

Although all SM proteins interact with their cognate syntaxin partners, there is considerable heterogeneity in binding modes that have thwarted efforts to identify a unifying mechanism of SM protein function (23, 32, 39). These modes include SM interactions with closed syntaxin (Fig. 7.3A), with an N-terminal syntaxin peptide (Fig. 7.3B), with t-SNARE dimers, and with assembled SNARE complexes (Fig. 7.3C). However, recent advancements are beginning to elucidate specific functions for some of these binding modes and hint at a conserved mechanism of SM action in promoting SNARE complex assembly and membrane fusion.

In part the difficulty in assigning a conserved function to SM proteins stems from the existence of a neuron-specific, high-affinity interaction between Munc18-1 and monomeric syntaxin 1a, in which the cavity formed by the Munc18-1 horseshoe envelopes syntaxin, locking it in a closed configuration incompatible with SNARE complex formation (14, 47). This binding mode is thus predicted to negatively regulate exocytosis, a hypothesis supported by impaired secretion observed upon overexpression of *Drosophila* Rop (48) and squid Sec1 (49) but contradicted by enhanced release observed upon Munc18-1 overexpression in chromaffin cells (36) and mammalian neurons (37). Heterologous expression studies suggest that Munc18-1–closed syntaxin complexes are

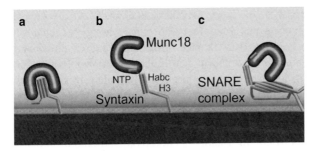

Fig. 7.3 The binding modes of SM proteins to syntaxin. Several configurations have been described for the binding of SM proteins to their corresponding syntaxin partner. These include SM interactions with closed syntaxin (A), with an N-terminal syntaxin peptide (B), and with assembled SNARE complexes (C). H3 denotes the H3 SNARE domain within syntaxin. NTP, N-terminal peptide

predominantly localized to intracellular compartments rather than the plasma membrane, leading to speculation that Munc18-1 binding to closed syntaxin may perform a chaperone function preventing nonspecific SNARE complex assembly on route to the plasma membrane or stabilizing syntaxin during transit (50). This latter possibility is supported by observed reductions in syntaxin levels in Munc18-1 and UNC-18 null mutants (34, 35). The Munc-18–closed syntaxin interaction may also be important for vesicle docking, as mutated Munc18-1 with reduced affinity for closed syntaxin *in vitro* attenuates the rescue of vesicle docking in Munc18-1 null chromaffin cells (51). This docking defect may represent specific loss of weakly tethered vesicles (discussed earlier), as vesicle priming is well supported by this mutated form of Munc18-1. Thus, binding of Munc18-1 to closed syntaxin appears to stimulate a vesicle-tethering step that is distinct from Munc18-1 involvement in the priming process (51). Munc18-2 can also support vesicle docking in Munc18-1 null mutants, but is less efficient in priming vesicles, likely because it is adapted to function with syntaxin-3. Interestingly, Munc18-2 overexpression is able to compete with wild-type levels of Munc18-1 for binding to closed syntaxin, inhibiting progression to the priming step (51). This experiment implies that there are two sequential binding modes between Munc18-1 and syntaxin, a monomeric interaction between Munc18-1 and closed syntaxin required for tethering and a subsequent interacting mode that renders vesicles primed.

A recently described binding mode between Munc18-1 and the N-terminus of open syntaxin 1a may serve this priming function (50). This N-peptide binding mode is a feature of many SM-syntaxin binding partners (29, 30, 52, 53), requiring a conserved short peptide sequence at the syntaxin N-terminus that fits into a conserved hydrophobic pocket on the external side of the SM horseshoe structure in domain 1 (29, 30). Heterologous expression studies suggest that Munc18-1–syntaxin N-peptide binding occurs preferentially at the plasma membrane and appears to be important in promoting SNARE complex assembly once syntaxin has adopted the open conformation (50). Specifically open syntaxin–Munc18-1 dimers readily form complexes with SNAP-25 either alone or with synaptobrevin, whereas open syntaxin lacking the N-peptide is unable to bind Munc18-1 *in vitro* and fails to assemble SNARE complexes (50). These observations indicate that Munc18-1 can remain associated with syntaxin during sequential stages of SNARE complex formation. However, on native plasma membranes, recombinant synaptobrevin can displace Munc18-1 from syntaxin–SNAP-25 dimers, leading to the suggestion that Munc18-1 may promote SNARE complex assembly by generating a syntaxin–SNAP-25 acceptor complex for synaptobrevin (54). *In vitro* liposome fusion assays similarly indicate that Munc18-1 facilitates vesicle fusion by promoting SNARE complex assembly via a syntaxin N-peptide interaction. Furthermore, the ability of Munc18-1 to promote liposome fusion is successful only when cognate SNAREs are present (55). This suggests that one of the functions of Munc18-1 and by extension other SM proteins in promoting fusion is to ensure the specificity of the SNARE assembly reaction at each trafficking compartment.

While current models suggest that the SM-syntaxin N-peptide binding mode plays a critical role in generating fusion competent vesicles, additional interactions between Munc18-1 and the SNARE complex also appear to be important for this function. Specifically, the N-peptide region of syntaxin alone does not stably bind to Munc18-1, and evidence suggests the SNARE domains of syntaxin, synaptobrevin, and SNAP-25 that constitute the SNARE complex bundle provide additional functionally important binding sites for Munc18-1 (56).

In summary, recent observations position Munc18-1 in two distinct and sequential steps of the vesicle cycle. The first specialized interaction with closed syntaxin may be important in trafficking of vesicles to the plasma membrane, the second stabilizing SNARE complex assembly via multiple interactions between Munc18-1 and open syntaxin as well as the other SNARE complex components (50, 55, 56). The SM-SNARE complex binding mode has now been established for SMs involved in various cellular trafficking events, including regulated exocytosis (Munc18-1), constitutive secretion (Sec1p), endocytosis (Vps45), and endoplasmic reticulum (ER) to Golgi trafficking (Sly1p), suggesting this interaction underlies a conserved vesicle trafficking function (57–61).

UNC-13/Munc13

Identification

Similar to UNC-18, UNC-13 was first identified in *C. elegans* via a forward genetic screen selecting for uncoordinated mutants, null mutants being essentially paralyzed (21). UNC-13 is a conserved protein encoded by a single gene with at least three splice variants in *C. elegans*. UNC-13 homologues are found only in organisms that have nervous systems. The *Drosophila* homologue Dunc13 is encoded by a single locus that gives rise to three isoforms (62; also go to FlyBase.org), whereas mice encode four homologous genes, Munc13-1, -2, -3, and -4, which may also exhibit alternative splicing (63, 64). UNC-13 (65) and Dunc13 (66) are expressed primarily in neurons, and Munc13-1, -2, and -3 exhibit tissue and temporal expression specificity (63, 67–70) whereas Munc13-4 is ubiquitously expressed.

Structure

UNC-13/Munc13 proteins are large (1500 to 2000 amino acids) multidomain proteins. In general, UNC-13/Munc13 isoforms are grouped into two classes, long (L) and short (S), based on the presence or absence of an extended amino terminus (Fig. 7.4A). All UNC-13/Munc13 isoforms contain a C1 domain, two C2 domains, and two Munc homology domains (MHDs). Most contain an N-terminal extension that has a third C2 domain, a Rim interacting domain (RID) and a calmodulin binding domain (CBD).

Function

Mutational perturbation of UNC-13 and its homologues results in very similar synaptic transmission defects: a nearly complete block of neurotransmitter release from presynaptic nerve terminals (45, 66, 68, 70, 71). In all mutants examined to date, the severe reduction in evoked neurotransmitter release (Fig. 7.4B) is associated with loss of the readily releasable vesicle pool (Fig. 7.4C), suggesting that UNC-13/Munc13 is required for vesicle priming. Consistent with this notion, overexpression of Munc13-1 in chromaffin cells results in an increase in the pool of readily releasable dense-core vesicles (72).

At synapses, UNC-13/Munc13 localizes near electron-dense presynaptic specializations (13) termed dense projections, which are thought to be presynaptic organizers containing many of the proteins required for neurotransmitter release, such as voltage-gated calcium channels, liprin, bassoon, piccolo, CAST, and Rim (73). UNC-13/Munc13 localization to sites near dense projections may ensure vesicle priming occurs at appropriate sites near calcium channels (13). Consistent with this notion, ultrastructural analyses of synapses fixed by high-pressure freezing show loss of plasma membrane contacting vesicles within 150 nm of the dense projection in *unc-13* mutants (12,13,20) (Fig. 7.4D). This is the same contacting vesicle pool that is abolished in syntaxin mutant synapses (12), suggesting that these vesicles represent both UNC-13–dependent and syntaxin-dependent primed vesicles. TIRFM analyses of chromaffin cells with enhanced Munc13-dependent vesicle priming show a corresponding increase in docked vesicles with restricted mobility, which likely reflects the behavior of primed vesicles in live images (40).

Interaction with Syntaxin

To define the region of UNC-13/Munc13 required for vesicle priming, attempts to identify a minimal UNC-13/Munc13 rescuing fragment have been conducted. Using this approach, a large fragment of Munc13-1, spanning virtually the entire region between C_2B and C_2C (amino acids 859 to 1531) encompassing both MHDs, was found to rescue synaptic transmission in cultured hippocampal neurons derived from Munc13-1/2 double knockout mice (74). The partial rescue of evoked release

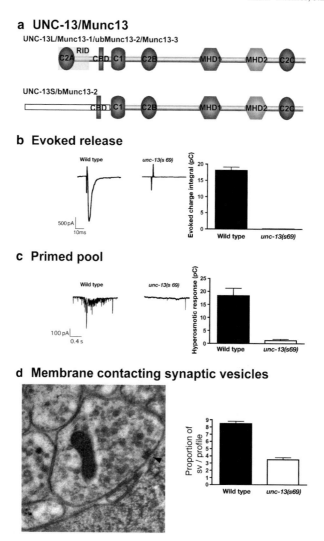

Fig. 7.4 The function of UNC-13/Munc13 in synaptic transmission. (A) UNC-13 and its homologues contain several functional domains, including C2 domains (C2A, C2B, and C2C), a rim-binding domain (RBD), a calmodulin-binding domain (CBD), a C1 domain (C1), and Munc-13 homology domains (MHD1 and MHD2). Munc13–2 has two splice variants, brain specific (bMunc13–2) and ubiquitous (ubMunc-13–2). (B,C) Loss of UNC-13 function nearly abolishes evoked neurotransmitter release and is accompanied by a loss of readily releasable (primed) synaptic vesicles as assayed by hyperosmotic stimulation. (D) At the ultrastructural level, few synaptic vesicles contact the plasma membrane in *unc-13* mutants. Black arrowhead indicates the dense-projection within the presynaptic terminal. (Adapted from Weimer et al [13].)

at excitatory synapses produced by this fragment was due to ~50% recovery of the fusion competent vesicle pool.

In chromaffin cells, overexpression of full-length Munc13-1 can double the size of the primed pool of dense-core vesicles. To elevate dense-core vesicle priming, a Munc13-1 fragment (amino acids 1100 to 1735) spanning the MHDs and the third C2 domain is required (75). This suggests that for Munc13 to be fully functional in priming, a domain encompassing both MHDs and C2C is required. Consistent with this premise, rescue of *C. elegans unc-13* mutants requires a similar region of UNC-13 (amino acids 676 to 1420) including C2C as well as both MHDs (18).

A study using the C-terminal region of Munc13-1 (amino acids 1181 to 1736) as bait in a yeast two-hybrid screen identified syntaxin 1B as a binding partner (17). The clones isolated in this screen encoded the first two alpha-helices (Ha and Hb) of syntaxin, suggesting that UNC-13/Munc13's role in vesicle priming is through its interaction with the syntaxin N-terminus. Consistent with this hypothesis, point mutations that disrupt syntaxin binding in the Munc13-1 minimally rescuing fragment abolish Munc13-1 dependent dense-core vesicle priming (75). Similarly, mutations introduced into *C. elegans* UNC-13 MHD2 that disrupt syntaxin binding also reduce evoked neurotransmitter release (18). Together, these experiments indicate that UNC-13/Munc13 promotes synaptic vesicle exocytosis through its interaction with syntaxin.

The observed interaction between Munc13 and syntaxin led to the speculation that UNC-13/Munc13 may facilitate vesicle priming by promoting or stabilizing the open conformation of syntaxin to expose its SNARE domain (76). Mutation of two residues in the linker region between the Habc and SNARE domains of vertebrate syntaxin 1a (LE165/166AA) are known to destabilize the closed conformation, rendering the protein constitutively open (14). Expression of the corresponding mutant form of open syntaxin in *C. elegans* (syntaxin LE166/167AA) was found to partially bypass the requirement for UNC-13 in synaptic vesicles priming (12,77), suggesting that UNC-13/Munc13 may promote vesicle priming by opening syntaxin (Fig. 7.1A). It should be noted that evoked synaptic transmission and behavior are not fully rescued in these animals (77,78), suggesting UNC-13 may play additional roles in exocytosis (78,79).

TOM-1/Tomosyn

Identification

Tomosyn was first identified as a novel syntaxin binding partner in pull-down assays from rat brain cytosol, *tomo* being Japanese for friend and *tomosyn* meaning "friend of syntaxin" (19). This ~130-kDa cytosolic protein is a member of a larger protein family with homologues in *Drosophila* (CG17762/FBgn0030412), *C. elegans* (*tom-1*, also know as *tomo-1*), and mammals (tomosyn-1 and -2) (80). More divergent members include the yeast proteins Sro7p and Sro77p (81,82), the *Drosophila* tumor suppressor lethal giant larvae (l(2)gl) (83), and mammalian Mlgl (84) and amysin (85).

Structure

Tomosyn has a large conserved N-terminal domain with multiple WD40 repeats separated by a regulatory linker to a C-terminal coiled domain that resembles the SNARE motif of synaptobrevin (VAMP-2) (86,87) (Fig. 7.5A). The crystal structure of yeast Sro7p indicates that the WD40 repeats that are conserved among other tomosyn family members form two β-propellers. These protein-interacting domains form a skewed clam shell structure, joined by a hinge region (87).

Function

The first tomosyn mutant (*tom-1*) was isolated in C. *elegans* in a screen selecting for mutants exhibiting enhanced cholinergic signaling (88). Although behaviorally *tom-1* mutants appear relatively normal, synaptic recordings reveal a dramatic increase in the size and duration of evoked release leading to a larger evoked charge integral (20,78) (Fig. 7.5B). This enhanced secretion is attributable to a larger pool of primed synaptic vesicles based on hyperosmotic data (Fig. 7.5C) as well as ultrastructural analysis (Fig. 7.5D). A similar increase in secretion following tomosyn RNA interference (RNAi) has also been observed in pancreatic beta cells (89). These studies suggest that tomosyn acts as a negative regulator of secretion. Consistent with this interpretation, overexpression of tomosyn in a variety of endocrine cells (adipocytes, PC12, chromaffin, and beta cells) as well as neurons decreases vesicle fusion events (20, 89–93). However, contradictory results showing that tomosyn RNAi inhibits release in pancreatic beta cells (94), and cultured neurons (93) have also been reported, suggesting that tomosyn may exert a permissive effect under some conditions.

Interestingly, perturbations of tomosyn function in cultured neurons also produce changes in neurite outgrowth, which may alter the number of synapses formed in culture, possibly complicating the interpretation of functional changes in synaptic strength observed in culture (95). Tomosyn is proposed to regulate neurite outgrowth by selectively binding and inhibiting vesicle secretion in growth cone palms, leaving vesicle fusion only at the growth cone leading edge. Sro7p is also implicated in polarized vesicle fusion leading to growth at the bud tip preceding yeast cell division, through interactions with the Q-SNARE Sec-9p (82). Similarly, both l(2)gl and Mlgl are implicated in establishing cell polarity, interactions between Mlgl and syntaxin-4 suggesting that this role may involve regulation of basolateral exocytosis (84,96). The fact that several tomosyn family members have been implicated in the regulation of secretory pathways suggests that they may act through a conserved molecular mechanism possibly involving interactions with SNARE proteins.

a TOM-1/Tomosyn

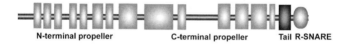

N-terminal propeller   C-terminal propeller   Tail R-SNARE

b Evoked synaptic release

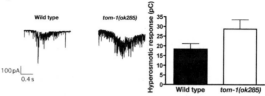

c Primed pool

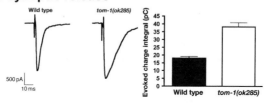

d Membrane contacting synaptic vesicles

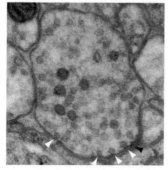
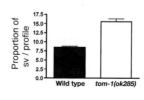

Fig. 7.5 Negative-regulation of synaptic transmission by TOM-1/tomosyn. (A) TOM-1/tomosyn contains 14 WD40 repeats, including seven closest to the amino-terminal forming one β-propeller and seven downstream forming the carboxy-terminal β-propeller. The protein also contains a putative auto inhibitory domain, referred to as Tail, and a SNARE motif. (B,C) Loss of TOM-1 function results in enhanced evoked neurotransmitter release due to an increase in the size of the primed pool of vesicles, as suggested by the prolonged evoked responses at the *C. elegans* NMJ and increased hyperosmotic responses. (D) The increase in primed vesicles in *tom-1* mutants correlates with an increase in the number of synaptic vesicles contacting the plasma membrane. Black arrowhead points to the dense projection within the presynaptic terminal, white arrows point to membrane contacting synaptic vesicles. (Adapted from Gracheva et al. [20].)

Interaction with Syntaxin

Tomosyn forms a tertiary complex with syntaxin and SNAP-25 that can also include synaptotagmin (19). The formation of this tomosyn SNARE complex requires the tomosyn C-terminal SNARE domain, which, like that of synaptobrevin, possesses an arginine residue (R) at the zero layer position (86). Experiments on PC12 membrane sheets show that the tomosyn SNARE domain competes with the synaptobrevin SNARE domain for syntaxin binding (90). Given the sequence similarity between the tomosyn and synaptobrevin SNARE domains, it is not surprising that the crystal structure of the recombinant tomosyn SNARE complex is virtually identical to that of the four-alpha-helical bundle formed by the synaptobrevin SNARE complex (90,97). There are subtle but likely important differences between the structures of these two core complexes. For example, tomosyn SNARE complexes do not bind tightly to complexin, a protein implicated in the regulation of exocytosis through interactions with the synaptobrevin SNARE complex (97,98). The formation of tomosyn SNARE complexes are not expected to bring vesicles into close apposition with the plasma membrane since tomosyn does not have a vesicle transmembrane domain. Thus tomosyn SNARE complexes are predicted to interfere with the formation of fusogenic SNARE complexes and therefore vesicle priming. In agreement with this model, overexpression of full-length tomosyn in chromaffin cells specifically reduces the fast phase of exocytosis that corresponds to the primed vesicle pool (92). Similarly the observed reduction of docked vesicles in TOM-1–overexpressing *C. elegans* synapses and the increase of membrane-associated/primed synaptic vesicles in *tom-1* deletion mutants are also consistent with a model in which tomosyn negatively regulates vesicle priming (20).

What remains to be established is the precise mechanism by which tomosyn inhibits vesicle priming. In this regard, it is interesting to note that overexpression of either amisyn or tomosyn carrying SNARE domain mutations that greatly diminish their syntaxin binding affinity retain their ability to inhibit release from PC12 cells (99). Furthermore, overexpression of tomosyn completely lacking the SNARE domain was recently shown to be as potent an inhibitor of dense core vesicle priming in PC12 cells as full-length tomosyn (100). These results suggest that the interaction of the tomosyn SNARE domain with syntaxin may be dispensable for the inhibitory function of this protein. It is also worth noting that several of the proteins that share homology to the large N-terminal of tomosyn do not have a conserved C-terminal SNARE domain, and yet still regulate secretion, possibly through other interactions with SNARE proteins. For example Mlgl, which lacks a C-terminal SNARE domain, binds specifically to syntaxin-4 and SNAP-23 (84). Similarly, Sro7, which also lacks a conserved C-terminal SNARE motif, binds to the yeast SNAP-25 homologue Sec9p via multiple interactions with its two N-terminal β-propellers (87). These considerations suggest that the molecular events underlying the inhibitory and perhaps also permissive regulatory roles of tomosyn in secretion likely involve additional domains other than the SNARE motif.

Interactions Among SNAREs, UNC-18/Munc18, UNC-13/Munc13, and TOM-1/Tomosyn

UNC-18–UNC-13 Interactions

The fact that *C. elegans unc-18* and *unc-13* mutants are similarly paralyzed with reduced evoked release and fewer docked/primed vesicles suggests that UNC-18 and UNC-13 act in the same pathway. The likelihood that these two proteins function in the same signaling cascade is further supported by their mutual interactions with the N-terminal of syntaxin (17). Furthermore, the observation that an UNC-13 protein fragment can interact directly with UNC-18 and displace UNC-18 from syntaxin *in vitro* suggests that the binding of UNC-18 and UNC-13 to syntaxin may be convergent or sequential events (16). The notion that Munc13 and Munc18 act in the same process is further supported by the recent observation that diacylglycerol (DAG)/phorbol ester–induced synaptic potentiation requires both activation of Munc13-1 and protein kinase C (PKC)-dependent phosphorylation of Munc18-1 (101). Specifically, binding of phorbol ester to the C1 domain of Munc13-1 potentiates release only if phorbol ester-mediated PKC-dependent phosphorylation of Munc18-1 precedes it (101,102).

Mechanistically it is still unclear what sequence of events underlies the actions of Munc13 and Munc18 in either basal or potentiated synaptic transmission. An essential role of UNC-13/Munc13 appears to be in promoting the availability of open syntaxin, possibly through a direct interaction with the syntaxin N-terminus (12, 18, 75, 77, 79). If this model is correct, at what point does UNC-18 become involved? Accumulating evidence indicates that all SM proteins may interact with assembled SNARE complexes, suggesting that this is the key event underlying their conserved permissive role. If so, UNC-18 binding to the SNARE complex must occur after UNC-13 renders the syntaxin SNARE domain accessible for SNARE complex assembly. Given that Munc18 binding to the N-terminal of syntaxin promotes SNARE assembly and vesicle fusion in *in vitro* fusion assays, Munc13 might have to relinquish or share its interaction with syntaxin to allow Munc18 function to proceed. Precisely how the interaction between Munc18-1 and the SNARE complex then promotes fusion has yet to be determined.

This hypothetical model does not adequately address the fact that Munc18-1 also binds to the closed conformation of syntaxin. One possibility is that the action of UNC-13/Munc13 in promoting the opening of syntaxin causes a conformational rearrangement that disrupts the high-affinity Munc18-1/syntaxin dimer, to allow syntaxin to unfold. The model above also fails to incorporate other roles of UNC-13/Munc13-1 in the regulation of exocytosis that are independent of the MHDs, such as vesicle targeting via Rim/Rab interactions (13, 103), synaptic potentiation via the C1 and CMB domains, as well as regulation involving interactions with DOC-2 and C2 domain activity. Similarly, this model does not address other roles for UNC-18/Munc18-1 in the transport or stabilization of syntaxin, vesicle delivery, and PKC-dependent synaptic potentiation. Both Munc13 and Munc18 are multidomain proteins capable of interacting with several other proteins, which may provide mechanisms to regulate their central roles in exocytosis to meet various physiologic demands.

UNC-13–TOM-1 Interactions

Whereas *C. elegans unc-13* mutants have severely impaired synaptic release due to a reduction in primed vesicles, *tom-1* mutants have enhanced release due to a larger primed vesicle pool (20, 78). These observations suggest that UNC-13 and TOM-1 have antagonistic actions in vesicle priming. This conclusion is further supported by observations that overexpression of membrane-bound UNC-13 electrophysiologically phenocopies the enhanced release of *tom-1* mutants (authors' unpublished results), and Munc13 overexpression enhances the priming of dense core vesicles (72), whereas tomosyn overexpression in *C. elegans* and several other cell types inhibits release by reducing the size of the primed vesicle pool (92). Furthermore, combining *tom-1* mutants with *unc-13* mutants partially restores the deficiencies in locomotion, synaptic transmission, and priming associated with *unc-13* mutants (20, 78).

Mechanistically, the negative-regulation of priming by tomosyn is thought to be the result of interactions with syntaxin and SNAP-25, interfering with the assembly of synaptobrevin-containing SNARE complexes. The precise nature of this inhibitory interaction remains to be elucidated. The leading hypothesis is that tomosyn inhibits secretion by forming complexes with syntaxin and SNAP-25 (90). Although the C-terminal SNARE domain of tomosyn binds to syntaxin, this domain may be dispensable for its inhibitory function, based on several recent studies demonstrating that tomosyn lacking the SNARE domain (or mutants that disrupt syntaxin-tomosyn SNARE domain binding) retains much of its ability to inhibit release (99, 100, 104). It seems likely, although not yet established, that an interaction between the tomosyn N-terminal and SNAP-25 may be important in this inhibitory mechanism, based on established interactions between the N-terminal β-propellers of yeast Sro7p and Sec9p (87).

What molecular model could explain the finding that *tom-1* mutants alleviate the *unc-13* priming defect? If UNC-13 promotes the open configuration of syntaxin to allow SNARE complex assembly, it is expected that the open conformation of syntaxin will also encounter and interact with tomosyn. Thus, SNARE complex formation in *unc-13* mutants may be hindered not only by a decreased probability of open syntaxin but also by the presence of tomosyn. Thus by eliminating tomosyn, the chance of SNARE complex formation might be marginally increased, explaining the observed increase in vesicle priming in *tom-1unc-13* double mutants. Consistent with this model, combining *tom-1unc-13* double mutants with a constitutively open form of syntaxin further improves the level of synaptic release (78).

While this model provides a plausible explanation for the basic antagonistic actions of UNC-13 and tomosyn, the ability of tomosyn to negatively regulate priming also appears to be subject to modulation by various kinases that change the affinity of tomosyn for syntaxin (93, 95, 105). In addition, tomosyn negatively regulates peptide secretion from dense core vesicles, a function that may indirectly modulate synaptic vesicle release through G-protein–mediated signaling cascades(106).

UNC-18–TOM-1 Interactions

In the initial characterization of tomosyn, Fujita *et al* (19) observed that tomosyn was capable of dissociating Munc18-1 from syntaxin. Recently, Gladycheva *et al* (105) observed a similar competition between Munc18 and tomosyn for syntaxin binding using fluorescence resonance energy transfer imaging. In these experiments, the interaction of Munc18-1 with syntaxin was shown to be important for the membrane trafficking of syntaxin, whereas that of tomosyn with syntaxin was not. However, tomosyn successfully competed with Munc18-1 for interactions with membrane-associated syntaxin, and formed tomosyn complexes with syntaxin and SNAP-25. These data are consistent with a model in which Munc18-1–syntaxin dimers facilitate the initial membrane localization of syntaxin, after which tomosyn successfully competes with Munc18 to establish tomosyn ternary SNARE complexes that are nonfusogenic. Thus Munc-18 and tomosyn might play antagonistic roles in vesicle priming based on observations that interactions between Munc18 and the assembled SNARE complex are essential for vesicle priming and fusion, whereas tomosyn negatively regulates priming. Analyses of genetic interactions between *C. elegans unc-18* and *tom-1* mutants may allow an independent verification of this model. Given the similar phenotypes of *unc-13* and *unc-18* mutants and the possible antagonistic roles of Munc-18 and tomosyn, we predict that *tom-1;unc-18* double mutants will exhibit a partial rescue of synaptic function compared with the *unc-18* single mutant, similar to that observed in *tom-1;unc-13* mutants.

Conclusion

The consensus of recent findings indicates that UNC-18/Munc18 and UNC-13/Munc13 act in concert to promote vesicle priming by promoting SNARE complex assembly. These events lead to the stable association of vesicles with the plasma membrane in a fusion competent state. Tomosyn, on the other hand, restricts priming through interactions with SNARE proteins. There are many details that remain to be elucidated regarding the temporal sequence, mechanics, and modulation of events conducted by these fascinating regulatory proteins in the execution of neurotransmission.

References

1. Ceccarelli B, Grohovaz F, Hurlbut WP. Freeze-fracture studies of frog neuromuscular junctions during intense release of neurotransmitter. II. Effects of electrical stimulation and high potassium. J Cell Biol 1979;81(1):178–192.
2. Heuser JE, Reese TS, Dennis MJ, Jan Y, Jan L, Evans L. Synaptic vesicle exocytosis captured by quick freezing and correlated with quantal transmitter release. J Cell Biol 1979;81(2):275–300.
3. Sabatini BL, Regehr WG. Timing of neurotransmission at fast synapses in the mammalian brain. Nature 1996;384(6605):170–172.
4. Sollner T, Whiteheart SW, Brunner M, et al. SNAP receptors implicated in vesicle targeting and fusion. Nature 1993;362(6418):318–324.
5. Broadie K, Prokop A, Bellen HJ, O'Kane CJ, Schulze KL, Sweeney ST. Syntaxin and synaptobrevin function downstream of vesicle docking in *Drosophila*. Neuron 1995;15(3):663–673.
6. Hanson PI, Roth R, Morisaki H, Jahn R, Heuser JE. Structure and conformational changes in NSF and its membrane receptor complexes visualized by quick-freeze/deep-etch electron microscopy. Cell 1997;90(3):523–535.
7. Lonart G, Sudhof TC. Assembly of SNARE core complexes prior to neurotransmitter release sets the readily releasable pool of synaptic vesicles. J Biol Chem 2000;275(36): 27703–27707.
8. Chen YA, Scales SJ, Scheller RH. Sequential SNARE assembly underlies priming and triggering of exocytosis. Neuron 2001;30(1):161–170.
9. Chen YA, Scheller RH. SNARE-mediated membrane fusion. Nat Rev Mol Cell Biol 2001;2(2):98–106.
10. Lin RC, Scheller RH. Structural organization of the synaptic exocytosis core complex. Neuron 1997;19(5):1087–1094.
11. Sutton RB, Fasshauer D, Jahn R, Brunger AT. Crystal structure of a SNARE complex involved in synaptic exocytosis at 2.4 A resolution. Nature 1998;395(6700):347–353.
12. Hammarlund M, Palfreyman MT, Watanabe S, Olsen S, Jorgensen EM. Open syntaxin docks synaptic vesicles. PLoS Biol 2007;5(8):e198.
13. Weimer RM, Gracheva EO, Meyrignac O, Miller KG, Richmond JE, Bessereau JL. UNC-13 and UNC-10/rim localize synaptic vesicles to specific membrane domains. J Neurosci 2006;26(31):8040–8047.
14. Dulubova I, Sugita S, Hill S, et al. A conformational switch in syntaxin during exocytosis: role of munc18. EMBO J 1999;18(16):4372–4382.
15. Pevsner J, Hsu SC, Scheller RH. n-Sec1: a neural-specific syntaxin-binding protein. Proc Natl Acad Sci USA 1994;91(4):1445–1449.
16. Sassa T, Harada S, Ogawa H, Rand JB, Maruyama IN, Hosono R. Regulation of the UNC-18–*Caenorhabditis elegans* syntaxin complex by UNC-13. J Neurosci 1999;19(12):4772–4777.
17. Betz A, Okamoto M, Benseler F, Brose N. Direct interaction of the rat unc-13 homologue Munc13-1 with the N terminus of syntaxin. J Biol Chem 1997;272(4):2520–2526.
18. Madison JM, Nurrish S, Kaplan JM. UNC-13 interaction with syntaxin is required for synaptic transmission. Curr Biol 2005;15(24):2236–2242.
19. Fujita Y, Shirataki H, Sakisaka T, et al. Tomosyn: a syntaxin-1–binding protein that forms a novel complex in the neurotransmitter release process. Neuron 1998;20(5):905–915.
20. Gracheva EO, Burdina AO, Holgado AM, et al. Tomosyn inhibits synaptic vesicle priming in Caenorhabditis elegans. PLoS Biol 2006;4(8):e261.
21. Brenner S. The genetics of *Caenorhabditis elegans*. Genetics 1974;77(1):71–94.
22. Saifee O, Wei L, Nonet ML. The *Caenorhabditis elegans unc-64* locus encodes a syntaxin that interacts genetically with synaptobrevin. Mol Biol Cell 1998;9(6):1235–1252.
23. Toonen RF, Verhage M. Vesicle trafficking: pleasure and pain from SM genes. Trends Cell Biol 2003;13(4):177–186.

24. Novick P, Schekman R. Secretion and cell-surface growth are blocked in a temperature-sensitive mutant of Saccharomyces cerevisiae. Proc Natl Acad Sci USA 1979;76 (4):1858–1862.

25. Hata Y, Slaughter CA, Sudhof TC. Synaptic vesicle fusion complex contains unc-18 homologue bound to syntaxin. Nature 1993;366(6453):347–351.

26. Harrison SD, Broadie K, van de Goor J, Rubin GM. Mutations in the *Drosophila Rop* gene suggest a function in general secretion and synaptic transmission. Neuron 1994;13(3):555–566.

27. Misura KM, Scheller RH, Weis WI. Three-dimensional structure of the neuronal-Sec1–syntaxin 1a complex. Nature 2000;404(6776):355–362.

28. Bracher A, Weissenhorn W. Crystal structures of neuronal squid Sec1 implicate inter-domain hinge movement in the release of t-SNAREs. J Mol Biol 2001;306(1):7–13.

29. Bracher A, Weissenhorn W. Structural basis for the Golgi membrane recruitment of Sly1p by Sed5p. EMBO J 2002;21(22):6114–6124.

30. Hu SH, Latham CF, Gee CL, James DE, Martin JL. Structure of the Munc18c/Syntaxin4 N-peptide complex defines universal features of the N-peptide binding mode of Sec1/Munc18 proteins. Proc Natl Acad Sci U S A 2007;104(21):8773–8778.

31. Rizo J, Sudhof TC. SNAREs and Munc18 in synaptic vesicle fusion. Nature Rev Neurosci 2002;3(8):641–653.

32. Gallwitz D, Jahn R. The riddle of the Sec1/Munc-18 proteins - new twists added to their interactions with SNAREs. Trends Biochem Sci 2003;28(3):113–116.

33. Schekman R, Novick P. 23 genes, 23 years later. Cell 2004;116(2 suppl):S13–15, 1 p. following S9.

34. Weimer RM, Richmond JE, Davis WS, Hadwiger G, Nonet ML, Jorgensen EM. Defects in synaptic vesicle docking in *unc-18* mutants. Nat Neurosci 2003;6(10):1023–1030.

35. Verhage M, Maia AS, Plomp JJ, et al. Synaptic assembly of the brain in the absence of neurotransmitter secretion. Science 2000;287(5454):864–869.

36. Voets T, Toonen RF, Brian EC, et al. Munc18–1 promotes large dense-core vesicle docking. Neuron 2001;31(4):581–591.

37. Toonen RF, Wierda K, Sons MS, et al. Munc18–1 expression levels control synapse recovery by regulating readily releasable pool size. Proc Natl Acad Sci USA 2006;103(48):18332–18337.

38. Rostaing P, Real E, Siksou L, et al. Analysis of synaptic ultrastructure without fixative using high-pressure freezing and tomography. Eur J Neurosci 2006;24(12):3463–3474.

39. Wojcik SM, Brose N. Regulation of membrane fusion in synaptic excitation-secretion coupling: speed and accuracy matter. Neuron 2007;55(1):11–24.

40. Nofal S, Becherer U, Hof D, Matti U, Rettig J. Primed vesicles can be distinguished from docked vesicles by analyzing their mobility. J Neurosci 2007;27(6):1386–1395.

41. Toonen RF, Kochubey O, de Wit H, et al. Dissecting docking and tethering of secretory vesicles at the target membrane. EMBO J 2006;25(16):3725–3737.

42. de Wit H, Cornelisse LN, Toonen RF, Verhage M. Docking of secretory vesicles is syntaxin dependent. PLoS ONE 2006;1:e126.

43. Marsal J, Ruiz-Montasell B, Blasi J, et al. Block of transmitter release by botulinum C1 action on syntaxin at the squid giant synapse. Proc Natl Acad Sci USA 1997;94(26): 14871–14876.

44. O'Connor V, Heuss C, De Bello WM, et al. Disruption of syntaxin-mediated protein interactions blocks neurotransmitter secretion. Proc Natl Acad Sci USA 1997;94(22):12186–12191.

45. Richmond JE, Davis WS, Jorgensen EM. UNC-13 is required for synaptic vesicle fusion in *C. elegans*. Nat Neurosci 1999;2(11):959–964.

46. Kidokoro Y. Roles of SNARE proteins and synaptotagmin I in synaptic transmission: studies at the Drosophila neuromuscular synapse. Neurosignals 2003;12(1):13–30.

47. Yang B, Steegmaier M, Gonzalez LC, Jr., Scheller RH. nSec1 binds a closed conformation of syntaxin1A. J Cell Biol 2000;148(2):247–252.

48. Schulze KL, Littleton JT, Salzberg A, et al. *rop*, a *Drosophila* homolog of yeast Sec1 and vertebrate n-Sec1/Munc-18 proteins, is a negative regulator of neurotransmitter release *in vivo*. Neuron 1994;13(5):1099–1108.

49. Dresbach T, Burns ME, O'Connor V, DeBello WM, Betz H, Augustine GJ. A neuronal Sec1 homolog regulates neurotransmitter release at the squid giant synapse. J Neurosci 1998;18 (8):2923–2932.

50. Rickman C, Medine CN, Bergmann A, Duncan RR. Functionally and spatially distinct modes of munc18–syntaxin 1 interaction. J Biol Chem 2007;282(16):12097–12103.

51. Gulyas-Kovacs A, de Wit H, Milosevic I, et al. Munc18–1: sequential interactions with the fusion machinery stimulate vesicle docking and priming. J Neurosci 2007;27(32):8676–8686.

52. Dulubova I, Yamaguchi T, Gao Y, et al. How Tlg2p/syntaxin 16 'snares' Vps45. EMBO J 2002;21(14):3620–3631.

53. Yamaguchi T, Dulubova I, Min SW, Chen X, Rizo J, Sudhof TC. Sly1 binds to Golgi and ER syntaxins via a conserved N-terminal peptide motif. Dev Cell 2002;2(3):295–305.

54. Zilly FE, Sorensen JB, Jahn R, Lang T. Munc18–bound syntaxin readily forms SNARE complexes with synaptobrevin in native plasma membranes. PLoS Biol 2006;4(10):e330.

55. Shen J, Tareste DC, Paumet F, Rothman JE, Melia TJ. Selective activation of cognate SNAREpins by Sec1/Munc18 proteins. Cell 2007;128(1):183–195.

56. Dulubova I, Khvotchev M, Liu S, Huryeva I, Sudhof TC, Rizo J. Munc18–1 binds directly to the neuronal SNARE complex. Proc Natl Acad Sci USA 2007;104(8):2697–2702.

57. Carr CM, Grote E, Munson M, Hughson FM, Novick PJ. Sec1p binds to SNARE complexes and concentrates at sites of secretion. J Cell Biol 1999;146(2):333–344.

58. Peng R, Gallwitz D. Multiple SNARE interactions of an SM protein: Sed5p/Sly1p binding is dispensable for transport. Embo J 2004;23(20):3939–3949.

59. Scott BL, Van Komen JS, Irshad H, Liu S, Wilson KA, McNew JA. Sec1p directly stimulates SNARE-mediated membrane fusion in vitro. J Cell Biol 2004;167(1):75–85.

60. Carpp LN, Ciufo LF, Shanks SG, Boyd A, Bryant NJ. The Sec1p/Munc18 protein Vps45p binds its cognate SNARE proteins via two distinct modes. J Cell Biol 2006;173(6):927–936.

61. Togneri J, Cheng YS, Munson M, Hughson FM, Carr CM. Specific SNARE complex binding mode of the Sec1/Munc-18 protein, Sec1p. Proc Natl Acad Sci USA 2006;103 (47):17730–17735.

62. Xu XZ, Wes PD, Chen H, et al. Retinal targets for calmodulin include proteins implicated in synaptic transmission. J Biol Chem 1998;273(47):31297–31307.

63. Brose N, Hofmann K, Hata Y, Sudhof TC. Mammalian homologues of *Caenorhabditis elegans unc-13* gene define novel family of C2–domain proteins. J Biol Chem 1995;270(42):25273–25280.

64. Koch H, Hofmann K, Brose N. Definition of Munc13–homology-domains and characterization of a novel ubiquitously expressed Munc13 isoform. Biochem J 2000;349(pt 1):247–253.

65. Kohn RE, Duerr JS, McManus JR, et al. Expression of multiple UNC-13 proteins in the *C. elegans* nervous system. Mol Biol Cell 2000;11(10):3441–3452.

66. Aravamudan B, Fergestad T, Davis WS, Rodesch CK, Broadie K. *Drosophila* UNC-13 is essential for synaptic transmission. Nat Neurosci 1999;2(11):965–971.

67. Augustin I, Betz A, Herrmann C, Jo T, Brose N. Differential expression of two novel Munc13 proteins in rat brain. Biochem J 1999;337(pt 3):363–371.

68. Augustin I, Korte S, Rickmann M, et al. The cerebellum-specific Munc13 isoform Munc13–3 regulates cerebellar synaptic transmission and motor learning in mice. J Neurosci 2001;21(1):10–17.

69. Yang CB, Zheng YT, Li GY, Mower GD. Identification of Munc13–3 as a candidate gene for critical-period neuroplasticity in visual cortex. J Neurosci 2002;22(19):8614–8618.

70. Varoqueaux F, Sigler A, Rhee JS, et al. Total arrest of spontaneous and evoked synaptic transmission but normal synaptogenesis in the absence of Munc13–mediated vesicle priming. Proc Natl Acad Sci USA 2002;99(13):9037–9042.

71. Augustin I, Rosenmund C, Sudhof TC, Brose N. Munc13–1 is essential for fusion competence of glutamatergic synaptic vesicles. Nature 1999;400(6743):457–461.

72. Ashery U, Varoqueaux F, Voets T, et al. Munc13–1 acts as a priming factor for large dense-core vesicles in bovine chromaffin cells. EMBO J 2000;19(14):3586–3596.

73. Zhen M, Jin Y. Presynaptic terminal differentiation: transport and assembly. Curr Opin Neurobiol 2004;14(3):280–287.

74. Basu J, Shen N, Dulubova I, et al. A minimal domain responsible for Munc13 activity. Nat Struct Mol Biol 2005;12(11):1017–1018.
75. Stevens DR, Wu ZX, Matti U, et al. Identification of the minimal protein domain required for priming activity of Munc13-1. Curr Biol 2005;15(24):2243–2248.
76. Brose N, Rosenmund C, Rettig J. Regulation of transmitter release by Unc-13 and its homologues. Curr Opin Neurobiol 2000;10(3):303–311.
77. Richmond JE, Weimer RM, Jorgensen EM. An open form of syntaxin bypasses the requirement for UNC-13 in vesicle priming. Nature 2001;412(6844):338–341.
78. McEwen JM, Madison JM, Dybbs M, Kaplan JM. Antagonistic regulation of synaptic vesicle priming by Tomosyn and UNC-13. Neuron 2006;51(3):303–315.
79. Basu J, Betz A, Brose N, Rosenmund C. Munc13-1 C1 domain activation lowers the energy barrier for synaptic vesicle fusion. J Neurosci 2007;27(5):1200–1210.
80. Groffen AJ, Friedrich R, Brian EC, Ashery U, Verhage M. DOC2A and DOC2B are sensors for neuronal activity with unique calcium-dependent and kinetic properties. J Neurochem 2006;97(3):818–833.
81. Kagami M, Toh-e A, Matsui Y. Sro7p, a Saccharomyces cerevisiae counterpart of the tumor suppressor l(2)gl protein, is related to myosins in function. Genetics 1998;149(4):1717–1727.
82. Lehman K, Rossi G, Adamo JE, Brennwald P. Yeast homologues of tomosyn and lethal giant larvae function in exocytosis and are associated with the plasma membrane SNARE, Sec9. J Cell Biol 1999;146(1):125–140.
83. Mechler BM, McGinnis W, Gehring WJ. Molecular cloning of lethal(2)giant larvae, a recessive oncogene of Drosophila melanogaster. EMBO J 1985;4(6):1551–1557.
84. Musch A, Cohen D, Yeaman C, Nelson WJ, Rodriguez-Boulan E, Brennwald PJ. Mammalian homolog of Drosophila tumor suppressor lethal (2) giant larvae interacts with basolateral exocytic machinery in Madin-Darby canine kidney cells. Mol Biol Cell 2002;13(1):158–168.
85. Scales SJ, Hesser BA, Masuda ES, Scheller RH. Amisyn, a novel syntaxin-binding protein that may regulate SNARE complex assembly. J Biol Chem 2002;277(31):28271–28279.
86. Masuda ES, Huang BC, Fisher JM, Luo Y, Scheller RH. Tomosyn binds t-SNARE proteins via a VAMP-like coiled coil. Neuron 1998;21(3):479–480.
87. Hattendorf DA, Andreeva A, Gangar A, Brennwald PJ, Weis WI. Structure of the yeast polarity protein Sro7 reveals a SNARE regulatory mechanism. Nature 2007;446(7135):567–571.
88. Dybbs M, Ngai J, Kaplan JM. Using microarrays to facilitate positional cloning: identification of tomosyn as an inhibitor of neurosecretion. PLoS Genet 2005;1(1):6–16.
89. Zhang W, Lilja L, Mandic SA, et al. Tomosyn is expressed in beta-cells and negatively regulates insulin exocytosis. Diabetes 2006;55(3):574–581.
90. Hatsuzawa K, Lang T, Fasshauer D, Bruns D, Jahn R. The R-SNARE motif of tomosyn forms SNARE core complexes with syntaxin 1 and SNAP-25 and down-regulates exocytosis. J Biol Chem 2003;278(33):31159–31166.
91. Widberg CH, Bryant NJ, Girotti M, Rea S, James DE. Tomosyn interacts with the t-SNAREs syntaxin4 and SNAP23 and plays a role in insulin-stimulated GLUT4 translocation. J Biol Chem 2003;278(37):35093–35101.
92. Yizhar O, Matti U, Melamed R, et al. Tomosyn inhibits priming of large dense-core vesicles in a calcium-dependent manner. Proc Natl Acad Sci U S A 2004;101(8):2578–2583.
93. Baba T, Sakisaka T, Mochida S, Takai Y. PKA-catalyzed phosphorylation of tomosyn and its implication in Ca2+-dependent exocytosis of neurotransmitter. J Cell Biol 2005;170(7):1113–1125.
94. Cheviet S, Bezzi P, Ivarsson R, et al. Tomosyn-1 is involved in a post-docking event required for pancreatic beta-cell exocytosis. J Cell Sci 2006;119(pt 14):2912–2920.
95. Sakisaka T, Baba T, Tanaka S, Izumi G, Yasumi M, Takai Y. Regulation of SNAREs by tomosyn and ROCK: implication in extension and retraction of neurites. J Cell Biol 2004;166(1):17–25.
96. Manfruelli P, Arquier N, Hanratty WP, Semeriva M. The tumor suppressor gene, lethal(2)giant larvae (1(2)gl), is required for cell shape change of epithelial cells during Drosophila development. Development 1996;122(7):2283–2294.

97. Pobbati AV, Razeto A, Boddener M, Becker S, Fasshauer D. Structural basis for the inhibitory role of tomosyn in exocytosis. J Biol Chem 2004;279(45):47192–47200.
98. Reim K, Mansour M, Varoqueaux F, et al. Complexins regulate a late step in Ca2+-dependent neurotransmitter release. Cell 2001;104(1):71–81.
99. Constable JR, Graham ME, Morgan A, Burgoyne RD. Amisyn regulates exocytosis and fusion pore stability by both syntaxin-dependent and syntaxin-independent mechanisms. J Biol Chem 2005;280(36):31615–31623.
100. Yizhar O, Lipstein N, Gladycheva SE, et al. Multiple functional domains are involved in tomosyn regulation of exocytosis. J Neurochem 2007;103(2):604–616.
101. Wierda KD, Toonen RF, de Wit H, Brussaard AB, Verhage M. Interdependence of PKC-dependent and PKC-independent pathways for presynaptic plasticity. Neuron 2007;54(2):275–290.
102. Palfreyman M, Jorgensen EM. PKC defends crown against Munc13. Neuron 2007;54(2):179–180.
103. Dulubova I, Lou X, Lu J, et al. A Munc13/RIM/Rab3 tripartite complex: from priming to plasticity? EMBO J 2005;24(16):2839–2850.
104. Gladycheva SE, Ho CS, Lee YY, Stuenkel EL. Regulation of Syntaxin1A/Munc18 complex for SNARE Pairing. J Physiol 2004;558(Pt3):857–871.
105. Gladycheva SE, Lam AD, Liu J, et al. Receptor-mediated regulation of tomosyn-syntaxin 1A interactions in bovine adrenal chromaffin cells. J Biol Chem 2007;282(31):22887–22899.
106. Gracheva EO, Burdina AO, Touroutine D, Berthelot-Grosjean M, Parekh H, Richmond JE. Tomosyn negatively regulates both synaptic transmitter and neuropeptide release at the C. elegans neuromuscular junction. J Physiol 2007;585(Pt3):705–709.

Chapter 8
Roles of the ELKS/CAST Family and SAD Kinase in Neurotransmitter Release

Toshihisa Ohtsuka and Yoshimi Takai

Contents

Abstract The active zone (AZ) is a specialized site for docking and fusion of synaptic vesicles in the nerve terminal. AZ-specific proteins include CAST, ELKS, RIMs, Munc13-1, Bassoon, and Piccolo. CAST interacts with these proteins, forming a large molecular complex at the AZ. Moreover, the direct interaction of CAST with RIM1 and Bassoon is involved in neurotransmitter release. Thus, CAST may play organizational and functional roles at the AZ. Furthermore, SAD kinase, a master kinase for axon/dendrite polarization in early synapse formation, has recently been identified as an AZ-associated kinase that directly phosphorylates RIM1. SAD regulates neurotransmitter release in a kinase activity-dependent manner. This chapter focuses on recent findings about the structure and function of the ELKS/CAST family and SAD, and discusses the roles of these proteins in neurotransmitter release.

Toshihisa Ohtsuka
Department of Clinical and Molecular Pathology, Graduate School of Medicine/Faculty of Medicine, University of Toyama, Sugitani 2630, Toyama 930-0194, Japan

Yoshimi Takai
Division of Molecular and Cellular Biology, Department of Biochemistry and Molecular Biology, Kobe University Graduate School of Medicine/Faculty of Medicine, Kusunoki-cho, Chuo-ku, Kobe 650-0017, Japan
e-mail: ytakai@molbio.med.osaka-u.ac.jp

Z.-W. Wang (ed.) *Molecular Mechanisms of Neurotransmitter Release,*
© Humana Press 2008 a part of Springer Science+Business Media, LLC

Keywords Active zone, synaptic vesicle, CAST, ELKS, SAD, neurotransmitter release.

Neurotransmitter release is regulated in a spatially and temporally coordinated manner at a specialized site in presynaptic nerve terminals, the active zone (AZ) (1). After docking to the AZ, synaptic vesicles (SVs), containing appropriate neurotransmitters, undergo a perfusion step or priming. Upon arrival of an action potential to the nerve terminal and the subsequent rise of the intracellular Ca^{2+} concentration, SVs fuse with the membrane and release their transmitters from the AZ into the synaptic cleft (2). The AZ thus plays a pivotal role in neurotransmitter release by determining the timing and site of the SV docking and fusion (3). As described in Chapter 1, the AZ appears as a slightly electron-dense region on electron microscopy (1, 4). The cytomatrix at the AZ is thus believed to contain various kinds of proteins implicated in signal transduction, cytoskeletal organization, and cell–cell adhesion as well as neurotransmitter release.

Recent biochemical and molecular biological approaches have allowed researchers to identify and characterize several AZ-specific proteins including Bassoon (5), Piccolo/Aczonin (6–8), RIM1 (9), Munc13-1 (10), ELKS (11–14), and CAST (13,15). These proteins are all relatively large and contain various significant domains such as coiled-coil, PDZ (PSD-95, Dlg, and ZO1), zinc finger, C2, and C1 domains. In addition, SAD kinase, a regulator of axon/dendrite polarization (16), has more recently been identified as an AZ- and SV-associated serine/threonine kinase (17). This chapter presents the current research on the roles of the ELKS/CAST family and SAD in neurotransmitter release, and we correlate the findings with the AZ structure and function.

Molecular Components of the Presynaptic Active Zone

CAST and ELKS

CAST (cytomatrix at the AZ-associated structural protein) was first purified and identified from the biochemically isolated postsynaptic density (PSD) fraction of rat brain (15). Since the biochemically isolated PSD fraction contains not only PSD components but also AZ proteins, it is reasonable that CAST is found in the PSD fraction. CAST is also called ERC2, which was subsequently isolated by yeast two hybrid screening as a RIM1 interactor (13). In vertebrates, CAST has ELKS as a family member (Fig. 8.1) (11–14). ELKS was originally identified as a gene with its 5" terminus fused to the *ret* tyrosine kinase oncogene in a papillary thyroid carcinoma (11). ELKS also has several other names including Rab6IP2 (12), ERC1 (13), and CAST2 (14). However, since ELKS was the first name give to this protein, we call it ELKS throughout this chapter to avoid confusion. While CAST is brain-specific, ELKS is ubiquitously expressed in various tissues and has a number of splicing isoforms (18). Among them, ELKSα is predominantly expressed in the brain (13,14,18). CAST and ELKSα show a relatively

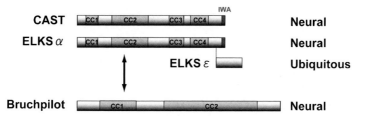

Fig. 8.1 Molecular structure of the ELKS/CAST family. ELKS/CAST contains four coiled-coil regions and a C-terminal IWA motif, which is required for binding to RIM1 PDZ domain. ELKS has at least five alternatively spliced isoforms, ELKSα, ELKSβ, ELKSγ, ELKSδ, and ELKSε (18). ELKSα is expressed mainly in the brain. Note that the longer isoform ELKSε lacks the IWA motif. The N-terminal region of *Drosophila* Bruchpilot resembles that of mammalian ELKS/CAST, but the C-terminal region is homologous to cytoskeletal proteins

high homology at the protein level (~70% identity). Both CAST and ELKSα are proteins of ~120 kDa with four coiled-coil regions and a unique COOH-terminal amino acid motif, IWA (symbols for amino acids Isoleucine, Tryptophan, and Alanine) (Fig. 8.1). In *C. elegans* (19) and *Drosophila* (Fig. 8.1) (20,21), only one gene product of the ELKS/CAST family has been identified and characterized.

In the mouse hippocampus, CAST is localized closed to the presynaptic plasma membrane (Fig. 8.2A) (15). Like CAST and Bassoon, ELKSα is localized at the vicinity of the presynaptic plasma membrane in the mouse cerebellum (Fig. 8.2B) (14). In mammalian retina, there is an equivalent of the AZ cytomatrix, called the synaptic ribbon, where photoreceptor cells and bipolar cells release glutamate as a neurotransmitter (22). At the immunoelectron microscopy level, CAST is localized at the base of the ribbon, whereas ELKSα is around the ribbon (23). In addition, a ubiquitous isoform of ELKS regulates exocytosis of insulin from pancreatic β-cells (24) and, in nonneural fibroblasts, is involved in the microtubule stabilization through its complex formation with the microtubule-binding protein CLASP and LL5β (25).

Other AZ Proteins

Bassoon and Piccolo are very large proteins structurally homologous to each other, except for the additional C2 and PDZ domains in Piccolo (6–8). They are expressed in most brain regions with overlapping localization. Their zinc-finger domains bind to the prenylated Rab3A-associated protein-1(Pra1) *in vitro*. The physiological significance of this interaction is currently unknown. Because Bassoon and Piccolo are major components of AZ precursor vesicles (26,27), their interactions with Pra1 may regulate trafficking of these vesicles in the axon during early synapse formation.

RIM1 and Munc13-1 directly interact with each other, and are known to be essential factors for priming in the SV cycling (28). RIM1 was originally identified as a Rab3A-binding protein (9). RIM1 also contains various domain structures, such as zinc-finger, PDZ, and C2 domains, suggesting that RIM1 functions as a

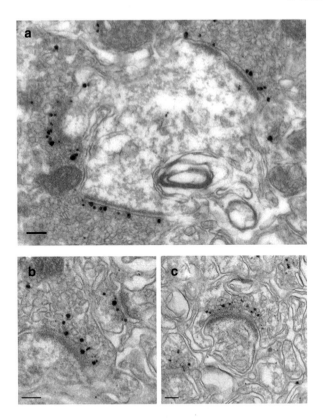

Fig. 8.2 Subsynaptic localization of ELKS/CAST. (a) CAST in the mouse hippocampus. (b) ELKS in the mouse cerebellum. (c) Bassoon in the mouse cerebellum. Localization of these proteins was determined by immunoelectron microscopy. The sections were reacted with the anti-CAST, anti-ELKS, or anti-Bassoon antibody, incubated with immunogold particles (1.4 nm) conjugated with goat immunoglobulin G (IgG) against rabbit and mouse IgGs, and silver enhanced. The black dots represent immunoreactivities of these antibodies against the specific AZ proteins. They are localized to the vicinity of the presynaptic plasma membranes. Scale bars = 100 nm. (From Deguchi-Tawarada et al [14] and Ohtsuka et al [15], with permission.)

scaffold protein at the AZ. Munc13-1 is a mammalian homologue of *Caenorhabditis elegans* UNC-13 (10). Munc13-1 regulates neurotransmitter release through interaction with syntaxin, a component of the SNARE (soluble *N*-ethylmaleimide–sensitive factor attachment protein receptor) complex (29–31).

Before the discovery of CAST in 2002, only four proteins—Bassoon, Piccolo, RIM1, and Munc13-1—were known as AZ-specific proteins, and the molecular mechanisms underlying their AZ localization were poorly understood. However, we now have a much better idea about the molecular mechanisms of AZ-specific protein localization. In the next section, we present a network of protein–protein interactions mediated by CAST at the AZ.

CAST-Dependent Molecular Complex at the Active Zone

The AZ cytomatrix is highly complex and resistant to extraction with nonionic detergents, such as Triton X-100, which makes it difficult to biochemically analyze the structure and function of the AZ. Thus, we first treated the PSD fraction containing the AZ components with SDS (sodium dodecyl sulfate), followed by dilution with Triton X-100, and then performed immunoprecipitation by an anti-CAST antibody. Intriguingly, all the known AZ proteins were coimmunoprecipitated with CAST, which was the first evidence that there is a network of protein–protein interactions among AZ proteins (Fig. 8.3) (15). CAST and ELKSα directly bind Bassoon, Piccolo, and RIM1, and further indirectly bind Munc13-1, forming a large molecular complex at the AZ. Exogenously expressed RIM1 without the PDZ domain, a CAST-binding domain shows a diffuse distribution in the axon of primary cultured rat hippocampal neurons, whereas CAST, lacking the IWA motif, a RIM1-binding motif, is correctly localized to the AZ (15). These observations suggest that CAST may play a role in anchoring RIM1 to the AZ. On the other hand, both CAST and Bassoon can localize to the AZ independent of each other in primary cultured neurons (32). At present, the targeting signal of Bassoon to the AZ appears to reside in several regions of

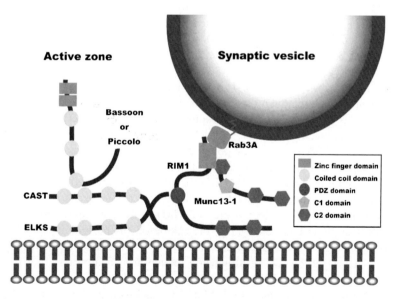

Fig. 8.3 A network of protein–protein interactions among the AZ proteins. CAST and ELKS can form homo- and hetero-oligomers. In addition, the second coiled-coil region of ELKS/CAST binds the third coiled-coil region of Bassoon/Piccolo. The C-terminal IWA motif of ELKS/CAST is required for binding the PDZ domain of RIM1. RIM1 and Munc13-1 bind to each other via the zinc-finger domain of RIM1 and the N-terminal C2 domain of Munc13-1

Bassoon, including amino acids 1692 to 2087, 2565 to 2714, and 3015 to 3263, which do not include a coiled-coil region that binds CAST (32,33).

Although such large AZ proteins may often be the cause of nonspecific binding, it is assumed, in accord with the following lines of evidence, that this CAST-dependent complex formation is specific: (1) these proteins are well colocalized at the AZ; (2) the binding of CAST and RIM1 is highly specific; (3) the binding of CAST and Bassoon is also specific; and (4) electrophysiological studies show that these bindings are implicated in synaptic transmission as described below. Currently, a full molecular structure of the AZ still remains unknown, but this CAST-dependent large protein complex may be a molecular basis for the electron density of the AZ. At the core of the AZ, CAST and ELKS may serve as "a nucleation site" for the assembly of the AZ by capturing Bassoon, Piccolo, RIM1, and Munc13-1 (Fig. 8.3).

CAST Implicated in Neurotransmitter Release

Using genetic deletion studies, RIM1, Munc13-1, and Bassoon have been shown to regulate neurotransmitter release at the priming step, although the gross synapse structure including the AZ structure in these knockout (KO) mice is intact (34–37). In the retina of Bassoon KO mice, the synaptic ribbon cannot attach to the presynaptic plasma membrane and is floating in the cytoplasm, and ectopic synapses are formed (38). The proper ribbon formation requires the interaction of Bassoon and a ribbon-specific protein, RIBEYE (39).

The role of CAST in neurotransmitter release has been examined using rat superior cervical ganglion neurons (SCGNs), in which well-characterized cholinergic synapses are formed (40). This is an ideal system because proteins can be introduced into the relatively large (30–40 μm) presynaptic cell bodies by microinjection, the injected proteins can rapidly diffuse to nerve terminals, and the effect on stimulated release of acetylcholine can be accurately monitored by recording excitatory postsynaptic potentials (EPSPs) evoked by action potentials in presynaptic neurons. Microinjection of the RIM1-binding domain of CAST or the CAST-binding domain of RIM1 significantly impairs neurotransmission (32). Because the direct binding of RIM1 and Munc13-1 is involved in the priming of SVs (28) and because the localization of RIM1 at the AZ appears to be CAST-dependent as described above (15), the inhibition of the binding of RIM1 to CAST likely affects the RIM1–Munc13-1 pathway, presumably by the mislocalization of RIM1 at the AZ, resulting in a reduction of neurotransmitter release. Consistent with this, ELKS regulates Ca^{2+}-dependent exocytosis of human growth hormone through the RIM1–Munc13-1 pathway in PC12 cells (CAST is not expressed in PC12 cells) (41). Moreover, inhibition of the CAST-Bassoon binding significantly impairs neurotransmission (32). It is currently unclear whether the impairment of synaptic transmission by the inhibition between CAST-Bassoon binding is due to mislocalization of CAST or Bassoon at the AZ since their localization to the AZ might be independent. A functional linkage between RIM1 and Bassoon is currently unclear, too, but, by forming the ternary complex with RIM1 and Bassoon, CAST may play a role as a "platform" on which the signaling pathways of Bassoon and RIM1 could be molecularly coupled. It is also possible that the impairment of synaptic transmission is due to the disruption of the binding of Piccolo to CAST, because Bassoon and Piccolo share the same binding site in CAST (the third coiled-coil region of Bassoon/Piccolo directly binds to the second coiled-coil region of CAST). Piccolo is structurally homologous to Bassoon but has additional PDZ and C2 domains (7,8), suggesting that Piccolo could play similar but not identical roles at the presynaptic site compared with Bassoon.

The specific localization of CAST and ELKS to the AZ and their association with the other AZ proteins suggest that ELKS/CAST might be involved in the formation or maintenance of the AZ. This notion is favored by results of two recent genetic studies in *Drosophila* (20,21). The monoclonal antibody NC82 has long been known to label the AZ of almost all the synapses in *Drosophila* (42,43). The groups led by Drs. Buchner and Sigrist have identified a gene product, Bruchpilot (BRP) (Fig. 8.1), that is recognized by NC82 (20). BRP is a ~190-kDa protein containing an N-terminal domain with significant homology to vertebrate ELKS/CAST and a large C-terminal domain rich in coiled-coil structures. *brp* mutants are defective in locomotor activity and show unstable flight behaviors (hence, "*bruchpilot*," meaning "crash pilot"). At the electron microscopic level, *brp* mutant neuromuscular junctions (NMJs) appear to have normal density of synapses and proper pre- and postsynaptic contacts; however, electron-dense matrix (T-bar) is completely lost, and clustering of Ca^{2+} channels is reduced at the nerve terminal (20,21). This is the first example that deletion of one molecule has resulted in the disappearance of the AZ cytomatrix or T-bar in *Drosophila*. At the NMJ of *brp* mutants, the amplitude of evoked postsynaptic currents is reduced to ~25% of the normal; however, spontaneous neurotransmitter release is unaffected, suggesting that the efficacy of synaptic exocytosis is impaired but the fundamental mechanism of exocytosis is still preserved in these mutants. Therefore, *Drosophila* BRP may play a role in clustering Ca^{2+} channels to the AZ, which would explain the deficiency of evoked synaptic transmission in *brp* mutants, but is not essential for synapse formation or normal spontaneous neurotransmitter release. Conceivably, vertebrate proteins that are structurally related to BRP, such as CAST and ELKS, might play a similar role in presynaptic structure.

BRP is expressed exclusively in the nervous system, suggesting that BRP may be functionally more similar to CAST than ELKS since CAST expression is restricted to the brain, whereas ELKS is ubiquitously expressed. Intriguingly, a *C. elegans* null mutant of *elks-1*, which encodes the only worm ELKS/CAST homologue, shows no significant changes in either synaptic ultrastructure or synaptic transmission (19). Thus, despite their structural similarities, it remains an open question whether proteins of the ELKS/CAST family play similar roles in vertebrates and invertebrates.

Phosphorylation Network at the AZ

Molecular components and protein–protein interactions at the AZ have progressively been revealed in the last decade. But, as to the signal transduction at the AZ, such as phosphorylation, lipid modification, and ubiquitination of the AZ proteins in the formation, maintenance, and function of the AZ, we are only at the beginning of understanding their underlying mechanisms. In this section, we present a current view on phosphorylation of AZ proteins by the serine/threonine kinase SAD.

SAD: Its Molecular Structure and Localization at Synapses

The serine/threonine kinase SAD-1 was originally identified by genetic screens to isolate mutants in *C. elegans* that affect SV clusters in sensory neurons (44). *sad-1* mutant animals show several distinct features in synaptic structure and function, such as diffuse and disorganized distribution of SVs at synapses and a failure to develop normal synapses in sensory axons. Most mutations occur in the kinase domain, suggesting that this domain of SAD-1 may play an important role in the formation of synapses. Recently, KO mice for SAD-1 orthologues (SAD kinases, named SAD-A and SAD-B) have been reported (16). Analysis of the mutant animals shows that mammalian SAD is required for the proper neural polarity that produces axons and dendrites, and that this function is promoted at least in part by SAD-dependent phosphorylation of the microtubule-associated protein Tau (16). These mutant animals die immediately after birth due to a lack of synapse formation, which makes it impossible to study a role of SAD in mature neurons. Independently, we isolated human homologues of SAD-1, and named them SAD-A and SAD-B (Fig. 8.4A). Both the proteins

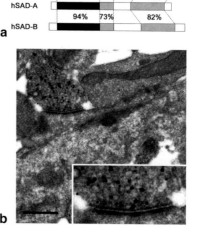

Fig. 8.4 Molecular structure and subsynaptic localization of SAD-B. (a) Comparison of structures between *C. elegans* SAD-1 (CeSAD-1), human SAD-A (hSAD-A), and human SAD-B (hSAD-B). One serine/threonine kinase domain (STK) and two short conserved regions (SCR) are conserved. (b) Immunoelectron microscopy of SAD-B. The SAD-B signals (black dots), which are silver-enhanced, are mainly detected in the presynaptic nerve terminal. Some of the signals are detected very close to the presynaptic plasma membrane. Scale bar = 500 nm. (From Inoue et al. [17], with permission.)

are mainly expressed in the brain, especially in the axon (17). They contain an N-terminal kinase domain and two short conserved regions (SCR1 and SCR2) in the middle and C-terminal portions. At the electron microscopic level, SAD-B is associated with SVs, and is also tightly associated with the AZ cytomatrix (Fig. 8.4B). By overexpressing various truncated forms of SAD-B in primary cultures of rat hippocampal neurons, SCR2 has been shown to be essential for the synaptic localization of SAD-B in neurons. But it is currently unknown whether this region is required for SAD-B localization to SVs or the AZ cytomatrix. Besides SAD, a number of kinases such as protein kinase A (PKA), protein kinase C (PKC), and CaMKII have been characterized in synapses, but they show ubiquitous distribution and are localized at both pre- and postsynaptic sides. Therefore, SAD is unique in that it is predominantly associated with SVs and the AZ cytomatrix in the nerve terminals.

SAD Implicated in Neurotransmitter Release

Such a unique localization of SAD-B at synapses allows us to easily imagine that SAD-B presynaptically regulates neurotransmitter release at the AZ. Overexpression of SAD-B in primary cultures of neurons significantly enhances the frequency but not amplitude of miniature excitatory postsynaptic currents (mEPSCs) (17). In contrast, a kinase dead mutant, in which lysine 64 in the adenosine triphosphate (ATP)-binding site is substituted by alanine, has no effect on the frequency of mEPSCs at $2\,mM\ Ca^{2+}$ concentration but dominant-negatively inhibits the frequency at $10\,mM\ Ca^{2+}$ concentration (17). These observations suggest that SAD-B is involved in spontaneous release of neurotransmitters. Moreover, microinjection of SCR2, which is required for SAD synaptic localization, or of a polyclonal anti-SCR2 antibody into a presynaptic cell of paired SCGNs significantly inhibits evoked neurotransmission. But acceleration of the SV cycle by increasing the frequency of stimulation from 0.05 to 0.2 Hz has no effect on SCR2-induced reduction of the EPSP amplitude. These observations suggest that the reduction of neurotransmitter release induced by SCR2 injection is not attributable to the activity-dependent cycling of SVs in presynaptic nerve terminals. Microinjection of SCR2 indeed inhibits the size of readily releasable pool (RRP), which is estimated by the size of postsynaptic currents evoked by application of a hypertonic sucrose solution. SCR2 appears to play a role in localizing SAD-B to the presynaptic terminal; it is possible that abnormal localization of endogenous SAD-B or disruption of endogenous SAD-B interaction with unidentified protein(s) in the presence of SCR2 may result in an inability of SAD-B to properly phosphorylate its substrate(s) such as RIM1 (see below) that are essential for proper maintenance of the size of the RRP.

Phosphorylation of RIM1 and Other AZ Proteins by SAD

The function of RIM1 may be altered depending on its phosphorylation state. A recent study showed that RIM1 is phosphorylated by PKA at serine 413, and this phosphorylation is critical to induction of presynaptic long-term potentiation by

RIM1 at cerebellar parallel fiber synapses (45). Interestingly, the degree of RIM1 phosphorylation in response to the PKA activator forskolin was less than that caused by the phosphatase inhibitor okadaic acid, suggesting that RIM1 is also phosphorylated by other kinase(s) (45). SAD-B is a candidate kinase for phosphorylating RIM1 because it closely associates with the AZ as RIM1 does. Indeed, our recent study showed that RIM1 but not Munc13-1 may be directly phosphorylated by SAD-B at least *in vitro* (17). The phosphorylation site of SAD-B in RIM1 is distinct from that of PKA (45), and is located near the C-terminal C2B domain (17). Because this domain interacts with a number of synaptic proteins including synaptotagmin, phosphorylation of this region by SAD-B may affect RIM1 interaction with these proteins. RIM1 has been shown to play multiple roles in neurotransmitter release including regulation of the RRP size, short-term plasticity, and evoked asynchronous release (46). However, it is still unknown how phosphorylation of RIM1 by SAD-B contributes to RIM1 function at the molecular level.

When SAD is overexpressed, it may potentially phosphorylate physiological as well as nonphysiological substrates. However, RIM1 but not Munc13-1 is phosphorylated by SAD-B *in vitro*, suggesting that SAD-B phosphorylates specific substrates. The localization of both SAD-B and RIM1 to the AZ cytomatrix also suggests that RIM1 is likely a physiological substrate of SAD-B *in vivo*. These findings argue against the possibility that the change in mEPSC frequency in cultured neurons transfected with SAD-B (17) was an artificial effect resulting from overexpression of the kinase. Like other serine/threonine kinases, SAD might also have multiple regulation targets. Other proteins localized on SVs or in the AZ are attractive candidates. Our preliminary data revealed that in addition to RIM1, SAD-B directly phosphorylates Bassoon, Piccolo, and CAST. Moreover, an antibody against a phosphorylated AZ protein by SAD-B showed specific immunoreactivity in intact brain tissues (unpublished). These observations suggest that SAD-B might modulate neurotransmitter release by phosphorylating a variety of proteins within the AZ cytomatrix.

To fully understand the function of SAD, it is essential to identify and characterize its upstream regulators as well as downstream substrates. Recently, a serine/threonine kinase, LKB1 (also known as STK1), has been reported as a candidate SAD-B activator. LKB1 is a critical regulator of cell polarity in non-neural tissues of nematodes, insects, and vertebrates (47–49). Specific deletion of LKB1 in mouse brain causes a defect in axon/dendrite polarity during early synapse development, which resembles the phenotype of SAD KO mice (50). Furthermore, activated LKB1 directly phosphorylates SAD-A and -B at specific residues in an activation loop of the SAD kinase domain. This phosphorylation enhances the kinase activity of SAD, resulting in phosphorylation of a microtubule-associated protein Tau by SAD (50). Thus, in immature neurons, a signaling pathway consisting of LKB1-SAD-Tau appears to be critical for the axon/dendrite polarization (Fig. 8.5). It is yet to be determined whether and how this signaling pathway is related to or contributes to a role of SAD in the AZ function.

Fig. 8.5 Neural polarity and the active zone function. In immature neurons, LKB1 phosphorylates SAD-B. Activated SAD-B in turn phosphorylates the microtubule-associated protein Tau, resulting in proper axon/dendrite formation. It is currently unknown whether and how LKB1 contributes to the SAD-B–mediated phosphorylation of the AZ proteins.

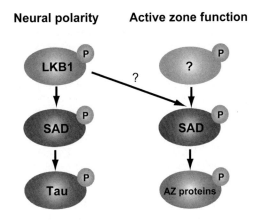

Conclusion

Our higher brain functions, such as learning and memory, emotion, and consciousness, definitely rely on the precise regulation of neural network that is communicated by synapses formed between neurons. As a specialized structure at the presynaptic terminal, the AZ has attracted great interest from many scientists since its discovery in 1960s. A future trend in this exciting field would be to reveal how the structure and function of the AZ are related to our brain function and behavior, and to elucidate the molecular and cellular mechanisms underlying this relationship.

Evidence suggests that the ELKS/CAST family and SAD play crucial roles in synaptic structure and function in nerve terminals. CAST may provide a platform for the assembly of a large molecular complex at the AZ, which could be a molecular basis for AZ formation. In addition, SAD can phosphorylate the AZ proteins including CAST, suggesting that there may be a phosphorylation network of the AZ proteins in the nerve terminals. Therefore, further studies on CAST and SAD would definitely shed new light on not only their roles in neurotransmitter release but also the relationship between the AZ and higher brain functions.

References

1. Landis DMD, Hall AK, Weinstein LA, Reese TS. The organization of cytoplasm at the presynaptic active zone of a central nervous system synapse. Neuron 1988;1:201–209.
2. Südhof TC. The synaptic vesicle cycle. Annu Rev Neurosci 2004;27:509–547.
3. Garner CC, Kindler S, Gundelfinger ED. Molecular determinants of presynaptic active zones. Curr Opin Neurobiol 2000;10:321–327.

4. Hirokawa N, Sobue K, Kanda K, Harada A, Yorifuji H. The cytoskeletal architecture of the presynaptic terminal and molecular structure of synapsin 1. J Cell Biol 1989;108:111–126.

5. tom Dieck S, Sanmarti-Vila L, Langnaese K, et al. Bassoon, a novel zinc-finger CAG/ glutamine-repeat protein selectively localized at the active zone of presynaptic nerve terminals. J Cell Biol 1998;142:499–509.

6. Cases-Langhoff C, Voss B, Garner AM, et al. Piccolo, a novel 420 kDa protein associated with the presynaptic cytomatrix. Eur J Cell Biol 1996;69:214–223.

7. Wang X, Kibschull M, Laue MM, Lichte B, Petrasch-Parwez E, Kilimann MW. Aczonin, a 550-kD putative scaffolding protein of presynaptic active zones, shares homology regions with Rim and Bassoon and binds Profilin. J Cell Biol 1999;147:151–162.

8. Fenster SD, Chung WJ, Zhai R, et al. Piccolo, a presynaptic zinc finger protein structurally related to bassoon. Neuron 2000;25:203–214.

9. Wang,Y, Okamoto M, Schmitz F, Hofmann K, and Südhof TC. Rim is a putative Rab3 effector in regulating synaptic vesicle fusion. Nature 1997;388:593–598.

10. Brose N, Hofmann K, Hata Y, Südhof TC. Mammalian homologues of C. elegans unc-13 gene define novel family of C2-domain proteins. J Biol Chem 1995;270:25273–25280.

11. Nakata T, Kitamura Y, Shimizu K, et al. Fusion of a novel gene, ELKS, to RET due to translocation t(10;12)(q11;p13) in a papillary thyroid carcinoma. Genes Chromosomes Cancer 1999;25:97–103.

12. Monier S, Jollivet F, Janoueix-Lerosey I, Johannes L, Goud B. Characterization of novel Rab6–interacting proteins involved in endosome-to-TGN transport. Traffic 2002;3:289–297.

13. Wang Y, Liu X, Biederer T, Südhof TC. A family of RIM-binding proteins regulated by alternative splicing: implications for the genesis of synaptic active zones. Proc Natl Acad Sci U S A 2002;99:14464–14469.

14. Deguchi-Tawarada M, Inoue E, Takao-Rikitsu E, Inoue M, Ohtsuka T, Takai Y. CAST2 : identification and characterization of a protein structurally related to the presynaptic cytomatrix protein CAST. Genes Cells 2004;9:15–23.

15. Ohtsuka T, Takao-Rikitsu E, Inoue E, et al. CAST: a novel protein of the cytomatrix at the active zone of synapses that forms a ternary complex with RIM1 and Munc13-1. J Cell Biol 2002;158:577–590.

16. Kishi M Pan YA, Crump JG, Sanes JR. Mammalian SAD kinases are required for neuronal polarization. Science 2005;307:929–932.

17. Inoue E, Mochida S, Takagi H, et al. SAD: a presynaptic kinase associated with synaptic vesicles and the active zone cytomatrix that regulates neurotransmitter release. Neuron 2006; 50:261–275.

18. Nakata T, Yokota T, Emi M, Minami S. Differential expression of multiple isoforms of the ELKS mRNAs involved in a papillary thyroid carcinoma. Genes Chromosomes Cancer 2002;35:30–37.

19. Deken SL, Vincent R, Hadwiger G, Liu Q, Wang ZW, Nonet ML. Redundant localization mechanisms of RIM and ELKS in Caenorhabditis elegans. J Neurosci 2005;25:5975–5983.

20. Wagh DA, Rasse T., Asan E, et al. Bruchpilot, a protein with homology to ELKS/CAST, is required for structural integrity and function of synaptic active zones in Drosophila. Neuron 2006;49:833–844.

21. Kittel RJ, Wichmann C, Rasse TM, et al. Bruchpilot promotes active zone assembly, Ca2+ channel clustering, and vesicle release. Science 2006;312:1051–1054.

22. Kalloniatis M, Tomisich G.. Amino acid neurochemistry of the vertebrate retina. Prog Retin Eye Res 1999;18:811–866.

23. Deguchi-Tawarada M, Inoue E, Takao-Rikitsu E, et al. The active zone protein CAST is a component of conventional and ribbon synapses in mouse retina. J Comp Neurol 2006;495:480–496.

24. Ohara-Imaizumi M, Ohtsuka T, Matsushima S, et al. ELKS, a protein structurally related to the active zone-associated protein CAST, is expressed in pancreatic beta cells and functions in insulin exocytosis: interaction of ELKS with exocytotic machinery analyzed by total internal reflection fluorescence microscopy. Mol Biol Cell 2005;16:3289–3300.

25. Lansbergen G, Grigoriev I, Mimori-Kiyosue Y, et al. CLASPs attach microtubule plus ends to the cell cortex through a complex with LL5beta. Dev Cell 2006;11:21–32.
26. Ahmari SE, Buchanan J, Smith SJ. Assembly of presynaptic active zones from cytoplasmic transport packets. Nat Neurosci 2000;3:445–451.
27. Shapira M, Zhai RG., Dresbach T, et al. Unitary assembly of presynaptic active zones from Piccolo-Bassoon transport vesicles. Neuron 2003;38:237–252.
28. Betz A, Thakur P, Junge HJ, et al. Functional interaction of the active zone proteins Munc13-1 and RIM1 in synaptic vesicle priming. Neuron 2001;30:183–196.
29. Brose N, Rosenmund C, Rettig J. Regulation of transmitter release by Unc-13 and its homologues. Curr Opin Neurobiol 2000;10:303–311.
30. Koushika SP, Richmond JE, Hadwiger G, et al. A post-docking role for active zone protein Rim. Nat Neurosci 2001;4:997–1005.
31. Richmond JE, Weimer RM, Jorgensen EM. An open form of syntaxin bypasses the requirement for UNC-13 in vesicle priming. Nature 2001;412:338–341.
32. Takao-Rikitsu E, Mochida S, Inoue E, et al. Physical and functional interaction of the active zone proteins, CAST, RIM1, and Bassoon, in neurotransmitter release. J Cell Biol 2004;164:301–311.
33. Dresbach T, Hempelmann A, Spilker C, et al. Functional regions of the presynaptic cytomatrix protein bassoon: significance for synaptic targeting and cytomatrix anchoring. Mol Cell Neurosci 2003;23:279–291.
34. Augustin I, Rosenmund C, Südhof T.C., Brose N. Munc13-1 is essential for fusion competence of glutamatergic synaptic vesicles. Nature 1999;400:457–461.
35. Castillo PE, Schoch S, Schmitz,F, Sudhof TC, Malenka RC. RIM1alpha is required for presynaptic long-term potentiation. Nature 2002;415:327–330.
36. Schoch S, Castillo PE, Jo T, et al. RIM1alpha forms a protein scaffold for regulating neurotransmitter release at the active zone. Nature 2002;415:321–326.
37. Altrock WD, tom Dieck S, Sokolov M, et al. Functional inactivation of a fraction of excitatory synapses in mice deficient for the active zone protein bassoon. Neuron 2003;37:787–800.
38. Dick O, tom Dieck S, Altrock WD, et al. The presynaptic active zone protein bassoon is essential for photoreceptor ribbon synapse formation in the retina. Neuron 2003;37:775–786.
39. tom Dieck S, Altrock WD, Kessels MM, et al. Molecular dissection of the photoreceptor ribbon synapse: physical interaction of Bassoon and RIBEYE is essential for the assembly of the ribbon complex. J Cell Biol 2005;168:825–836.
40. Mochida S, Sheng ZH, Baker C, Kobayashi H, Catterall WA. Inhibition of neurotransmission by peptides containing the synaptic protein interaction site of N-type Ca^{2+} channels. Neuron 1996;17:781–788.
41. Inoue E, Deguchi-Tawarada M, Takao-Rikitsu E, et al. ELKS, a protein structurally related to the active zone protein CAST, is involved in Ca2+-dependent exocytosis from PC12 cells. Genes Cells 2006;11:659–672.
42. Hofbauer A. Eine Bibliothek monoklonaler Antikorper gegen das Gehin van Drosophila melanogaster. Habilitation thesis. University of Wurzburg, Wurzburg, Germany, 1991.
43. Rein K, Zockler M, Heisenberg M. A quantitative three-dimensional model of the Drosophila optic lobes. Curr Biol 1999;9:93–96.
44. Crump JG, Zhen M, Jin Y, Bargmann CI. The SAD-1 kinase regulates presynaptic vesicle clustering and axon termination. Neuron 2001;29:115–129.
45. Lonart G, Schoch S, Kaeser PS, Larkin CJ, Südhof TC, Linden DJ. Phosphorylation of RIM1alpha by PKA triggers presynaptic long-term potentiation at cerebellar parallel fiber synapses. Cell 2003;115:49–60.
46. Calakos N, Schoch S, Südhof TC, Malenka RC. Multiple roles for the active zone protein RIM1alpha in late stages of neurotransmitter release. Neuron 2004;42:889–896.
47. Baas AF, Boudeau J, Sapkota GP, et al. Activation of the tumour suppressor kinase LKB1 by the STE20–like pseudokinase STRAD. EMBO J 2003;22:3062–3072.
48. Martin SG, St Johnston D. A role for Drosophila LKB1 in anterior-posterior axis formation and epithelial polarity. Nature 2003;421:379–384.

49. Watts JL, Morton DG., Bestman J, Kemphues KJ. The C. elegans par-4 gene encodes a putative serine-threonine kinase required for establishing embryonic asymmetry, Development 2000;127:1467–1475.
50. Barnes AP, Lilley BN, Pan YA, et al. LKB1 and SAD kinases define a pathway required for the polarization of cortical neurons. Cell 2007;129:459–460.

Chapter 9
The Role of Potassium Channels in the Regulation of Neurotransmitter Release

Laurence O. Trussell and Michael T. Roberts

Contents

Abstract Neurotransmitter release is critically dependent on the duration of the presynaptic action potential. A variety of K$^+$ channels play key roles in determining spike width. Moreover, K$^+$ channels control how readily terminals can spike, and also suppress aberrant firing. Finally, K$^+$ channels, through their control of the presynaptic resting potential, may impact presynaptic calcium levels and the spontaneous and evoked release of transmitter.

Keywords Axon, exocytosis, transmitter release, synapse, potassium channel.

Laurence O. Trussell
Oregon Hearing Research Center / Vollum Institute, Portland, OR 97239, USA
e-mail: trussell@ohsu.edu

Importance of Spike Width

A major role of K⁺ channels in excitable cells is to repolarize the cell membrane potential during an action potential; in this regard they help define the unit of neural coding. But in nerve terminals, these channels take on additional essential functions. Beginning with work on neuromuscular junction and squid giant synapse (1–4), studies over nearly 50 years have shown that neurotransmitter release is acutely sensitive to K⁺ channel antagonists and to the duration of the presynaptic spike; thus, K⁺ channels are essential determinants of synaptic strength. Since the relation between the spike and release is so critical, we will examine it in some detail, in order to better appreciate the roles of particular types of K⁺ channels.

Ca^{2+} enters the nerve terminal during the repolarizing phase of the spike and is the primary chemical messenger triggering exocytosis. The spike thus serves both to activate Ca^{2+} channels while the voltage is positive and to provide electrical driving force for Ca^{2+} entry upon repolarization. In the squid giant synapse and in the mammalian calyx of Held, where careful presynaptic voltage-clamp recordings have been made, it is clear that the peak of Ca^{2+} channel activation occurs just after the crest of the spike (5,6). Although in mammals the spike appears to activate a large fraction of the available Ca^{2+} channels (7), slowing the decay of the spike (i.e., broadening it) increases total Ca^{2+} entry by prolonging the length of time the channels are active. There is a third to fourth power cooperative relationship between Ca^{2+} concentration and vesicle release probability (5,8,9). Consequently, small increments in Ca^{2+} resulting from small changes in spike width can lead to a proportionally greater increase in release. For example, in the squid, an increase of only 30% in spike width, observed with partial inhibition of voltage-gated K⁺ channels, led to a 190% increase in the postsynaptic response (10). An added factor that contributes to this steep sensitivity is the brief duration of Ca^{2+} entry, which limits saturation of the release process (11–13). Thus, by setting spike width K⁺ channels play a critical role in controlling the efficacy of synaptic transmission. Moreover, because the Ca^{2+} influx is greatest upon repolarization, spike width also impacts the synaptic delay (1,2,4,14). Cases should be noted in which spike broadening *reduced* transmitter output (14–16), presumably due to reduced Ca^{2+} driving force (15), but these cases only emphasize the key role of channels that control presynaptic potential changes.

Analysis of Presynaptic K⁺ Channels

Most voltage-gated K⁺ channels can be functionally classified by the voltage range over which they become active and whether or not they inactivate during prolonged or repeated depolarization (17). Further insight into their roles is obtained through the use of channel blockers and genetic deletion. Moreover, some K⁺ channels are activated by Ca^{2+}, and so are dependent on factors regulating Ca^{2+} influx. In studies of the role of K⁺ channels in transmission, a variety of techniques have been applied, but only in a handful of cases have definitive results been obtained. This reflects the fact that K$^+$ channels can alter diverse aspects of synaptic function and that direct assessment of function is difficult to obtain in tiny central nervous system (CNS) synapses. For example, immunolocalization of channels can indicate where they are, but not what they do (18). Application of nonselective K$^+$ channel blockers, such as tetraethylammonium (TEA) (3,4,10) or either 4-aminopyridine (4-AP) or 3,4-diaminopyridine (DAP) (10,19) have long been known to alter evoked exocytosis; however, their usefulness in terms of their ability to identify specific channel subtypes is limited unless other channel subtypes can be excluded with other blockers. Drugs may also change the frequency of spontaneous activity (20), but this does not indicate whether the target channel is axonal or synaptic, or whether the effect of the blocker is to modify the action potential or the resting membrane potential. The most convincing work has explored the presynaptic role of different channel subtypes by using a battery of channel blockers in direct presynaptic recordings of electrical activity. These and other studies are reviewed below (see also refs. 21 and 22).

Role of Kv3 Channels in Presynaptic Spike Repolarization

The Kv3 family of channels comprises four gene products (Kv3.1 to 3.4), many of which are expressed in nerve terminals. Kv3.1 to 3.3 code for weakly inactivating, high-voltage–activated (HVA) channels with rapid gating kinetics, ideal features for enabling consistent spike repolarization during high-frequency activity (17). Indeed, it is now clear that these channels are expressed in subpopulations of neurons that fire at high rates during long depolarizations or fire reliably in phase with high-frequency stimulation (23). In the calyx of Held, voltage-step experiments reveal an HVA outward current sensitive to the same concentrations of extracellular TEA that block postsynaptic Kv3.1 channels or Kv3.1 channels in heterologous expression systems (24). Moreover, subunits for Kv3.1 and 3.3 show strong expression in the calyx of Held, colocalizing with presynaptic markers. At the electron microscopy (EM) level, antibodies to Kv3.1b label the presynaptic membranes away from the synaptic cleft. TEA both widened the presynaptic spike and increased the postsynaptic excitatory postsynaptic current (EPSC) amplitude and time course, the latter presumably because more transmitter was released over a longer time (24,25). Kv3.4 is localized at many nerve terminals (26), encodes an inactivating channel when expressed heterologously (17), and is also found in the calyx of Held (24). However, there is little evidence so far for a fast inactivating TEA-sensitive channel in the calyx; in addition, repetitive action potential trains, which might be expected to generate cumulative inactivation of K$^+$ current, exhibit little spike broadening (25). Thus, it may be that Kv3.4 channels form a heteromultimeric complex with other Kv3 subunits (27). Although TEA also blocks several other Kv channel subunits, additional studies with selective antagonists to the Kv1 family subunits indicated different roles for those channels in the calyx (as discussed in the following section).

Direct presynaptic recordings have been made from terminals of cerebellar basket cells, a γ–aminobutyric acid (GABA)ergic interneuron, revealing an HVA outward current blocked by TEA (28). It seems, however, that these channels do not alter the presynaptic spike or transmitter release in basket cell terminals, as moderate bath concentrations of TEA did not affect presynaptic Ca^{2+} transients and only moderately increased IPSC amplitude (29,30). This points to an important caveat in interpreting studies in this field: the presence of a channel, determined either by immunohistochemical or even physiologic means, cannot by itself be taken as evidence that the channel plays a functional role!

Immunolocalization studies place Kv3 channels in a wide variety of nerve terminals, suggesting that their functional role as revealed in the calyx may be true for many brain regions (18,26,31,32). Rarely has this been confirmed with functional studies. A particularly compelling case was made by Goldberg et al (33). Recording from fast-spiking neocortical interneurons and their targets, these authors observed that the amplitudes of inhibitory postsynaptic currents (IPSCs) were increased by 1 mM TEA and that paired-pulse ratios decreased, a sign of elevated transmitter release probability. This effect was absent in double knockout mice lacking the Kv3.1 and 3.2 genes. Moreover, imaging studies revealed that TEA enhanced Ca^{2+} transients in boutons made by interneurons. Dendrotoxin, a blocker of Kv1 channels, had little effect. In another study, the double knockout mice were used to examine cerebellar function, finding that transmission in parallel fibers was impaired and postsynaptic responses to parallel fiber activation showed reduced paired-pulse ratios, consistent with a broadened presynaptic spike (34).

Kv1-Family Channels: Diverse Actions on Presynaptic Function

This family comprises seven genes, Kv1.1 to 1.7 (17). Channels composed of tetrameric subsets of Kv1 subunits, particularly Kv1.1, 1.2 and 1.4, are associated with a slowly inactivating outward current that activates at potentials relatively hyperpolarized to that of Kv3 channels (the so-called low-voltage–activated [LVA] channel). Immunolocalization studies clearly place members of this family in axonal and preterminal membranes (18). However, their roles in presynaptic function divide into two quite distinct (but not mutually exclusive) categories.

Adjustment of Presynaptic Membrane Potential and Excitability

Kv1.1 and 1.2 channels localize to the preterminal membrane of the calyx of Held, and calyx recordings revealed LVA outward currents blocked by the Kv1 antagonists dendrotoxin-I or -K, margatoxin, and tityustoxin (21,24,35). Experiments using mixtures of antagonists suggest that these currents are generated by mixtures of channels, including 1.1/1.2 heteromers and 1.2 homomers (21). Excised patch studies, in which membrane from the calyceal terminal was excised using the out-side-out patch configuration, showed that some Kv1 channels are also in the nerve terminal itself (35). Interestingly, the cell bodies generating the calyx possess a different channel subset, indicating that specific K^+ channels are selectively tar-geted to axonal/synaptic membrane (21). What is the function of these Kv1 chan-nels in synaptic "performance"? In studies of the calyx carried out at room temperature, application of the Kv1 blockers margatoxin or tityustoxin did not alter the width of the presynaptic spike but rather enhanced the likelihood of spiking, both reducing threshold and increasing the number of spikes per stimulus (21,24,35). Such an action is consistent with the idea that an LVA channel helps modify the membrane potential and conductance near rest, and dampens excitability after an action potential.

This proposed role in setting excitability is echoed by studies in several other synapses. The terminals of cerebellar basket cells express a Kv1 current and block of these channels with α-dendrotoxin increases the frequency and amplitude of spontaneous IPSCs in Purkinje cells (28,30). The complement of Kv channels in the terminals was different from that of the parent cell body (36). Kv1.1-null mice have enhanced axonal firing in basket cells, motor nerves, and hippocampus (37,38). The picture then is that K^+ channels that activate near the resting potential serve a "stabilizing" role in presynaptic activity (21). In the cases discussed above, they do not determine spike width, either because they activated too slowly or because they are not expressed at sufficiently high density, relative to Kv3-family ion channels. This point is made clear in experiments in which Kv3 channels were first blocked by TEA; upon subsequent block of Kv1 channels, the presynaptic spike width and the size of the EPSC increased (24).

Spike Broadening and Enhancement of Release

Inactivation of K^+ channels has long been thought to control presynaptic spike width in a use-dependent fashion. Studies on *Drosophila* showed that the product of the *Shaker* gene encoded an inactivating K^+ channel (39) that critically deter-mined the duration of the presynaptic spike (40). In terminals of the posterior pitui-tary, repetitive stimulation increased the output of the hormones oxytocin and vasopressin. Presynaptic recordings revealed that these stimuli resulted in cumula-tive inactivation of an A-type K^+ channel, with a frequency-dependence similar to that of the enhanced hormone release (41). The molecular identity of this channel in pituitary terminals is not clear, however (42).

Definitive evidence for a role for inactivating Kv1 channels in setting spike width at conventional fast synapses comes from the landmark study of Geiger and Jonas (43). Recordings were made from hippocampal mossy fiber boutons in brain slices at near-physiologic temperature. Repetitive stimuli, at rates known to be experienced *in vivo*, elicited presynaptic spikes that broadened dramatically upon increase in duration or frequency of the train. The spike voltage waveforms elicited a dendrotoxin-sensitive outward current showing cumulative inactivation (although the authors did not show that actual presynaptic spikes were broadened by dendrotoxin). Finally, such changes in spike width were shown to increase both presynaptic Ca^{2+} flux and neurotransmitter release. This study shows that short-term synaptic plasticity can be elicited not only by mechanisms such as residual Ca^{2+} and vesicle depletion but also by use-dependent change in spike width.

This scenario is probably also true of cortical pyramidal cells. In direct recordings from axons of layer 5 pyramidal cells of prefrontal cortex, a dendrotoxin-sensitive inactivating K^+ current determined the width of the axonal, but not somatic, spike (44). Weak depolarization of the cell body led to both broadening of the axon spike and enhancement of excitatory postsynaptic potentials (EPSPs) dependent on Kv1 channels. Bursts of EPSPs were passively transmitted to the axon and could therefore provide a means of adjusting axonal membrane potential and spike width (45). A very different picture of the consequences of changes in axonal membrane potential will be discussed below (see Presynaptic Resting Membrane Potential).

Ca^{2+}-Activated K^+ Channels

Big and small conductance, Ca^{2+}-activated, K^+ channels (BK and SK channels, respectively) activate in response to increases in intracellular Ca^{2+} concentration and also, in the case of BK channels, in response to membrane depolarization (46,47). With these properties, BK and SK channels seem particularly well suited to roles in the presynaptic terminal. In the simplest scenario, Ca^{2+}-activated K^+ channels might detect the same Ca^{2+} influx that induces neurotransmitters to release, activate, and conduct outward currents that rapidly repolarize the terminal, limiting action potential width and terminating release. The most direct criteria for establishing the presence of Ca^{2+}-activated K^+ channels involves detection of a K^+ current that increases with increasing cytosolic Ca^{2+} concentrations, or more commonly, requires extracellular Ca^{2+} and is blocked by selective antagonists. Below we focus on presynaptic BK channels, where there is abundant, and controversial, evidence for physiologic roles in fast synaptic transmission. Roles for BK channels in endocrine secretion are not discussed (see refs. 22 and 48).

BK Channels in the Central Nervous System

The presence of BK channels in mammalian central terminals was first suggested by flux studies of rat brain synaptosomes (49). Subsequent immunolocalization and EM studies indicate that BK channel α-subunits achieve significant expression levels in axons and terminals of neurons in hippocampus, cerebellum, and other brain regions (50–54). In the hippocampus, there are conflicting data about the function of presynaptic BK channels. Hu and colleagues (50) examined glutamatergic CA3 synapses onto CA1 pyramidal neurons in rat hippocampal slices. Electron microscopy immunogold labeling demonstrated that BK channel α-subunits were expressed in presynaptic terminals located in CA1 stratum radiatum, where they were generally found adjacent to postsynaptic densities expressing N-methyl-D-aspartate (NMDA) receptor subunits. Application of iberiotoxin (IbTX) both increased postsynaptic potentials and broadened presynaptic spikes. However, this IbTX effect occurred only in the presence of the voltage-gated K^+ channel blocker 4-AP, which significantly broadened presynaptic action potentials on its own. The interpretation of this result was that presynaptic BK channels generally do not affect terminal excitability, but that under extreme, possibly even pathologic, circumstances they may limit excitability.

A later examination of CA3 to CA3 synapses arrived at a different conclusion. Raffaelli and colleagues (55), using rat hippocampal slice cultures, found that IbTX and paxilline (another BK blocker) increased the frequency, but not the amplitude, of spontaneous EPSCs. In dual recordings from synaptically connected CA3 pyramidal cells in the absence of 4-AP, paxilline and IbTX decreased the transmission failure rate, increased the amplitude of EPSCs, and decreased the paired-pulse ratio. Showing that BK blockers broadened somatic action potentials, the authors proposed that presynaptic BK channels limit the excitability of terminals under physiologic conditions. Differences in preparation (culture vs. acute slice), recording temperatures, or developmental stages might explain these conflicting results. It is notable that the postsynaptic cells in the two studies were different; perhaps subunit-specific differences in BK kinetics or expression level vary among terminals of the same neuron.

While immunohistochemistry indicates that basket cell terminals of the cerebellum express high levels of BK channel α-subunits (52), physiologic studies have failed to uncover a functional role. Conflicting results exist regarding whether the BK blocker charybdotoxin (CTX) blocks somatic K^+ currents of basket cells (28,30). CTX increased the frequency of spontaneous (TTX-dependent) IPSCs recorded in Purkinje cells, the postsynaptic target of basket cells, and increased spike-evoked Ca^{2+} transients in basket cell terminals; however, the latter effect was only seen when CTX was coapplied with 4-AP. Since IbTX did not alter the frequency of spontaneous IPSCs and since CTX may also block some Kv1 channels (56), it is likely that the CTX effects in basket cells were not caused by BK channel block.

At the rat calyx of Held, an IbTX-sensitive current contributes 12% of total presynaptic K^+ current (24). IbTX, however, had no effect on evoked EPSCs recorded from postsynaptic medial nucleus of the trapezoid body (MNTB) neurons. It was suggested that this was due to the kinetics of BK channel activation, which may be too slow in the calyx to allow BK channels to contribute to action potential repolarization, a conclusion also applied to the presynaptic Ca^{2+}-dependent K^+ current of squid giant synapse (10). An investigation of developmental changes in calyx K^+ currents occurring over the second postnatal week found that BK current densities remained constant over this period (35), in contrast to Kv1 and Kv3 channels, which increased markedly. Finally, IbTX had no effect on the ability of the calyx to follow high-frequency trains of action potentials.

BK Channels at the Neuromuscular Junction

As with CNS synapses, BK channels are present in many motor nerve terminals, but reports conflict as to their functional roles. Mallart (57) first identified a Ca^{2+}- and TEA-sensitive K^+ current in extracellular recordings from mouse triangularis sterni nerve endings. Similar currents were soon recorded from terminals at the frog and lizard neuromuscular junction (NMJ) and found to be blocked by CTX (58–60). However, studies of frog, lizard, and mouse NMJ have suggested that prior block of voltage-gated K^+ channels by diaminopyridine is required to resolve clear effects of CTX (58–60). Moreover, in zebrafish NMJ, neither IbTx, CTX, nor paxilline altered EPSCs in control conditions (14).

Several reports examined voltage changes in the preterminal axon of NMJ using intracellular microelectrodes. In recordings from lizard NMJ (61), reduction of bath Ca^{2+} had no effect on the spike unless presumptive delayed rectifier channels (possibly Kv1) were first blocked with 4-AP. The authors found that under these conditions a BK component probably played a role in spike repolarization while SK channels may generate a slow afterhyperpolarization. Thus, two Ca^{2+}-activated K^+ channel subtypes are present, but it remains uncertain from this work what their role is under physiologic conditions. In crayfish NMJ, intraterminal recordings showed components of the spike sensitive to blockers of both delayed rectifier and Ca^{2+}-activated K^+ channels (62,63). When delayed rectifiers were preblocked, subsequent addition of TEA potently lengthened the spike, increased transmitter release, and altered the relation between presynaptic potential and synaptic facilitation.

Robitaille and colleagues (64,65) used the frog NMJ to examine the effect of BK channels on neurotransmitter release, finding that CTX and IbTX increased the amplitude of end-plate potentials elicited by motor nerve stimulation. Using a Ca^{2+} sensitive dye, it was found that CTX increased the magnitude of terminal Ca^{2+} transients. Bath application of membrane permeant forms of the fast Ca^{2+} buffer 1,2-bis (o-aminophenoxy)ethane-N,N,N′,N′-tetraacetic acid (BAPTA), but not the slow buffer ethyleneglycoltetraacetic acid (EGTA), increased end-plate potentials when loaded into terminals. Labeling of the NMJ with a CTX-biotin conjugate revealed colocalization of BK channels and Ca^{2+} channels in terminals, suggesting that BK channels are activated by high, local concentrations of Ca^{2+}.

A presynaptic role of BK channels has been studied in nerve-muscle cultures from *Xenopus* embryos, which makes possible simultaneous recordings of presynaptic currents and postsynaptic potentials. Using this preparation, it was shown that CTX and IbTX block a presynaptic outward current that is activated during the rising phase of the action potential (66). Ca^{2+} influx through an ω-CgTx sensitive Ca^{2+} current was necessary to activate the BK current. In fact, the coupling between this Ca^{2+} current and presynaptic BK currents was so tight that a subsequent study was able to utilize BK currents to estimate the time course and peak concentrations of Ca^{2+} occurring at the active zone during an action potential (67). Further experiments with this preparation showed that block of terminal BK channels caused a paradoxical *decrease* in end-plate current amplitudes (15). The authors explained this result by demonstrating that action potential broadening could, under very specific conditions, decrease peak Ca^{2+} influx, presumably by decreasing the Ca^{2+} driving force. It should be noted that effectiveness of CTX in the *Xenopus* work and the work of Robitaille and colleagues (64,65) compared to previous work suggests that batch-dependent variation in drug quality or selectivity might account for why pre-block of other K^+ channels was sometimes necessary.

Interestingly, a genetic approach in *Caenorhabditis elegans* also found a central role for BK channels in neuromuscular transmission. Undertaking a genome-wide screen for mutations able to rescue a *C. elegans* mutant paralyzed by a deficiency in synaptic transmission, Wang and colleagues (68) identified loss-of-function mutations in the *slo-1* BK channel gene as the only K^+ channel mutations able to increase synaptic release and restore movement. Consistent with a role for BK channels at motor nerve terminals, immunolocalization of wild-type BK channels demonstrated expression at the NMJ, and recordings from body-wall muscle cells showed that the *slo-1* mutants exhibited prolonged EPSCs and increased quantal content when compared to wild type worms.

BK Channels in Sensory Receptors

Hair Cells

Cochlear and vestibular hair cells convert the force of displacement of their stereo-cilia into electrical potentials, leading to neurotransmitter release onto afferent fibers. Unlike conventional CNS synapses, most mature hair cells do not fire action potentials. Instead, direct current (DC) or phase-locked changes in membrane potential trigger exocytosis (69–71). The functions of BK channels in hair cells of mammalian and nonmammalian vertebrates appear to differ. Localization studies show that BK channel α-subunits are expressed along with Ca^{2+} channels at the hair cell active zone in several nonmammalian species (72–74). In turtle, frog, and chick, the balance of BK and voltage-gated Ca^{2+} channels allows hair cells to be electrically tuned to specific frequencies of stereociliary vibration; systematic variation in BK channel properties along the cochlear tonotopic axis contributes to hair cell tuning across the sound frequency spectrum (69,75). This modulation seems to result from tonotopically regulated changes in alternative splicing, association with accessory subunits, and phosphorylation.

In mammals, BK currents comprise a large portion of inner hair cell K^+ current and significantly lower the membrane time constant, enabling rapid signal transduction (76). CTX and IbTX perfusion into the cochlea significantly block sound-evoked, compound action potentials recorded from guinea pig auditory nerve, although this is likely due to direct block of BK channels in the auditory nerve (77,78). Immunostaining revealed that BK channels are localized to the apical region of mammalian hair cells, away from the basal active zone (79). Surprisingly, gene knockout studies indicate that transmitter release by hair cells is not much affected by loss of BK function (77,80), as compared to release from their nonmammalian counterparts.

Retinal Synapses

The earliest functional evidence for expression of Ca^{2+}-activated K^+ channels at presynaptic terminals came from studies of barnacle photoreceptor neurons (81,82). More recent studies have examined BK channel contributions to terminal excitability at two vertebrate retinal synapses. Goldfish bipolar cell terminals are large enough to permit direct, whole-cell recordings. Terminals severed from bipolar cell somata exhibited a large, CTX- and TEA-sensitive outward current (83,84). The rapid activation kinetics and BAPTA resistance of this BK current indicated that most terminal BK channels reside in close proximity to voltage-gated Ca^{2+} channels (84). Cell-attached recordings revealed a correlation between membrane patches exhibiting exocytosis and those expressing BK currents (85). Terminals of the Mb1 class of bipolar cells give rise to Ca^{2+}-dependent action potentials for which BK channels provide most of the repolarizing current (86). These action potentials reliably induce neurotransmitter release, as demonstrated by capacitance measurements.

Like cochlear hair cells, salamander rod photoreceptors use membrane depolarization, but not action potentials, to elicit neurotransmitter release. Conflicting reports indicate that the majority of rod BK channels are expressed in either terminals (87) or the soma (88). BK channel blockers were found to inhibit rod Ca^{2+} currents and decrease EPSC amplitudes in postsynaptic cells, suggesting that rod terminal BK channels normally promote release (87). This might occur through a mechanism in which BK-mediated K^+ accumulation in the synaptic cleft leads to an enhancement of Ca^{2+} channel function.

Presynaptic Resting Membrane Potential

Many studies indicate that transmitter release can be modulated by relatively small changes in the resting membrane potential of nerve terminals. For example, in the calyx of Held, subthreshold depolarization weakly activates Ca^{2+} channels, which, over time, leads to enhancement of release probability (89). Such studies highlight the need to explore an area that has received very little attention thus far: the ion channels that underlie the resting potential of a synapse. Typically, the resting potential reflects the sum of several inward and outward currents that may be voltage dependent and independent; however, the particular complement of channels serving these roles may vary widely with cell type. In octopus cell bodies of the cochlear nucleus, the resting potential is determined by the resting level of activation of Kv1 and HCN ("I_H") channels (90,91). In sympathetic neurons, the resting potential is generated by a balance of inward rectifying K^+ channels, leak K^+ channels, and electrogenic activity of the Na-K–adenosine triphosphatase (ATPase) (92). Recent studies have pointed to the roles of two-pore K^+ channels, which comprise a large family of channels with varying types of modulation (93); these may account in part for K^+ leak currents. Indeed, in cerebellar granule cells, these channels may contribute a voltage independent leak that sets the resting potential (94). However, little information is available on which channels are open at rest in a synapse. In the calyx of Held, the resting potential may reflect a balance in activity of HCN and Na-K-ATPase (95); however, the role of resting K$^+$ channels has not been explored at this synapse. One indirect approach that has been used at less accessible synapses is to test K$^+$ channel blockers on the frequency of miniature synaptic currents, which reflect spike-independent release. In neurons isolated from substantia nigra, Kv1 antagonists increased the spontaneous synaptic release rate, indicating that these channels must contribute to the resting presynaptic conductance, such that blocking them depolarized the terminal (20). However this approach, when applied to more intact tissue, must be viewed with caution, as subthreshold voltage changes in the axon or even cell body may be passively transmitted to nerve terminals (45,96). The latter observations also suggest that modulation of K$^+$ channels far from a terminal may have consequences for synaptic function.

Conclusion

Kv1, Kv3, and BK channels have proven roles in controlling exocytosis, but do so in different ways in different terminals. Kv3 functions to repolarize the presynaptic spike and provides a consistent, use-independent tuning of presynaptic Ca^{2+} flux. The ability of Kv1 to inactivate during sequential spikes endows terminals with a mechanism for facilitating Ca^{2+} influx during high-frequency activity. In other terminals, these same channels serve as a brake, preventing multiple back-firings when a single spike invades the terminal. BK channels have a broad distribution but seem to repolarize spikes mainly in subsets of neuromuscular junctions; perhaps modulation of these channels dynamically enhances or diminishes their contribution to spike repolarization and accounts for inconsistencies in the ability to detect their function.

Acknowledgments We wish to thank Drs. Paul Brehm, Hai Huang, and Sid Kuo for comments on the manuscript. This work was supported by National Institutes of Health (NIH) grants NS28901 and DC04450.

References

1. Katz B, Miledi R. A study of synaptic transmission in the absence of nerve impulses. J Physiol 1967;192(2):407–436.
2. Katz B, Miledi R. The release of acetylcholine from nerve endings by graded electric pulses. Proc R Soc Lond B Biol Sci 1967;167(6):23–38.
3. Koketsu K. Action of tetraethylammonium chloride on neuromuscular transmission in frogs. Am J Physiol 1958;193(1):213–218.
4. Kusano K, Livengood DR, Werman R. Tetraethylammonium ions: effect of presynaptic injection on synaptic transmission. Science 1967;155(767):1257–1259.

5. Borst JG, Sakmann B. Calcium influx and transmitter release in a fast CNS synapse. Nature 1996;383(6599):431–434.
6. Llinas R, Sugimori M, Simon SM. Transmission by presynaptic spike-like depolarization in the squid giant synapse. Proc Natl Acad Sci U S A 1982;79(7):2415–2419.
7. Borst JG, Sakmann B. Calcium current during a single action potential in a large presynaptic terminal of the rat brainstem. J Physiol 1998;506(pt 1):143–157.
8. Augustine GJ, Charlton MP, Smith SJ. Calcium entry into voltage-clamped presynaptic terminals of squid. J Physiol 1985;367:143–162.
9. Dodge FA Jr, Rahamimoff R. Co-operative action a calcium ions in transmitter release at the neuromuscular junction. J Physiol 1967;193(2):419–432.
10. Augustine GJ. Regulation of transmitter release at the squid giant synapse by presynaptic delayed rectifier potassium current. J Physiol 1990;431:343–364.
11. Bollmann JH, Sakmann B. Control of synaptic strength and timing by the release-site Ca2+ signal. Nat Neurosci 2005;8(4):426–434.
12. Fedchyshyn MJ, Wang LY. Developmental transformation of the release modality at the calyx of Held synapse. J Neurosci 2005;25(16):4131–4140.
13. Yang YM, Wang LY. Amplitude and kinetics of action potential-evoked Ca2+ current and its efficacy in triggering transmitter release at the developing calyx of held synapse. J Neurosci 2006;26(21):5698–5708.
14. Wen H, Brehm P. Paired motor neuron-muscle recordings in zebrafish test the receptor blockade model for shaping synaptic current. J Neurosci 2005;25(35):8104–8111.
15. Pattillo JM, Yazejian B, DiGregorio DA, Vergara JL, Grinnell AD, Meriney SD. Contribution of presynaptic calcium-activated potassium currents to transmitter release regulation in cultured Xenopus nerve-muscle synapses. Neuroscience 2001;102(1):229–240.
16. Spencer AN, Przysiezniak J, Acosta-Urquidi J, Basarsky TA. Presynaptic spike broadening reduces junctional potential amplitude. Nature 1989;340(6235):636–638.
17. Coetzee WA, Amarillo Y, Chiu J, et al. Molecular diversity of K+ channels. Ann N Y Acad Sci 1999;868:233–285.
18. Trimmer JS, Rhodes KJ. Localization of voltage-gated ion channels in mammalian brain. Annu Rev Physiol 2004;66:477–519.
19. Thesleff S. Aminopyridines and synaptic transmission. Neuroscience 1980;5(8): 1413–1419.
20. Shimada H, Uta D, Nabekura J, Yoshimura M. Involvement of Kv channel subtypes on GABA release in mechanically dissociated neurons from the rat substantia nigra. Brain Res 2007; 1141:74–83.
21. Dodson PD, Forsythe ID. Presynaptic K+ channels: electrifying regulators of synaptic terminal excitability. Trends Neurosci 2004;27(4):210–217.
22. Jackson MB. Presynaptic excitability. Int Rev Neurobiol 1995;38:201–251.
23. Li W, Kaczmarek LK, Perney TM. Localization of two high-threshold potassium channel subunits in the rat central auditory system. J Comp Neurol 2001;437(2):196–218.
24. Ishikawa T, Nakamura Y, Saitoh N, Li WB, Iwasaki S, Takahashi T. Distinct roles of Kv1 and Kv3 potassium channels at the calyx of Held presynaptic terminal. J Neurosci 2003; 23(32):10445–10453.
25. Wang LY, Kaczmarek LK. High-frequency firing helps replenish the readily releasable pool of synaptic vesicles. Nature 1998;394(6691):384–388.
26. Brooke RE, Atkinson L, Batten TF, Deuchars SA, Deuchars J. Association of potassium channel Kv3.4 subunits with pre- and post-synaptic structures in brainstem and spinal cord. Neuroscience 2004;126(4):1001–1010.
27. Baranauskas G, Tkatch T, Nagata K, Yeh JZ, Surmeier DJ. Kv3.4 subunits enhance the repolarizing efficiency of Kv3.1 channels in fast-spiking neurons. Nat Neurosci 2003;6(3):258–266.
28. Southan AP, Robertson B. Electrophysiological characterization of voltage-gated K(+) currents in cerebellar basket and Purkinje cells: Kv1 and Kv3 channel subfamilies are present in basket cell nerve terminals. J Neurosci 2000;20(1):114–122.

29. Southan AP, Robertson B. Modulation of inhibitory post-synaptic currents (IPSCs) in mouse cerebellar Purkinje and basket cells by snake and scorpion toxin K+ channel blockers. Br J Pharmacol 1998;125(6):1375–1381.
30. Tan YP, Llano I. Modulation by K+ channels of action potential-evoked intracellular Ca2+ concentration rises in rat cerebellar basket cell axons. J Physiol 1999;520(pt 1):65–78.
31. Brooke RE, Atkinson L, Edwards I, Parson SH, Deuchars J. Immunohistochemical localisation of the voltage gated potassium ion channel subunit Kv3.3 in the rat medulla oblongata and thoracic spinal cord. Brain Res 2006;1070(1):101–115.
32. Chang SY, Zagha E, Kwon ES, et al. Distribution of Kv3.3 potassium channel subunits in distinct neuronal populations of mouse brain. J Comp Neurol 2007;502(6):953–972.
33. Goldberg EM, Watanabe S, Chang SY, et al. Specific functions of synaptically localized potassium channels in synaptic transmission at the neocortical GABAergic fast-spiking cell synapse. J Neurosci 2005;25(21):5230–5235.
34. Matsukawa H, Wolf AM, Matsushita S, Joho RH, Knopfel T. Motor dysfunction and altered synaptic transmission at the parallel fiber-Purkinje cell synapse in mice lacking potassium channels Kv3.1 and Kv3.3. J Neurosci 2003;23(20):7677–7684.
35. Nakamura Y, Takahashi T. Developmental changes in potassium currents at the rat calyx of Held presynaptic terminal. J Physiol 2007;581(pt 3):1101–1112.
36. Southan AP, Robertson B. Patch-clamp recordings from cerebellar basket cell bodies and their presynaptic terminals reveal an asymmetric distribution of voltage-gated potassium channels. J Neurosci 1998;18(3):948–955.
37. Smart SL, Lopantsev V, Zhang CL, et al. Deletion of the K(V)1.1 potassium channel causes epilepsy in mice. Neuron 1998;20(4):809–819.
38. Zhang CL, Messing A, Chiu SY. Specific alteration of spontaneous GABAergic inhibition in cerebellar purkinje cells in mice lacking the potassium channel Kv1. 1. J Neurosci 1999;19(8):2852–2864.
39. Timpe LC, Schwarz TL, Tempel BL, Papazian DM, Jan YN, Jan LY. Expression of functional potassium channels from Shaker cDNA in Xenopus oocytes. Nature 1988;331(6152):143–145.
40. Jan YN, Jan LY, Dennis MJ. Two mutations of synaptic transmission in Drosophila. Proc R Soc Lond B Biol Sci 1977;198(1130):87–108.
41. Jackson MB, Konnerth A, Augustine GJ. Action potential broadening and frequency-dependent facilitation of calcium signals in pituitary nerve terminals. Proc Natl Acad Sci U S A 1991;88(2):380–384.
42. Bielefeldt K, Rotter JL, Jackson MB. Three potassium channels in rat posterior pituitary nerve terminals. J Physiol 1992;458:41–67.
43. Geiger JR, Jonas P. Dynamic control of presynaptic Ca(2+) inflow by fast-inactivating K(+) channels in hippocampal mossy fiber boutons. Neuron 2000;28(3):927–939.
44. Shu Y, Yu Y, Yang J, McCormick DA. Selective control of cortical axonal spikes by a slowly inactivating K+ current. Proc Natl Acad Sci U S A 2007;104(27):11453–11458.
45. Shu Y, Hasenstaub A, Duque A, Yu Y, McCormick DA. Modulation of intracortical synaptic potentials by presynaptic somatic membrane potential. Nature 2006;441(7094):761–765.
46. Bond CT, Maylie J, Adelman JP. SK channels in excitability, pacemaking and synaptic integration. Curr Opin Neurobiol 2005;15(3):305–311.
47. Latorre R, Brauchi S. Large conductance Ca2+-activated K+ (BK) channel: activation by Ca2+ and voltage. Biol Res 2006;39(3):385–401.
48. Solaro CR, Prakriya M, Ding JP, Lingle CJ. Inactivating and noninactivating Ca(2+)- and voltage-dependent K+ current in rat adrenal chromaffin cells. J Neurosci 1995;15(9):6110–6123.
49. Bartschat DK, Blaustein MP. Calcium-activated potassium channels in isolated presynaptic nerve terminals from rat brain. J Physiol 1985;361:441–457.
50. Hu H, Shao LR, Chavoshy S, et al. Presynaptic Ca2+-activated K+ channels in glutamatergic hippocampal terminals and their role in spike repolarization and regulation of transmitter release. J Neurosci 2001;21(24):9585–9597.
51. Knaus HG, Schwarzer C, Koch RO, et al. Distribution of high-conductance Ca(2+)-activated K+ channels in rat brain: targeting to axons and nerve terminals. J Neurosci 1996;16(3):955–963.

52. Misonou H, Menegola M, Buchwalder L, et al. Immunolocalization of the Ca2+-activated K+ channel Slo1 in axons and nerve terminals of mammalian brain and cultured neurons. J Comp Neurol 2006;496(3):289–302.
53. Sailer CA, Kaufmann WA, Kogler M, et al. Immunolocalization of BK channels in hippocampal pyramidal neurons. Eur J Neurosci 2006;24(2):442–454.
54. Sausbier U, Sausbier M, Sailer CA, et al. Ca2+ -activated K+ channels of the BK-type in the mouse brain. Histochem Cell Biol 2006;125(6):725–741.
55. Raffaelli G, Saviane C, Mohajerani MH, Pedarzani P, Cherubini E. BK potassium channels control transmitter release at CA3–CA3 synapses in the rat hippocampus. J Physiol 2004;557(pt 1):147–157.
56. MacKinnon R, Reinhart PH, White MM. Charybdotoxin block of Shaker K+ channels suggests that different types of K+ channels share common structural features. Neuron 1988;1 (10):997–1001.
57. Mallart A. A calcium-activated potassium current in motor nerve terminals of the mouse. J Physiol 1985;368:577–591.
58. Anderson AJ, Harvey AL, Rowan EG, Strong PN. Effects of charybdotoxin, a blocker of Ca2+-activated K+ channels, on motor nerve terminals. Br J Pharmacol 1988;95(4):1329–1335.
59. Hevron E, David G, Arnon A, Yaari Y. Acetylcholine modulates two types of presynaptic potassium channels in vertebrate motor nerve terminals. Neurosci Lett 1986;72(1):87–92.
60. Lindgren CA, Moore JW. Identification of ionic currents at presynaptic nerve endings of the lizard. J Physiol 1989;414:201–222.
61. Morita K, Barrett EF. Evidence for two calcium-dependent potassium conductances in lizard motor nerve terminals. J Neurosci 1990;10(8):2614–2625.
62. Sivaramakrishnan S, Bittner GD, Brodwick MS. Calcium-activated potassium conductance in presynaptic terminals at the crayfish neuromuscular junction. J Gen Physiol 1991;98(6): 1161–1179.
63. Sivaramakrishnan S, Brodwick MS, Bittner GD. Presynaptic facilitation at the crayfish neuromuscular junction. Role of calcium-activated potassium conductance. J Gen Physiol 1991;98(6):1181–1196.
64. Robitaille R, Charlton MP. Presynaptic calcium signals and transmitter release are modulated by calcium-activated potassium channels. J Neurosci 1992;12(1):297–305.
65. Robitaille R, Garcia ML, Kaczorowski GJ, Charlton MP. Functional colocalization of calcium and calcium-gated potassium channels in control of transmitter release. Neuron 1993;11(4):645–655.
66. Yazejian B, DiGregorio DA, Vergara JL, Poage RE, Meriney SD, Grinnell AD. Direct measurements of presynaptic calcium and calcium-activated potassium currents regulating neurotransmitter release at cultured Xenopus nerve-muscle synapses. J Neurosci 1997;17 (9):2990–3001.
67. Yazejian B, Sun XP, Grinnell AD. Tracking presynaptic Ca2+ dynamics during neurotransmitter release with Ca2+-activated K+ channels. Nat Neurosci 2000;3(6):566–571.
68. Wang ZW, Saifee O, Nonet ML, Salkoff L. SLO-1 potassium channels control quantal content of neurotransmitter release at the C. elegans neuromuscular junction. Neuron 2001;32(5): 867–881.
69. Fettiplace R, Fuchs PA. Mechanisms of hair cell tuning. Annu Rev Physiol 1999; 61:809–834.
70. Fuchs PA. Time and intensity coding at the hair cell's ribbon synapse. J Physiol 2005;566 (pt 1):7–12.
71. Moser T, Neef A, Khimich D. Mechanisms underlying the temporal precision of sound coding at the inner hair cell ribbon synapse. J Physiol 2006;576(pt 1):55–62.
72. Issa NP, Hudspeth AJ. Clustering of Ca2+ channels and Ca(2+)-activated K+ channels at fluorescently labeled presynaptic active zones of hair cells. Proc Natl Acad Sci U S A 1994;91(16):7578–7582.
73. Roberts WM, Jacobs RA, Hudspeth AJ. Colocalization of ion channels involved in frequency selectivity and synaptic transmission at presynaptic active zones of hair cells. J Neurosci 1990;10(11):3664–3684.

74. Samaranayake H, Saunders JC, Greene MI, Navaratnam DS. Ca(2+) and K(+) (BK) channels in chick hair cells are clustered and colocalized with apical-basal and tonotopic gradients. J Physiol 2004;560(pt 1):13–20.
75. Housley GD, Marcotti W, Navaratnam D, Yamoah EN. Hair cells–beyond the transducer. J Membr Biol 2006;209(2–3):89–118.
76. Kros CJ, Ruppersberg JP, Rusch A. Expression of a potassium current in inner hair cells during development of hearing in mice. Nature 1998;394(6690):281–284.
77. Oliver D, Taberner AM, Thurm H, et al. The role of BKCa channels in electrical signal encoding in the mammalian auditory periphery. J Neurosci 2006;26(23):6181–6189.
78. Skinner LJ, Enee V, Beurg M, et al. Contribution of BK Ca2+-activated K+ channels to auditory neurotransmission in the Guinea pig cochlea. J Neurophysiol 2003;90(1):320–332.
79. Pyott SJ, Glowatzki E, Trimmer JS, Aldrich RW. Extrasynaptic localization of inactivating calcium-activated potassium channels in mouse inner hair cells. J Neurosci 2004;24 (43):9469–9474.
80. Pyott SJ, Meredith AL, Fodor AA, Vazquez AE, Yamoah EN, Aldrich RW. Cochlear function in mice lacking the BK channel alpha, beta1, or beta4 subunits. J Biol Chem 2007;282 (5):3312–3324.
81. Edgington DR, Stuart AE. Properties of tetraethylammonium ion-resistant K+ channels in the photoreceptor membrane of the giant barnacle. J Gen Physiol 1981;77(6):629–646.
82. Stockbridge N, Ross WN. Localized Ca2+ and calcium-activated potassium conductances in terminals of a barnacle photoreceptor. Nature 1984;309(5965):266–268.
83. Burrone J, Lagnado L. Electrical resonance and Ca2+ influx in the synaptic terminal of depolarizing bipolar cells from the goldfish retina. J Physiol 1997;505(pt 3):571–584.
84. Sakaba T, Ishikane H, Tachibana M. Ca2+-activated K+ current at presynaptic terminals of goldfish retinal bipolar cells. Neurosci Res 1997;27(3):219–228.
85. Llobet A, Cooke A, Lagnado L. Exocytosis at the ribbon synapse of retinal bipolar cells studied in patches of presynaptic membrane. J Neurosci 2003;23(7):2706–2714.
86. Palmer MJ. Modulation of Ca(2+)-activated K+ currents and Ca(2+)-dependent action potentials by exocytosis in goldfish bipolar cell terminals. J Physiol 2006;572(pt 3):747–762.
87. Xu JW, Slaughter MM. Large-conductance calcium-activated potassium channels facilitate transmitter release in salamander rod synapse. J Neurosci 2005;25(33):7660–7668.
88. Macleish PR, Nurse CA. Ion channel compartments in photoreceptors: evidence from salamander rods with intact and ablated terminals. J Neurophysiol 2007;98(1):86–95.
89. Awatramani GB, Price GD, Trussell LO. Modulation of transmitter release by presynaptic resting potential and background calcium levels. Neuron 2005;48(1):109–121.
90. Bal R, Oertel D. Hyperpolarization-activated, mixed-cation current (I(h)) in octopus cells of the mammalian cochlear nucleus. J Neurophysiol 2000;84(2):806–817.
91. Bal R, Oertel D. Potassium currents in octopus cells of the mammalian cochlear nucleus. J Neurophysiol 2001;86(5):2299–2311.
92. Jones SW. On the resting potential of isolated frog sympathetic neurons. Neuron 1989;3(2):153–161.
93. Plant LD, Rajan S, Goldstein SA. K2P channels and their protein partners. Curr Opin Neurobiol 2005;15(3):326–333.
94. Aller MI, Veale EL, Linden AM, et al. Modifying the subunit composition of TASK channels alters the modulation of a leak conductance in cerebellar granule neurons. J Neurosci 2005;25(49):11455–11467.
95. Kim JH, Sizov I, Dobretsov M, von Gersdorff H. Presynaptic Ca2+ buffers control the strength of a fast post-tetanic hyperpolarization mediated by the alpha3 Na(+)/K(+)-ATPase. Nat Neurosci 2007;10(2):196–205.
96. Alle H, Geiger JR. Combined analog and action potential coding in hippocampal mossy fibers. Science 2006;311(5765):1290–1293.

Chapter 10
Modulation of Neurotransmitter Release and Presynaptic Plasticity by Protein Phosphorylation

Zu-Hang Sheng

Contents

Abstract Second-messenger regulation of protein interactions in the synaptic vesicle release machinery is one mechanism by which cellular events modulate synaptic transmission. Identification of protein kinases and their targets at nerve terminals, particularly those functionally regulated by synaptic activity or intracellular [Ca2+], is critical to understand the modulation of neurotransmitter release and synaptic plasticity. The phosphorylation and dephosphorylation states of soluble N-ethylmale-imide–sensitive factor attachment receptor (SNARE) proteins and their regulatory components can regulate the biochemical pathways leading from synaptic vesicle docking and priming to fusion. Recent advances in experimental tools, including genetic manipulation in murine models, expression of mutant proteins via transfec-

Zu-Hang Sheng
Synaptic Function Section, National Institute of Neurological Disorders and Stroke,
National Institutes of Health, Bethesda, Maryland 20892-3701, USA
e-mail: shengz@ninds.nih.gov

Z.-W. Wang (ed.) *Molecular Mechanisms of Neurotransmitter Release,*
© Humana Press 2008 a part of Springer Science+Business Media, LLC

tion and viral infection in primary neuronal cultures, and the generation of phospho-specific antibodies, have allowed the study of the functional involvement of protein phosphorylation in synaptic vesicle exocytosis. This chapter provides an overview of the candidate targets of the second messenger–activated protein serine-threonine kinases in the release machinery, and discusses the potential impact of these phosphorylation events in synaptic strength and presynaptic plasticity.

Keywords Synaptic vesicle, docking, priming, presynaptic, exocytosis, phosphorylation, calcium/calmodulin-dependent protein kinase II (CaMKII), cAMP-dependent protein kinase (PKA), protein kinase C (PKC), SNAREs, release machinery, synaptic plasticity.

Activity-dependent plasticity of synaptic transmission is central to the process of information storage in the brain. Synapses are composed of two functionally connected units: the presynaptic compartment, where there is a large number of proteins constituting the synaptic vesicle release machinery, and the postsynaptic apparatus, which detects transmitters and propagates signals. Neurotransmitter release involves a series of protein interactions between the membranes of synaptic vesicles and presynaptic terminals, culminating in the calcium-dependent fusion of the two membranes (see Chapter 3). The synaptic vesicle-associated membrane protein synaptobrevin (VAMP) interacts with two plasma membrane-associated proteins, synaptosome-associated protein of 25 kDa (SNAP-25) and syntaxin, to form a stable soluble N-ethylmaleimide–sensitive factor attachment receptor (SNARE) complex (also called core complex). Formation of the SNARE complex is proposed to bring the vesicular and plasma membranes into close apposition, providing the energy to drive mixing of the two lipid bilayers. The final stages of vesicle fusion, however, are strictly Ca^{2+}-dependent.

Calcium ions entering the nerve terminal via voltage-dependent calcium channels bind to synaptotagmin, a putative Ca^{2+} sensor of the release machinery (see Chapter 6). This results in fusion of the two membranes and release of neurotransmitters into the synaptic cleft. Presynaptic exocytosis is characterized by a rapid response and limited release with only a small percentage of morphologically docked synaptic vesicles completing fusion upon Ca^{2+} influx. These properties suggest that the function of the release machinery and the final steps of synaptic vesicle priming and fusion are tightly and finely regulated.

Protein phosphorylation represents an important mechanism for regulating protein–protein interactions and is implicated in modulation of synaptic transmission in response to a variety of extracellular signals and synaptic stimuli, including neurotransmitters, neurotrophic factors, hormones, and light. Most proteins within the release apparatus are the substrates of second messenger–activated protein serine-threonine kinases. The time interval between the arrival of the action potential at the nerve terminal and subsequent vesicle fusion is too brief to allow protein phosphorylation to play an acute role in a single round of vesicle

Fig. 10.1 Schematic diagram of protein phosphorylation by a protein kinase and the reversal of this reaction by a protein phosphatase. ADP, adenosine diphosphate; ATP, adenosine triphosphate

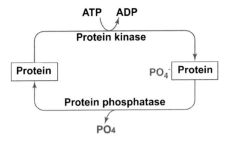

exocytosis. However, protein kinases may have significant effects on subsequent rounds of neurotransmitter release. In this chapter, an overview is provided on how phosphorylation of SNAREs and their regulatory proteins, in particular that by second messenger–activated serine/threonine kinases, modulates synaptic transmission.

Second Messenger–Activated Protein Serine/Threonine Kinases Enriched in Synapses

Phosphorylation of a protein introduces a negatively charged phosphate group, thus altering the conformation and functional activity of the protein. Given that the steady state of phosphorylation is regulated dynamically by protein kinases and phosphatases (Fig. 10.1), phosphorylation or dephosphorylation of presynaptic proteins may be achieved physiologically through activation or inactivation of either a protein kinase or phosphatase. Each of these mechanisms is found in synapses and plays a role in the modulation of synaptic transmission through the diverse signal transduction pathways. A prominent pathway is illustrated in Figure 10.2. The extracellular signals or first messengers act on plasma membrane receptors such as G-protein–coupled receptors for many neurotransmitters, hormones, and sensory stimuli. These ligand-receptor interactions regulate intracellular concentrations of second messengers in targeted neurons. Key second messengers that directly activate protein kinases include cyclic adenosine monophosphate (cAMP), cyclic guanosine monophosphate (cGMP), Ca^{2+}, and diacylglycerol (DAG). The activation of specific classes of protein serine-threonine kinases at nerve terminals by these second messengers then triggers the phosphorylation of synaptic proteins, leading to the modulation of biochemical pathways from synaptic vesicle docking and priming to fusion.

Second messenger-activated protein kinases including cAMP-dependent protein kinase A (PKA), Ca^{2+}/calmodulin-dependent kinase II (CaMKII), protein kinase C (PKC), casein kinase II (CKII), and cyclin-dependent kinase 5 (CDK5) are present at nerve terminals and implicated in short and long-term changes in synaptic efficacy (1–6). Furthermore, activation of these protein kinases at presynaptic terminals correlates with increased transmitter release. A number of SNARE components and their regulatory

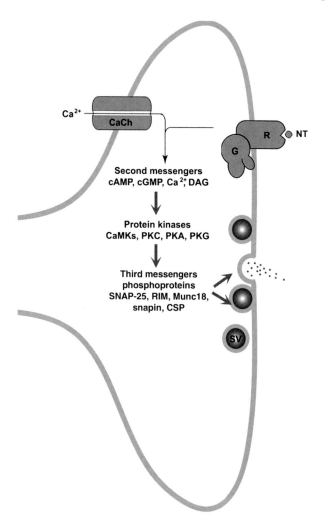

Fig. 10.2 Schematic diagram of second messenger–activated protein kinases at nerve terminals. Extracellular signals (first messengers), such as neurotransmitters (NT) and growth factors, bind specifically to their G protein-coupled (G) membrane receptors (R) at nerve terminals and produce biologic responses via a series of intracellular signals (second and third messengers). Cyclic adenosine monophosphate (cAMP) and cyclic guanosine monophosphate (cGMP) act as second messengers to activate protein kinase A (PKA) and protein kinase G (PKG), respectively. Ca^{2+} exerts many of its second-messenger actions through the activation of Ca^{2+}-dependent protein kinases such as CaMKs and protein kinase C (PKC). Not illustrated in the figure is that some protein phosphatases can also be regulated directly by second messengers. Such phosphorylation and dephosphorylation of SNAREs and their regulatory proteins may be part of the mechanisms underlying the regulation of synaptic vesicle exocytosis. DAG, diacylglycerol; SV, synaptic vesicle

proteins are potential substrates for these kinases, and the functional consequences of these phosphorylation events have been evaluated in a physiologic context (7).

cAMP-Dependent Protein Kinase (Protein Kinase A)

The inactive holoenzyme of PKA, which consists of a tetramer of two catalytic (C) and two regulatory (R) subunits, is activated by the binding of cAMP to its regulatory subunits and the release of its active catalytic subunits. There are three isoforms of C subunits (Cα, Cβ, and Cγ) and four isoforms of R subunits (RIα, RIβ, RIIα, and RIIβ); most of these isoforms are distributed in neurons. Protein kinase A is highly compartmentalized in the cells via the A kinase anchor proteins (AKAPs). Through its binding to the regulatory subunits of PKA, AKAP restricts the kinase in close proximity to the cAMP cascade of the signal transduction pathway and its substrates within subcellular regions of neurons.

Calcium/Calmodulin-Dependent Protein Kinase II

CaMKII, a major type of CaMKs in the brain, exhibits well-known substrate specificity and mediates many of the second messenger actions of Ca^{2+} in neurons. In basal Ca^{2+} conditions, its catalytic domain and autoinhibitory domain at the amino terminal are bound to each other to form an inactive kinase. The binding of Ca^{2+} and calmodulin (CaM) to CaMKII releases the inhibitory domain and allows autophosphorylation and activation of the catalytic domain.

Protein Kinase C

Protein kinase C is formed by a single polypeptide containing both regulatory and catalytic domains under physiologic conditions. In the resting state, the regulatory domain binds and inhibits the catalytic domain. This inhibition is relieved when Ca^{2+} or DAG binds to the regulatory domain. Multiple isoforms of PKC have been identified, and the brain contains at least seven isoforms of the enzyme. These isoforms of PKC vary in cellular distribution in the brain and possess distinct regulatory properties, such as variable sensitivities to activation by Ca^{2+} and DAG. PKC is predominantly a cytoplasmic protein under basal conditions. Upon activation by Ca^{2+} or DAG, the enzyme is translocated to the plasma membrane, likely via high-affinity binding to a number of membrane-associated proteins, called receptors for activated C kinase (RACKs). RACKs are thought to recruit these widely distributed PKCs from cytoplasma to specific subcellular membrane regions where the phosphorylation activity is required. PKC has broad substrate specificity and mediates numerous second-messenger functions of Ca^{2+} in synapses.

Presynaptic Modulation and Synaptic Plasticity

It is widely accepted that memory formation is dependent on changes in synaptic efficiency that permits strengthening of associations between neurons. Activity-dependent synaptic plasticity at appropriate synapses during memory formation is necessary for information storage. At least two forms of plasticity can be discerned: short-term plasticity that lasts at most for a few minutes, and long-term plasticity that persists for several days or longer (8,13). Synaptic strength can either be potentiated or depressed (8). The actual change that sustains the enhanced activity is less clear, however. Current evidence indicates a role for a postsynaptic change, likely an increase in the number of synaptic α-amino-3-hydroxy-5-methyl-4-isoxazole propionic acid (AMPA) receptors or an increase in their single-channel conductance. However, there is also evidence that synaptic potentiation can be expressed as a presynaptic increase in glutamate release. This could result from an enhanced probability of release (9) or in the quantity of glutamate released as a result of an alteration in fusion pore kinetics (10) or quantal content (11). There is also substantial evidence that gene expression leading to de novo protein synthesis and structural alterations of individual synapses or the formation of new synapses is important for the long-term maintenance of altered synaptic strength.

Certain forms of long-term plasticity can be induced by presynaptic mechanisms and depend on cAMP-activated PKA (12). Presynaptic mechanisms are also responsible for some short-term forms of plasticity such as facilitation, augmentation, and post-tetanic potentiation (13). The modulation of synaptic vesicle exocytosis is a major mechanism for regulating synaptic strength. Synaptic transmission is initiated when an action potential triggers neurotransmitter release in the presynaptic nerve terminal. The action potential induces the opening of voltage-gated Ca^{2+} channels, and the resulting Ca^{2+} influx triggers synaptic vesicle exocytosis and release of the neurotransmitter to the synaptic cleft. However, nerve terminals do not convert every action potential into synaptic vesicle exocytosis, but they do so with a certain probability, known as the release probability. The release probability is determined by the product of two parameters: the number of vesicles that are immediately available for release and the probability that each of these will be released in response to a single action potential. Neither of these parameters is fixed. The number of vesicles available is determined by a dynamic equilibrium between the docked, but immature, and the fully mature, referred to as "primed," vesicles. The docked vesicles in turn are in equilibrium with the remainder of the releasable pool that is not yet docked. The size of this pool is affected by its depletion during transmitter release and the rate at which it can be replenished. Thus, any change affecting one of these vesicle pools has the potential to change the release probability and thereby synaptic plasticity.

The SNARE-Based Release Machinery and Regulatory Mechanisms

Neurotransmitter release and vesicle pool dynamics are highly regulated by a series of molecular interactions among vesicular, plasma membrane, and cytosolic proteins. SNARE proteins are essential components of this machinery (see Chapter 3). In synaptic vesicle exocytosis, the three SNARE proteins synaptobrevin (VAMP2), syntaxin 1 and SNAP-25, form a four-helical bundle aligned in parallel. According to the current model, this configuration pulls the two membranes together in a so-called zipper-like fashion (14–16). Elevated Ca^{2+} then triggers the conformational or electrostatic change in a Ca^{2+} sensor that completes the fusion reaction. The proteins that act as the exocytotic Ca^{2+}-sensor are synaptotagmins, vesicle membrane proteins capable of binding Ca^{2+}, SNARE proteins, and phospholipids (17). After fusion, α-SNAP and N-ethylmaleimide–sensitive factor (NSF) are recruited from the cytoplasm, and subsequent adenosine triphosphate (ATP) hydrolysis by NSF causes dissociation of the SNARE complex, which is then free for recycling and a new round of exocytosis. As exocytosis of synaptic vesicles bears distinct features that are dictated by the special requirements of synaptic function, many additional regulatory proteins are utilized in order to meet these special needs. Over the past decade significant progress has been made in identifying these regulatory proteins and in characterizing their physiologic contributions to the modulation of neurotransmitter release. For instance, active zone proteins Munc13, Munc18, and RIM have been identified as important factors in synaptic vesicle priming steps (18–20), whereas complexins, snapin, and cysteine string protein (CSP) have been implicated in the direct modulation of synaptotagmin interactions with the SNARE complex (21–23).

One mechanism by which changes in synaptic strength could occur at nerve terminals involves second messenger–dependent regulation of protein interactions within the release machinery. Many studies in invertebrates and mammalian systems indicate that the regulation of synaptic strength can be controlled by protein phosphorylation. Slower changes, lasting from seconds to minutes, could be achieved by activation of Ca^{2+}-dependent kinases, such as CaMKII, which has been shown to phosphorylate synapsin and thereby regulates the availability of synaptic vesicles for release. Protein kinases implicated in different aspects of long-term changes in synaptic efficacy include CaMKII, PKA, PKC, CKII, mitogen-activated protein kinase (MAPK), and CDK5. All these second messenger–activated protein kinases are expressed in presynaptic terminals, and a number of the proteins implicated in synaptic vesicle release and recycling have been reported as *in vitro* substrates of these kinases (7,24,25). Some of those phosphorylation events, particularly by CaMKII, PKA, and PKC, were shown to affect exocytosis in a physiologic context, implicating them as important factors in presynaptic plasticity. Thus, it is conceivable that sustained neuronal activity and synaptic stimuli lead to kinase activation and subsequent phosphorylation of the particular proteins in the release machinery.

CaMKII-Mediated Regulation of Synaptic Vesicle Mobilization and Availability for Exocytosis

CaMKII is highly expressed in the hippocampus and is present at both the presynaptic terminals and postsynaptic density of neurons. Pharmacologic manipulations and genetic knockout and knock-in approaches have established that CaMKII is critical for the induction of synaptic plasticity (2,6,26). The ability of CaMKII to induce synaptic plasticity at the postsynaptic site has been extensively studied and is not discussed in this chapter. Although CaMKII was found to associate with synaptic vesicles at presynaptic terminals (27), very little is known about its role in the modulation of synaptic transmission and synaptic plasticity. Ninan and Arancio (28) provided direct evidence that presynaptic activation of CaMKII is necessary for inducing synaptic plasticity in cultured hippocampal neurons. They showed that application of the membrane-permeant CaMKII inhibitor KN93 blocked gluta-mate-induced increase in the number of active synapse, as revealed by activity-dependent labeling of presynaptic boutons with FM1-43, and that presynaptic injection of a CaMKII inhibitory peptide suppressed the potentiation of synaptic transmission induced by high-frequency stimulation. These observations suggest that presynaptic CaMKII is essential for glutamate-induced conversion of preexisting silent synapses into functional ones and for synaptic plasticity.

A key question remains to be addressed: What are the molecular targets for CaMKII at presynaptic terminals? Biochemical studies suggest that a number of pre-synaptic proteins serve as the substrates for CaMKII *in vitro*, including the SNARE components syntaxin, SNAP-25, and VAMP2, and synaptotagmin 1 (29,30). However, phosphorylation of VAMP2 by CaMKII did not show any significant effect on its binding to both syntaxin 1A and SNAP-25 *in vitro*. In addition, a mutant VAMP2 lacking the CaMKII phosphorylation sites functions normally in Ca^{2+}-induced exocytosis in insulin-secreting cells (31), suggesting that VAMP2 phosphor-ylation by CaMKII *in vivo* may not be of physiologic relevance. The juxtamembrane domain of synaptotagmin 1 contains a threonine residue (Thr-112) that may be phos-phorylated by either CaMKII or PKC. Phosphorylation of synaptotagmin 1 by PKC, in response to an elevation of $[Ca^{2+}]_i$ or phorbol ester treatment, increases syntaxin and SNAP-25 binding in PC12 cells (32,33). However, exocytosis is not modified by the phosphorylation of synaptotagmin 1 in chromaffin cells (34). The autophosphor-ylation of CaMKII has been reported to affect synaptic transmission through regula-tion of SNARE complex formation (35). The autophosphorylated CaMKII specifically binds to syntaxin at Ca^{2+} concentrations of >1 µM, and the bound CaMKII dissociates from syntaxin when the Ca^{2+} concentration decreases or the CaMKII is dephosphor-ylated. This interaction might provide new insight into the mechanism of presynaptic plasticity via Ca^{2+}-dependent autophosphorylation of CaMKII. A recent study further assessed the function of presynaptic CaMKII at the *Caenorhabditis elegans* neu-romuscular junction (36). Either loss-of-function or gain-of-function of the gene encoding CaMKII inhibited neurotransmitter release, and the inhibitory effect of the gain-of-function mutation could be abolished by blockade or mutations of the BK channel SLO-1. These observations suggest that presynaptic CaMKII is a bidirec-tional modulator of neurotransmitter release, and that its inhibitory effect on neuro-transmitter release is mediated by the BK channel.

One important CaMKII substrate at the nerve terminals is synapsin I, which is the only reported presynaptic substrate persistently phosphorylated at its CaMKII phospho-rylation sites during long-term potentiation (LTP) (37). Stimulation sufficient to induce LTP produced a long-lasting increase in the phosphorylation of synapsin I at its

CaMKII sites without affecting synapsin I levels. This result suggests that LTP expression is accompanied by, and may be dependent on, persistent changes in the activity of presynaptic CaMKII and the degree of synapsin I phosphorylation. Synapsin I is a neuronal phosphoprotein specifically associated with synaptic vesicles. Synapsins also associate with components of the cytoskeleton, such as actin, tubulin, and spectrin, and move dynamically in response to physiologic stimuli (24). Synapsin I is phosphorylated at two serine residues within its tail or filamentous domain by CaMKII. These phosphorylation events decrease its affinity for both synaptic vesicles and actin.

Synapsins have been implicated in the regulation of neurotransmitter release by controlling the number of vesicles available at release sites for exocytosis. A number of *in vitro* biochemical studies have demonstrated that synapsins dynamically associate with and dissociate from synaptic vesicles in response to synaptic activity in a CaMKII phosphorylation-dependent manner (38–40). Using real-time imaging approaches in living hippocampal synapses, Chi and colleagues (41) showed that synapsin I dissociated from vesicles and dispersed into the cytosol after the activation of CaMKII. Furthermore, synapsin carrying mutations in the CaMKII phosphorylation sites had slower dispersion rates, and concomitantly slower vesicle exocytosis, presumably because of reduced mobility of synaptic vesicles at the nerve terminals. Phosphorylation of synapsin I by CaMKII occurs in response to the Ca^{2+} influx during tetanic stimulation and enhances neurotransmitter release by enabling mobilization of a large number of synaptic vesicles to release sites. In contrast, the mutant mouse that lacks synapsin I is deficient in post-tetanic potentiation. Under resting conditions, synapsins tether synaptic vesicles to cytoskeletal elements and prevent neurotransmitter release; during synaptic activity, synapsins are phosphorylated, dissociate from synaptic vesicles, and allow vesicles to mobilize and fuse with the plasma membrane. Thus, synapsin I, through its dynamic association with synaptic vesicles and its ability to be phosphorylated by CaMKII, appears to control the rate of vesicle availability for exocytosis (Fig. 10.3).

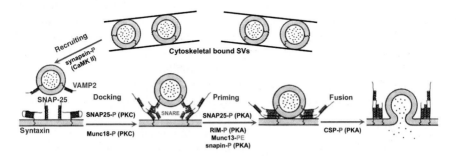

Fig. 10.3 Schematic diagram of multiple kinases and their targets in regulation of synaptic vesicle exocytosis. The SNAREs and regulatory proteins are proposed to be involved in presynaptic modulation via second messenger–dependent phosphorylation (P) by various kineses, including CaMKII, PKC, and PKA, or via modulation by phorbol ester (PE) receptor. The coexistence of multiple kinases with their targets at different steps of the synaptic vesicle cycle might underlie the robust effect of these signal cascades on synaptic vesicle release and synaptic plasticity

Activation of PKC is Implicated in Presynaptic Plasticity

Protein kinase C is an important second messenger–activated protein kinase in the regulation of synaptic transmission. Induction of LTP results in activation of PKC (42). Conversely, inhibition of this kinase prevents LTP (43). At both pre- and postsynaptic sites of synapses, phosphorylation of PKC substrates after LTP induction has been observed. Most of the early studies suggesting PKC involvement in the modulation of neurotransmitter release were based on the application of phorbol esters, which are potent DAG analogues. In the hippocampus, as in many other neuronal preparations, activation of PKC by phorbol ester treatment results in an enhanced glutamate release (44,45). The recent observation that phorbol esters appeared to increase the Ca^{2+} sensitivity of exocytosis without affecting the number of releasable vesicles or Ca^{2+}-binding sites implies that phorbol esters are affecting the priming or fusion of synaptic vesicles. Generally these effects of phorbol ester were attributed to PKC phosphorylation of presynaptic proteins. However, phorbol ester receptors other than PKC have recently been identified. One such phorbol ester receptor particularly important in neurotransmission is Munc13. Munc13s are a family of proteins encoded by three genes in mammals *(munc13-1, −2, and −3)*. They are specifically localized at presynaptic terminals, where they function to change syntaxin from a "closed" to an "open" conformation and thereby to allow SNARE complex formation (46–49). It is thought that Munc-13s are presynaptic DAG/phorbol ester receptors and translocate to the plasma membrane upon DAG or phorbol ester binding, which resembles the translocation of PKC in response to phorbol ester binding. Consistent with this notion, genetically modified mice that express mutant Munc13-1 lacking the phorbol ester–binding site fail to exhibit the robust increase in release in response to phorbol ester treatment (50).

Although the phorbol ester–mediated augmentation of synaptic vesicle priming in hippocampal neurons could be partially mediated by Munc13 proteins, PKC-specific phorbol ester effects on synaptic transmission are also well documented. For example, application of the PKC-specific inhibitor BIS (bisindolylmaleimide) blocks the increase in the size of the readily releasable pools in cultured hippocampal synapses (51) and chromaffin cells (52), and prevents the enhancement of neurotransmitter release in ciliary ganglion synapses and retinal bipolar cells in response to treatment by phorbol esters. This inhibitory role is likely mediated through a PKC-dependent mechanism as the PKC inhibitor BIS targets the ATP-binding site of PKC and should not affect the DAG-binding proteins such as Munc13. Furthermore, application of purified PKC into permeabilized chromaffin and PC12 cell enhances exocytosis. These data provide direct evidence that PKC modulates the activity of the exocytotic machinery and further imply that Ca^{2+} or DAG activation can affect multiple intracellular substrates and receptors, each capable of regulating specific components of the release machinery. It is unlikely that a single phosphorylation event of a particular protein could have such dramatic effects on multiple steps of synaptic vesicle exocytosis.

Recent work shows that a number of exocytotic proteins may serve as PKC substrates *in vitro*. However, relatively few of them can be phosphorylated in a cellular environment and even fewer have been tested for the physiologic relevance of PKC-dependent phosphorylation in the modulation of synaptic transmission. To reveal the detailed molecular mechanisms underling Ca^{2+}/DAG-induced changes in synaptic strength, it is necessary to use multiple approaches or tools, such as specific kinase inhibitors, phosphomimetic PKC substrates, and electrophysiologic analyses of vesicle fusion. SNAP-25 and Munc18 are two attractive candidate PKC substrates for which the physiologic role of PKC-dependent phosphorylation is relatively well supported by experimental evidence.

SNAP-25

Protein kinase C–mediated phosphorylation of SNAP-25 can be induced in PC12 cells by treatment with phorbol esters (53) and in hippocampal neurons by induction of LTP (54). A prominent PKC phosphorylation site in SNAP-25 has been mapped to a specific serine residue (Ser-187), which is located within the negatively charged C-terminal between the cleavage sites for botulinum toxins A and E. This region is of critical importance in calcium-triggered exocytosis. Neutralization of negatively charged residues within this region decreases vesicle secretion (55) and interferes with its interaction with synaptotagmin I (56). However, stimulation of PC12 cells with phorbol esters showed no correlation between the increase in secretion of dopamine and acetylcholine and the phosphorylation of SNAP-25 (57). These findings raise the question of whether the effect of phorbol ester 12-myristate 13-acetate (PMA) on vesicle release in particular PC12 cells was mediated via PKC phosphorylation of SNAP-25 or by direct activation of non-PKC phorbol ester receptors such as Munc13.

One piece of convincing evidence in support of SNAP-25 as a PKC target during the release process came from a study in which phosphomimetic mutants of SNAP-25 were expressed in chromaffin cells (58). To exclude the possibility that the presynaptic phorbol ester receptor Munc13 acts as a priming factor independently of PKC activation, Nagy and colleagues (58) avoided application of phorbol esters in the study and instead relied on the expression of SNAP-25 mutants and the endogenous PKC activation after calcium increases. By using a mutagenesis approach in combination with high time-resolution capacitance measurements, they found that expression of SNAP-25 mutants mimicking the phosphorylated state of Ser-187 accelerated vesicle recruitment after depletion of the releasable vesicle pools. However, expression of mutants simulating the nonphosphorylated state, or blocking PKC activity, decreased the refilling of the vesicle pools. Their biochemical studies further confirmed that the level of phosphorylated SNAP-25 in resting cells is low but that a partial phosphorylation occurs when $[Ca^{2+}]_i$ is increased. The PKC-mediated phosphorylation of SNAP-25 also plays an important role in synaptic vesicle release at sensory-motor synapses in *Aplysia* (59). The rates of synaptic depression were slowed when the cells expressed mutant SNAP-25 with the phosphomimetic residue Glu or Asp. Furthermore, the stimulatory effect of phorbol 12,13-dibutyrate (PDBu) on transmitter release was blocked in cells expressing nonphosphorylated mutant SNAP-25. These results further support the hypothesis that PKC phosphorylation of

SNAP-25 at Ser-187 is required to refill the releasable vesicle pool in response to synaptic activity or elevated intracellular calcium concentration.

The molecular mechanism underlying the PKC-mediated biochemical effect on the function of SNAP-25 remains to be elucidated. One hypothesis is that SNAP-25 phosphorylation at Ser-187 participates in the modulation of SNARE complex assembly, which is based on the biochemical observation that the phosphomimetic mutation of Ser-187 selectively increases the binding affinity of SNAP-25 for syntaxin (60). It is possible that phosphorylation of SNAP-25 accelerates the association of syntaxin and SNAP-25 heterodimers, a rate-limiting step in SNARE complex assembly, thereby favoring the formation of functional ternary complexes and making more releasable vesicles available after the preexisting vesicle pool has been depleted (Fig. 10.3). This model is consistent with the observed phenotype of the increased refilling rate after stimulation in chromaffin cells following expression of the S187E mutant (58) and the observed increase in the size of the highly Ca^{2+}-sensitive vesicle pool (60).

Munc18

Munc18 is a syntaxin-binding protein involved in neurotransmitter release by binding tightly to syntaxin, holding it in a closed conformation, and preventing its assembly into a SNARE complex (61,62). By an as yet unknown mechanism, Munc18 releases syntaxin in a state that is primed for its interaction with the other SNARE proteins, thus permitting the formation of the SNARE complexes. Although recent studies suggest that Munc18 may also play a syntaxin-independent role in exocytosis, modification of the interaction between Munc18 and syntaxin could be one of the important mechanisms for the regulation of neurotransmitter release. Munc18-1 can be phosphorylated by PKC in vitro; the phosphorylation was confirmed in chromaffin cells and in intact cortical synaptosomes in response to depolarization by KCl or 4-aminopyridine, and by PKC activation with phorbol ester (63). Using phospho-specific antisera, Munc18a could be phosphorylated at the residue Ser-313 in intact and permeabilized chromaffin cells in response to histamine and Ca^{2+} (64). Phosphorylation of Munc18 by PKC reduces the amount of Munc18 for binding to syntaxin (65) and expression of the phosphomimetic mutant of Munc18-1 leads to the accelerated kinetics of vesicle fusion in chromaffin cells (66). Interestingly, the PKC phosphorylation sites in Munc18-1 are not conserved in other members of the Munc18/Sec1 family, which are involved in general intracellular membrane fusion, suggesting that PKC phosphorylation of Munc18-1 is specific for regulated exocytosis. The finding of PKC phosphorylation of Munc18 in synaptosomes may indicate that this PKC-mediated phosphorylation represents one of the signal pathways in inducing presynaptic plasticity. Although the phosphorylation of Munc18-1 at the Ser-313 has been shown to reduce its binding to syntaxin, it is still not clear whether this biochemical effect alone could fully contribute to the increased rate of transmitter release observed in chromaffin cells.

Protein Kinase A Phosphorylation of Presynaptic Proteins and Synaptic Plasticity

Activation of PKA has been implicated in the presynaptic form of LTP that involves a modification of the release machinery (12) and is induced in hippocampal mossy fiber and cerebellar parallel fiber synapses (4,5,67). Presynaptic LTP is mediated by the activation of Ca^{2+}-sensitive adenylyl cyclase, leading to a rise in the concentration of cAMP and the consequent activation of PKA. An LTP-like effect can also be produced by bath application of the adenylyl cyclase activator forskolin or by membrane-permeant cAMP analogues, and LTP in cerebellum is impaired in type I adenylyl cyclase mutant mice (68). Furthermore, induction of LTP by tetanic stimulation is blocked when PKA inhibitors are applied in the bath or when presynaptic granule cells are transfected with an expression vector encoding a peptide inhibitor of PKA. Activation of cAMP-dependent PKA has been shown to enhance release probability at many synapses. Application of forskolin on adult rat and mouse hippocampal slices or hippocampal neuron cultures increases the frequency of spontaneous miniature excitatory postsynaptic currents (mEPSCs) without affecting their amplitude. Although the use of specific PKA inhibitors, such as Rp-cAMP, H89, KT5720, and PKI (PKA inhibitor peptide), have established PKA as a key target for the cAMP induced modulation of synaptic transmission at many synapses (69,70), a direct effect of cAMP on transmitter release cannot be excluded. For instance, forskolin-induced synaptic potentiation at the calyx of Held could not be blocked by PKA inhibitors (71). Recent studies have identified a direct cAMP-target, cAMP-GEFII (72), which is involved in PKA-independent regulation of exocytosis in PC12 cells.

In cultured hippocampal neurons, activation of PKA increases neurotransmitter release without changing the number of functional terminals or the number of docked vesicles within individual synapses after 3 minutes of treatment with forskolin, suggesting that the short-term effects of cAMP may directly affect the release machinery (70). The enhancement in release was proposed to be the result of the engagement of a step downstream from calcium influx via either increased calcium cooperativity for release or enhanced coupling of the calcium-sensing molecule(s) to the synaptic vesicle fusion apparatus (73). Potential targets for the cAMP/PKA signal cascade are the release machinery and its regulatory components including α-SNAP (30), cysteine string protein (74), snapin (75), rabphilin (76), RIM1 (77), SNAP-25 (31,78), and syntaphilin (79). Functional characterization of the PKA target(s) that regulates assembly/disassembly of the fusion machinery and the priming and recycling of docked synaptic vesicles is critical to the elucidation of the molecular mechanisms underlying synaptic plasticity.

RIM1

The recent demonstration that phosphorylation of RIM1α by PKA is necessary for induction of presynaptic LTP at cerebellar parallel fiber synapses raises the possibility that synaptic strength may be controlled by a small number of key PKA targets.

RIM1α serves as a substrate of PKA phosphorylation in the induction of presynaptic LTP (77). PKA directly phosphorylates RIM1α at two sites: Ser-413 between the N-terminal zinc finger and the central PDZ domain, and Ser-1548 at the C terminal. LTP is absent in cultured cerebellar granule and Purkinje neurons from RIM1α knockout mice but can be rescued by presynaptic expression of RIM1α. Mutant RIM1α lacking the N-terminal PKA phosphorylation site is unable to rescue LTP in RIM1α knockout neurons and selectively suppresses LTP in wild-type neurons. This suggests that PKA phosphorylation of RIM1α at a single N-terminal site is required for the induction of presynaptic LTP. One key question remains to be answered: How does PKA phosphorylation of RIM1α at Ser-413 mediate a long-lasting change in neurotransmitter release? Ser-413 is localized in a conserved sequence between the Zn^{2+} finger and the PDZ domain of RIM1α. It seems likely that RIM1α phosphorylation modulates release by regulating protein–protein interactions. One possible mechanism is that phosphorylation shifts the balance between Rab3 and Munc13 binding to the Zn^{2+} finger domain of RIM1α. Rab3 and Munc13 compete with one another for binding to RIM1α, and both interactions are physiologically important for RIM1α to regulate synaptic strength. However, expression of a RIM1α mutant (S413D) in an attempt to mimic the phosphorylated state did not suffice to increase the EPSC amplitude, leaving the unresolved question of whether phosphorylation of RIM1α at Ser-413 is sufficient to induce LTP in this system. Thus, further biochemical and physiologic tests of the proposed modulation of these protein interactions via PKA phosphorylation of RIM1α will be necessary to support this hypothesis.

SNAP-25

Besides being a substrate of PKC at residue Ser-187, SNAP-25 is also phosphorylated at Thr-138 by PKA both *in vitro* and *in vivo*. In chromaffin cells, PKA phosphorylation of SNAP-25 is necessary to maintain the release-ready and primed pool of vesicles. Chromaffin cells have two characterized releasable and primed vesicle pools—the slowly releasable pool (SRP) and the readily releasable pool (RRP)—which are released in slow and fast exocytotic burst upon stimulation, respectively. PKA and the phosphatase calcineurin have antagonistic effects on the size of both the SRP and the RRP. Using a phosphopeptide-specific antibody, Nagy and colleagues (80) showed that endogenous SNAP-25 in chromaffin cells is phosphorylated by PKA at Thr-138. Expression of the SNAP-25 mutant T138D, which mimics the PKA-phosphorylated state of SNAP-25, did not show a significant effect on secretion. In contrast, the mutant T138A caused a twofold decrease in both fast and slow exocytotic burst components. Furthermore, expression of either mutant eliminated the effect of PKA inhibitors on the SRP, but not on the RRP, suggesting that phosphorylation of SNAP-25 underlies PKA action on the SRP.

In chromaffin cells, as depletion of the RRP is followed by refilling from the SRP, phosphorylation of SNAP-25 not only regulates the size of the SRP, but also indirectly changes the size of the RRP. However, more detailed analyses revealed that PKA-dependent phosphorylation of SNAP-25 at Thr-138 occluded the effect of PKA inhibitors only on the SRP, implicating an additional downstream PKA target(s) in regulating the size of the RRP. Similar to chromaffin cells, neurons also exhibit multiple kinetic components of release; however, it is not clear whether they have a pool analogous to the SRP. The highly conserved function of SNARE proteins in both neurons and chromaffin cells suggests that PKA phosphorylation of SNAP-25 at Thr-138 should have a similar role in regulating the transition between distinct vesicle pools in neurons. Thus, in considering the already described findings of PKC phosphorylation of SNAP-25 (58), vesicle refilling and pool size in chromaffin cells are coordinately controlled by phosphorylation of SNAP-25 via two different signal pathways. PKA phosphorylation of SNAP-25 at Thr-138 controls the size of the releasable vesicle pools, whereas PKC phosphorylation of SNAP-25 at Ser-187 is involved in regulating refilling after the pools have been emptied. Given the relationship between the neuronal readily releasable pool and synaptic efficacy, further characterization of the combined effect of cophosphorylation of SNAP-25 by both PKC and PKA in neurons should clarify their potential contributions to the modulation of synaptic vesicle exocytosis via these two different signal pathways (Fig. 10.3).

Although phosphorylation of SNAP-25 by both PKC and PKA is well established, the biologic significance of the phosphorylation events in SNARE protein interactions is much less clear. Unlike PKC phosphorylation, PKA phosphorylation of SNAP-25 has been shown to play a less significant role in the formation of the ternary SNARE complex. Biochemical studies have demonstrated that PKA-dependent phosphorylation of SNAP-25 does not regulate the ternary SNARE complex assembly and that Thr-138 is not an essential residue for the formation or stability of the complex (31). Priming of vesicles, although still not fully understood, is usually described as the process of maturation from a docked vesicle with an assembled SNARE complex into a fusion competent complex. It is likely achieved by regulatory roles of SNARE interacting proteins. Modulation of these interactions via PKA phosphorylation of SNAP-25 could potentially be the mechanism responsible for the observed effects. Thus, more biochemical studies are necessary to elucidate how both PKC and PKA phosphorylation of SNAP-25 controls vesicle pool dynamics, which could provide insight into the presynaptic modulation of synaptic plasticity.

Snapin

The maturation of a docked synaptic vesicle into a release-ready vesicle requires synaptotagmin, which provides Ca^{2+}-dependent regulation of the fusion machinery. New evidence has emerged indicating that the interaction of synaptotagmin with SNAP-25 or the SNARE complex is critical for vesicle release and provides a clue as to how a calcium sensor is structurally and functionally coupled to the SNARE-based fusion machinery. However, the mechanisms underlying the regulation of this coupling during vesicle priming remain unclear. Snapin is a newly identified SNAP-25 and synaptotagmin-binding protein that enhances the association of synaptotagmin with the SNARE complex (81). Snapin is a ubiquitously expressed soluble protein detected in both cytosol and peripheral membrane-associated fractions. In addition to binding to SNAP-25, snapin also interacts with a number of other proteins including SNAP-23, and the postulated function of snapin has been expanded to include a broader range of intracellular membrane fusion and trafficking events. The physiologic role of snapin in vesicle exocytosis was established by microinjection of snapin into presynaptic superior cervical ganglion neurons (SCGNs) in culture, and by transient expression of snapin in both adrenal chromaffin cells (75) and hippocampal neurons (82). Genetic study showed that deletion of the snapin gene in mouse leads to a marked reduction in the amount of the synaptotagmin-SNARE complex. Exocytosis of large dense-core vesicles in *snapin* (−/−) chromaffin cells displayed a selective reduction in the exocytotic burst without a change in the sustained component of release, suggesting a reduction in the pool size of release-ready vesicles. This inhibitory effect could be fully rescued by expressing a wild-type *snapin* transgene in the mutant cells (22), suggesting that snapin is an important modulator for neuroexocytosis, possibly by stabilizing the structural coupling of synaptotagmin with the SNARE complex.

Snapin was identified as a PKA substrate, and phosphorylation of snapin at Ser-50 both *in vitro* and *in vivo* leads to increased binding of synaptotagmin to the SNARE complex. Substitution of Ser-50 with a negatively charged aspartate (S50D), a mutation that mimics the effect of phosphorylation, also resulted in an increased affinity of snapin for SNAP-25. Expression of snapin S50D in chromaffin cells enhances secretion, suggesting that PKA phosphorylation of snapin modulates the efficacy of its action on release (75). In addition, transient expression of snapin S50D in cultured hippocampal neurons resulted in an increased release probability of individual vesicles and faster synaptic depression during high-frequency stimulation at "autapses" (82). In contract, expression of snapin S50A, a mutant that cannot be phosphorylated, did not alter the size of the pool or the probability of release. These results establish snapin as an important target of PKA and indicate a role for snapin in the PKA-induced modulation of transmitter release.

Cysteine String Protein

Cysteine string protein (CSP) is a synaptic vesicle membrane protein that binds to both syntaxin and synaptotagmin (83) and is essential for a Ca^{2+}-dependent step of synaptic vesicle exocytosis (84). Like snapin, CSP is a PKA substrate *in vitro* and *in vivo*. However, PKA-mediated phosphorylation of CSP inhibits its interactions with syntaxin and synaptotagmin *in vitro* and in pull-down assays (74), while that of snapin enhances the coupling of synaptotagmin with the SNARE complex. Overexpression of wild-type CSP in chromaffin cells markedly slows release kinetics (85). When a nonphosphorylatable mutant CSP, CSP S10A, is expressed, the slowing effect upon release kinetics was absent, suggesting that the effect on release kinetics is a phosphorylation-dependent event. Since CSP is an *in vivo* PKA substrate whose phosphorylation alters release kinetics in chromaffin cells, this protein is another attractive candidate that may contribute to the cAMP/PKA signal cascade-dependent presynaptic plasticity in neurons.

Conclusion

Recent advances in experimental tools, including genetic manipulation in murine models, overexpression of mutant proteins via transfection and viral infection in primary neuronal cultures, and the generation of phospho-specific antibodies, have allowed us to address important questions concerning the regulation of neurotransmitter release and synaptic plasticity via activation of second messenger–dependent protein kinases. As reviewed in this chapter, promising progress has been made in the identification of *in vivo* protein kinase substrates and in characterizing their physiologic relevance in the regulation of synaptic vesicle release. The coexistence of multiple kinases with their targets at the nerve terminals might underlie the robust effects of second messenger signal cascades on synaptic vesicle release by acting on different steps of the vesicle cycle (Fig. 10.3). This would provide a molecular basis for functional heterogeneity of phosphorylation-mediated modulation of synaptic strength in different synapses. The next steps will be aimed at extending these findings to the various forms of synaptic plasticity. A challenging task facing synaptic physiologists in the future is to integrate all of the data on individual kinases and their substrates into a comprehensive model defining the cellular signal transduction pathways that might be responsible for presynaptic modulation of neurotransmission.

References

1. Charriaut-Marlangue C, Otani S, Creuzet C, Ben-Ari Y, Loeb J. Rapid activation of hippocampal casein kinase II during long-term potentiation. Proc Natl Acad Sci U S A 1991;88:10232–10236.
2. Silva AJ, Stevens CF, Tonegawa S, Wang Y. Deficient hippocampal long-term potentiation in alpha-calcium-calmodulin kinase II mutant mice. Science 1991;257:201–206.
3. Abeliovich A, Chen C, Goda Y, Silva AJ, Stevens CF, Tonegawa S. Modified hippocampal long-term potentiation in PKC γ-mutant mice. Cell 1991;75:1253–1262.
4. Huang YY, Li XC, Kandel ER. cAMP contributes to mossy fiber LTP by initiating both a covalently mediated early phase and macromolecular synthesis-dependent late phase. Cell 1991;79:69–79.
5. Weisskopf MG, Castillo PE, Zalutsky RA, Nicoll RA. Mediation of hippocampal mossy fiber long-term potentiation by cyclic AMP. Science 1991;265:1878–1882.
6. Mayford M, Bach ME, Huang YY, Wang L, Hawkins RD, Kandel ER. Control of memory formation through regulated expression of a CaMKII transgene. Science 1991;274:1678–1683.
7. Leedners AGM, Sheng Z-H. Modulation of neurotransmitter release by the second messenger-activated protein kinases: Implications for presynaptic plasticity. Pharmacol Ther 2005; 105:69–84.
8. Malenka RC, Nicoll RA. Long-term potentiation—a decade of progress? Science 1999;285:1870–1874.
9. Bolshakov VY, Siegelbaum SA. Regulation of hippocampal transmitter release during development and long-term potentiation. Science 1995;269:1730–1734.
10. Choi S, Klingauf J, Tsien RW. Postfusional regulation of cleft glutamate concentration during LTP at "silent synapses." Nat Neurosci 2000;3:330–336.
11. Burgoyne RD, Barclay JW. Splitting the quantum: regulation of quantal release during vesicle fusion. Trends Neurosci 2002;25:176–178.
12. Nicoll RA, Malenka RC. Contrasting properties of two forms of long-term potentiation in the hippocampus. Nature 1995;377:115–118.

13. Zucker RS, Regehr WG. Short-term synaptic plasticity. Annu Rev Physiol 2002;64:355–405.
14. Südhof TC. The synaptic vesicle cycle revisited. Neuron 2000;28:317–320.
15. Chen YA, Scheller RH. SNARE-mediated membrane fusion. Nat Rev Mol Cell Biol 2001;2:98–106.
16. Murthy VN, De Camilli P. Cell biology of the presynaptic terminal. Annu Rev Neurosci 2003;26:701–728.
17. Chapman ER. Synaptotagmin: a Ca^{2+} sensor that triggers exocytosis? Nat Rev Mol Cell Biol 2002;3:498–508.
18. Augustin I, Rosenmund C, Südhof TC, Brose N. Munc13–1 is essential for fusion competence of glutamatergic synaptic vesicles. Nature 1999;400:457–461.
19. Verhage M, et al. Synaptic assembly of the brain in the absence of neurotransmitter secretion. Science 2000;287:864–869.
20. Schoch S, Castillo PE, Jo T, et al. RIM1α forms a protein scaffold for regulating neurotransmitter release at the active zone. Nature 2002;415:321–326.
21. Reim K, Mansour M, Varoqueaux F, et al. Complexins regulate a late step in Ca2+-dependent neurotransmitter release. Cell 2001;104:71–81.
22. Tian JH, Wu ZX, Unzicker M, et al. The role of Snapin in neurosecretion: snapin knock-out mice exhibit impaired calcium-dependent exocytosis of large dense-core vesicles in chromaffin cells. J Neurosci 2005;25:10546–10555.
23. Evans GJO, Morgan A, Burgoyne RD. Tying everything together: the multiple roles of cysteine string protein (CSP) in regulated exocytosis. Traffic 2003;4:653–659.
24. Greengard P, Valtorta F, Czernik AJ, Benfenati F. Synaptic vesicle phosphoproteins and regulation of synaptic function. Science 1993;259:780–785.
25. Morgan A, Burgoyne RD, Barclay JW, et al. Regulation of exocytosis by protein kinase C. Biochem Soc Trans 2005;33,1341–1344.
26. Giese KP, Fedorov NB, Filipkowski RK, Silva AJ. Autophosphorylation at Thr286 of the calcium-calmodulin kinase II in LTP and learning. Science 1998;279:870–873.
27. Benfenati F, Valtorta F, Rubenstein JL, Gorelick FS, Greengard P, Czernik AJ. Synaptic vesicle-associated Ca2+/calmodulin-dependent protein kinase II is a binding protein for synapsin I. Nature 1992;359:417–420.
28. Ninan I, Arancio O. Presynaptic CaMKII is necessary for synaptic plasticity in cultured hippocampal neurons. Neuron 2004;42:129–141.
29. Nielander HB, Onofri F, Valtorta F, et al. Phosphorylation of VAMP/synaptobrevin in synaptic vesicles by endogenous protein kinases. J Neurochem 1995;65:1712–1720.
30. Hirling H, Scheller RH. Phosphorylation of synaptic vesicle proteins: modulation of the alpha SNAP interaction with the core complex. Proc Natl Acad Sci U S A 1996;93:11945–11949.
31. Risinger C, Bennett MK. Differential phosphorylation of syntaxin and synaptosome-associated protein of 25 kDa (SNAP-25) isoforms. J Neurochem 1999;72:614–624.
32. Hilfiker S, Pieribone VA, Nordstedt C, Greengard P, Czernik AJ. Regulation of synaptotagmin I phosphorylation by multiple protein kinases. J Neurochem 1999;73:921–932.
33. Verona M, Zanotti S, Schäfer T, Racagni G, Popoli M. Changes of synaptotagmin interaction with t-SNARE proteins in vitro after calcium/calmodulin-dependent phosphorylation. J Neurochem 2000;74:209–221.
34. Nagy G, Kim JH, Pang ZP, et al. Different effects on fast exocytosis induced by synaptotagmin 1 and 2 isoforms and abundance but not by phosphorylation. J Neurosci 2006;26:632–643.
35. Ohyama A, et al. Regulation of exocytosis through Ca2+/ATP-dependent binding of autophosphorylated Ca2+/calmodulin-activated protein kinase II to syntaxin 1A. J Neurosci 2002;22:3342–3351.
36. Liu Q, Chen B, Ge Q, Wang Z-W. Presynaptic CaMKII modulates neurotransmitter release by activating BK channels at C. elegans neuromuscular junction. J Neurosci 2007;27:10404–10413.
37. Nayak AS, Moore CI, Browning MD. Ca2+/calmodulin-dependent protein kinase II phosphorylation of the presynaptic protein synapsinI is persistently increased during long-term potentiation. Proc Natl Acad Sci U S A 1996;93:15451–15456.

38. Torri TF, Bossi M, Fesce R, Greengard P, Valtorta F. Synapsin I partially dissociates from synaptic vesicles during exocytosis induced by electrical stimulation. Neuron 1992;9:1143–1153.

39. Stefani G, Onofri F, Valtorta F, Vaccaro P, Greengard P, Benfenati F. Kinetic analysis of the phosphorylation-dependent interactions of synapsin I with rat brain synaptic vesicles. J Physiol 1997;504:501–515.

40. Hosaka M, Hammer RE, Südhof TC. A phospho-switch controls the dynamic association of synapsins with synaptic vesicles. Neuron 1999;24:377–387.

41. Chi P, Greengard P, Ryan TA. Synaptic vesicle mobilization is regulated by distinct synapsinI phosphorylation pathways at different frequencies. Neuron 2003;38:69–78.

42. Klann E, Chen SJ, Sweatt JD. Persistent protein kinase activation in the maintenance phase of long-term potentiation. J Biol Chem 1991;266:24253–24256.

43. Lovinger DM, Wong KL, Murakami K, Routtenberg A. Protein kinase C inhibitors eliminate hippocampal long-term potentiation. Brain Res 1987;436:177–183.

44. Malenka RC, Madison DV, Nicoll RA. (1986) Potentiation of synaptic transmission in the hippocampus by phorbol esters. Nature 1986;321:175–177.

45. Parfitt KD, Madison DV. Phorbol esters enhance synaptic transmission by a presynaptic, calcium-dependent mechanism in rat hippocampus. J Physiol 1993;471:245–268.

46. Brose N, Rosenmund C, Rettig J. Regulation of transmitter release by Unc-13 and its homologues. Curr Opin Neurobiol 2000;10:303–311.

47. Ashery U, Varoqueaux F, Voets T, et al. Munc13–1 acts as a priming factor for large dense-core vesicles in bovine chromaffin cells. EMBO. J 2000;19:3586–3596.

48. Richmond JE, Welmer RM, Jorgensen EM. An open form of syntaxin bypasses the requirement for UNC-13 in vesicle priming. Nature 2001;412:338–341.

49. Betz A, Ashery U, Rickmann M, et al. Munc13–1 is a presynaptic phorbol ester receptor that enhances neurotransmitter release. Neuron 1998;21:123–136.

50. Rhee JS, Betz A, Pyott S, et al. á Phorbol ester- and diacylglycerol-induced augmentation of transmitter release is mediated by Munc 13s and not by PKCs. Cell 2002;108,121–133.

51. Stevens CF, Sullivan JM. Regulation of the readily releasable vesicle pool by protein kinase C. Neuron 1998;21:885–893.

52. Gillis KD, Mossner R, Neher E. Protein kinase C enhances exocytosis from chromaffin cells by increasing the size of the readily releasable pool of secretory granules. Neuron 1996; 16:1209–1220.

53. Shimazaki Y, Nishiki T, Omori A, et al. Phosphorylation of 25–kDa synaptosome-associated protein; Possible involvement in protein kinase C-mediated regulation of neurotransmitter release. J Biol Chem 1996;271:14548–14553.

54. Genoud S, Pralong W, Riederer BM, Eder L, Catsicas S, Muller D. Activity-dependent phosphorylation of SNAP-25 in hippocampal organotypic cultures. J Neurochem 1999;72:1699–1706.

55. Sørensen JB, Matti U, Wei S, et al. The SNARE protein SNAP-25 is linked to fast calcium triggering of exocytosis. Proc Natl Acad Sci U S A 2002;99:1627–1632.

56. Zhang X, Kim-Miller MJ, Fukuda M, Kowalchyk JA, Martin TFJ. Ca2+-dependent synaptotagmin binding to SNAP-25 is essential for Ca2+-triggered exocytosis. Neuron 2002;34:599–611.

57. Iwasaki S, Kataoka M, Sekiguchi M, Shimazaki Y, Sato K, Takahashi M. Two distinct mechanisms underline the stimulation of neurotransmitter release by phorbol esters in clonal rat pheochromocytoma PC12 cells. J Biochem 2000;128:407–414.

58. Nagy G, Matti U, Nehring RB, et al. Protein kinase C-dependent phosphorylation of synaptosome-associated protein of 25kDa at Ser187 potentiates vesicle recruitment. J Neurosci 2002;22:9278–9286.

59. Houeland G, Nakhost A, Sossin WS, Castellucci VF. PKC modulation of transmitter release by SNAP-25 at sensory-to-motor synapses in aplysia. J Neurophysiol 2007;97:134–143.

60. Yang Y, Craig TJ, Chen X, et al. Phosphomimetic mutation of Ser-187 of SNAP-25 increases both syntaxin binding and highly Ca2+-sensitive exocytosis. J Gen Physiol 2007;129:233–244.

61. Dulubova I, Sugita S, Hill S, et al. A conformational switch in syntaxin during exocytosis: role of munc18. EMBO J 1999;18:4372–4382.

62. Misura KM, Scheller RH, Weis WI. Three-dimensional structure of the neuronal-Sec1–syntaxin 1a complex. Nature 2000;404:355–362.
63. De Vries KJ, Geijtenbeek A, Brian EC, de Graan PNE, Ghijsen WEJM, Verhage M. Dynamics of munc18–1 phosphorylation/dephosphorylation in rat brain nerve terminals. Eur J Neurosci 2000;12:385–390.
64. Craig TJ, Evans GJ, Morgan A. Physiological regulation of Munc18/ nSec1 phosphorylation on serine-313. J Neurochem 2003;86,1450–1457.
65. Fujita Y, Sasaki T, Fukui K, et al. Phosphorylation of Munc-18/n-Sec1/rbSec1 by protein kinase C: its implication in regulating the interaction of Munc-18/n-Sec1/rbSec1 with syntaxin. J Biol Chem 1996;271:7265–7268.
66. Barclay JW, Craig TJ, Fisher RJ, Ciufo LF, Evans GJ, Morgan A. Phosphorylation of Munc18 by protein kinase C regulates the kinetics of exocytosis. J Biol Chem 2003;278:10538–10545.
67. Salin PA, Malenka RC, Nicoll RA. cAMP mediates a presynaptic form of LTP at cerebellar parallel fiber synapses. Neuron 1996;16:797–803.
68. Storm DR, Hansel C, Hacker B, Parent A, Linden DJ. Impaired cerebellar long-term potentiation in type I adenylyl cyclase mutant mice. Neuron 1998;20:1199–1210.
69. Chavez-Noriega LE, Stevens CF. Increased transmitter release at excitatory synapses produced by direct activation of adenylate cyclase in rat hippocampal slices. J Neurosci 1994;14:310–317.
70. Trudeau LE, Emery DG, Haydon PG. Direct modulation of the secretory machinery underlies PKA-dependent synaptic facilitation in hippocampal neurons. Neuron 1996;17:789–797.
71. Sakaba T, Neher E. Preferential potentiation of fast-releasing synaptic vesicles by cAMP at the calyx of Held. Proc Natl Acad Sci U S A 2001;98:331–336.
72. Kaneko M, Takahashi T. Presynaptic mechanism underlying cAMP-dependent synaptic potentiation. J Neurosci 2004;24:5202–5208.
73. Trudeau LE, Fang Y, Haydon PG. Modulation of an early step in the secretory machinery in hippocampal nerve terminals. Proc Natl Acad Sci U S A 1998;95:7163–7168.
74. Evans GJO, Morgan A. Phosphorylation-dependent interaction of the synaptic vesicle proteins cysteine string protein and synaptotagmin I. Biochem J 2002;364:343–347.
75. Chheda MG, Ashery U, Thakur P, Rettig J, Sheng Z-H. Phosphorylation of Snapin by PKA modulates its interaction with the SNARE complex. Nat Cell Biol 2001;3:331–338.
76. Lonart G, Südhof TC. Region-specific phosphorylation of rabphilin in mossy fiber nerve terminals of the hippocampus. J Neurosci 1998;18:634–640.
77. Lonart G, Schoch S, Kaeser PS, Larkin CJ, Südhof TC, Linden DJ. Phosphorylation of RIM1alpha by PKA triggers presynaptic long-term potentiation at cerebellar parallel fiber synapses. Cell 2003;115:49–60.
78. Hepp R, Cabaniols J-P, Roche PA. Differential phosphorylation of SNAP-25 in vivo by protein kinase C and protein kinase A. FEBS Lett 2002;532:52–56.
79. Boczan J, Leenders AG, Sheng Z-H. Phosphorylation of syntaphilin by cAMP-dependent protein kinase modulates its interaction with syntaxin-1 and annuls its inhibitory effect on vesicle exocytosis. J Biol Chem 2004;279:18911–18919.
80. Nagy G, Reim K, Matti U, et al. Regulation of releasable vesicle pool sizes by protein kinase A-dependent phosphorylation of SNAP-25. Neuron 2004;41:417–429.
81. Ilardi JM, Mochida S, Sheng Z-H. Snapin: a SNARE-associated protein implicated in synaptic transmission. Nat Neurosci 1999;2:119–124.
82. Thakur P, Stevens DR, Sheng Z-H, Rettig J. Effects of PKA-mediated phosphorylation of Snapin on synaptic transmission in cultured hippocampal neurons. J Neurosci 2004; 24:6476–6481.
83. Nie Z, Ranjan R, Wenniger JJ, Hong SN, Bronk P, Zinsmaier KE. Overexpression of cysteine-string proteins in Drosophila reveals interactions with syntaxin. J Neurosci 1999;19: 10270–10279.
84. Dawson-Scully K, Bronk P, Atwood HL, Zinsmaier KE. Cysteine-string protein increases the calcium sensitivity of neurotransmitter exocytosis in Drosophila. J Neurosci 2000;20:6039–6047.
85. Graham ME, Burgoyne RD. Comparison of cysteine string protein (Csp) and mutant alpha-SNAP overexpression reveals a role for csp in late steps of membrane fusion in dense-core granule exocytosis in adrenal chromaffin cells. J Neurosci 2000;20:1281–1289.

Chapter 11
Synaptic Vesicle Endocytosis

Liesbet Smitz and Patrik Verstreken

Contents

Abstract Synapses locally recycle vesicles to ensure the maintenance of neuronal communication critical for normal brain function. While several modes of vesicle regeneration are thought to exist, clathrin-mediated endocytosis (CME) is the best studied mechanism of synaptic vesicle recycling. During CME, the membrane bends, invaginates, and forms a new vesicle that is pinched from the synaptic membrane. As this is not easily achieved, numerous proteins and lipids have been identified that orchestrate vesicle formation from the presynaptic membrane and by integrating structural, biochemical, and *in vivo* loss of function studies in various organisms a molecular description of the process is starting to emerge.

Keywords Clathrin-mediated endocytosis, synaptic vesicle recycling, adaptors, AP2, AP180, actin, amphiphysin, auxilin, calcineurin, cdk-5, clathrin heavy chain, clathrin light chain, dap160, intersectin, dynamin, endophilin, eps15, epsin, hsc70, phosphatidyl inositol kinase, talin, stonin, syndapin, synaptojanin and synaptotagmin.

Patrik Verstreken
VIB Department of Developmental Genetics, K.U.Leuven Center for Human Genetics,
Program in Molecular and Developmental Genetics, Program in Cognitive and Molecular
Neuroscience, 3000 Leuven, Belgium

In our brains, billions of neurons are organized into interconnected neuronal circuits optimized to transmit electrical pulses. The importance of maintaining neuronal communication is underscored by the numerous disorders, such as autism, epilepsy, and drug addiction, that arise from altered neurotransmission in specific circuits. During intense stimulation, neurons release massive amounts of neurotransmitter using synaptic vesicles. Since the number of synaptic vesicles at the nerve terminal is insufficient to account for the neurotransmitters released during bursts of intense stimulation, synapses need to be continuously supplied with fresh vesicles to avoid running out of ammunition. Since axonal transport of new vesicle proteins is too slow, efficient vesicle regeneration systems are put in place at the synapse. Hence, in order to understand the mechanisms of neuronal communication, we need to dissect the mechanisms of synaptic vesicle recovery at the synapse. The ultimate hope is to use this knowledge to understand normal as well as diseased brain function.

Following fusion, vesicles appear to be regenerated by different mechanisms: either they recycle locally by closing their fusion pore, without collapsing into the membrane, a process commonly referred to as "kiss-and-run," or they do collapse in the membrane and new vesicles recycle through clathrin-dependent or -independent invagination of a membrane patch. This chapter discusses the molecular mechanisms concerning clathrin-mediated vesicle retrieval, as in most neurons this is the predominant form of recycling. While clathrin-independent mechanisms of membrane invagination have also been proposed for the recycling of synaptic vesicles, the molecular components involved remain enigmatic, and its role in synaptic vesicle retrieval per se remains debated (1,2). Kiss-and-run–type recycling was discussed in Chapter 2.

Clathrin-mediated endocytosis (CME) initiates by sorting synaptic vesicle cargo (the proteins and lipids that should end up in the vesicle), followed by the polymerization of coat proteins, including clathrin and adaptors. Polymerization is accompanied by invagination of a membrane patch, eventually culminating in the formation of a coated pit (Fig. 11.1). This pit is detached from the membrane to form a new vesicle that is subsequently uncoated and refilled with transmitter, ready to take on a new round of release. Although coated vesicle formation is frequently viewed as a linear set of steps, energetic considerations indicate that the early phases of cargo concentration, membrane invagination, and coat assembly likely all occur in parallel (3). Nonetheless, for clarity we describe different steps of vesicle formation separately, highlighting the relevant molecular components important for each particular phase (Fig. 11.1).

Clathrin-Mediated Endocytosis

Early Endocytosis: Formation of a Shallow Pit

Clathrin-mediated endocytosis of synaptic vesicles initiates with the formation of clathrin-coated pits that consist of three layers. The inner membrane layer contains transmembrane cargo, while the outer layer is composed of lattices of clathrin triskelions that act as a mechanical scaffold. The intermediate layer contains adap-

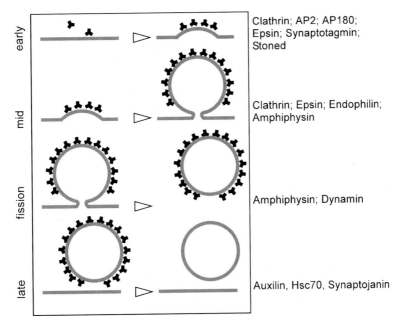

Fig. 11.1 Clathrin-mediated endocytosis. Steps involved in clathrin-mediated endocytosis and some of the proteins involved, as discussed in the text. Note that while this diagram shows sequential endocytic steps, current data suggest that early and mid-endocytic steps may occur in parallel, leading up to vesicle fission. The list of proteins shown is not meant to be complete but illustrates the involvement of some of the proteins during vesicle formation

tor proteins that link clathrin and the invaginating membrane together (4). This section highlights clathrin's structural properties and the importance of adaptor molecules, AP2, AP180, stoned, and epsin, to recruit and stabilize clathrin at the plasma membrane.

Clathrin and the Formation of Coated Vesicles

The abundance of clathrin-coated vesicles found in various eukaryotic cell types suggests it plays a central role in membrane trafficking (5–7). Clathrin is found in numerous species and the remarkable amino acid sequence identity suggests a common conserved function for the protein (8,9). While genetic perturbation of the gene does point to a critical role for the protein in cellular and organismal viability (10–13) (Table 11.1), detailed *in vivo* analyses of clathrin function in neurons and its role in the recycling of synaptic vesicles merits further investigation (2,14).

Biochemical and structural studies of clathrin reveal mechanisms of polymerization and cage formation (3,15–18). Three clathrin heavy chains (CHCs) and three clathrin light chains (CLCs) interact to form clathrin triskelia (Fig. 11.2A), three legged-structures

Table 11.1 Loss-of-function studies of some of the proteins implicated in synaptic vesicle endocytosis

Protein	Localization in the cell during endocytosis	Some of the organisms where loss-of-function studies show defects in synaptic clathrin-mediated endocytosis (CME)	Proposed function
α-Adaptin (AP2)	Vesicle coat and synaptic hot spots	*Drosophila* (31)	It assembles an endocytic complex and links the clathrin coat to the internalizing synaptic membrane patch
AP180	Vesicle coat	*Drosophila* (30) *C. elegans* (49) Squid (34)	It regulates synaptic vesicle size, likely by regulating the size of the clathrin basket that forms when a membrane patch internalizes
Protein	Localization in the cell during endocytosis	Some of the organisms where loss-of-function studies show defects in synaptic clathrin-mediated endocytosis (CME)	Proposed function
Amphiphysin	Nerve terminal, epithelial cells, and muscle cells	Mouse (143) Lamprey (142)	It binds several endocytic proteins, can bend membranes. and may recruit dynamin during vesicle formation; in muscles, the protein is involved in tubulating membranes
Auxilin	Clathrin-coated vesicles	Squid (182)	It recruits hsc70 to coated vesicles and facilitates clathrin uncoating following fission
Clathrin heavy chain	Membrane of budding vesicles	*Drosophila* (13)	Fly *chc* mutants are embryonic lethal but the function CHC in the fly nervous system has not been studied; however, RNAi and pharmacologic inhibition on neuron culture show reduced recycling (14,195).
dap160	Endocytic regions in the nerve terminal	*Drosophila* (68) Lamprey (161)	It may serve as a scaffold for endocytosis and maintains high dynamin levels by collaborating with eps15

(continued)

Table 11.1 (continued)

Protein	Localization in the cell during endocytosis	Some of the organisms where loss-of-function studies show defects in synaptic clathrin-mediated endocytosis (CME)	Proposed function
Dynamin	Endocytic regions in the nerve terminal. neck and head of forming synaptic vesicles	Drosophila (193) C. elegans (194) Mouse (67)	It is essential to separate newly formed vesicles from the plasma membrane; it might also play a role during early stages of endocytosis
Endophilin	Endocytic regions in the nerve terminal and coated vesicles	Drosophila (93–95) C. elegans (91) Lamprey (88,103)	It serves as an adaptor for synaptojanin and is critical for uncoating; it can also sense curvature and bend membrane facilitating the transition from early to late endocytic stages
eps15	On the rims of coated pits; not on coated vesicles	Drosophila (68,147,157) C. elegans (113) Squid (156)	It may serve as a scaffold for endocytosis and maintains high dynamin levels by collaborating with dap160
hsc70	Nerve terminal	Squid (182)	It promotes vesicle uncoating through an interaction with auxilin
Stoned/stonin	Nerve terminal	Drosophila (64,65)	It is a specialized sorting adaptor that cooperates with AP2 to ensure high-fidelity recycling of synaptic membrane
Synaptojanin	Nerve terminal	Drosophila (90) C. elegans (104) Mouse (43) Lamprey (103) Zebrafish (183)	It is a phosphoinositide phosphatase involved in endocytosis and cooperates with endophilin to promote vesicle uncoating
Synaptotagmin	Synaptic vesicles and synaptic membrane	Drosophila (78,80) C. elegans (79) Squid (81)	Synaptotagmin binds AP2, and, through this interaction, it may recruit the endocytic machinery to promote synaptic vesicle retrieval from the membrane

that can assemble into cages around invaginating synaptic membranes in a highly cooperative manner (19,20). Each heavy chain consists of an N-terminal β-propeller globular domain (TD) and a large linear domain with eight tandem repeats

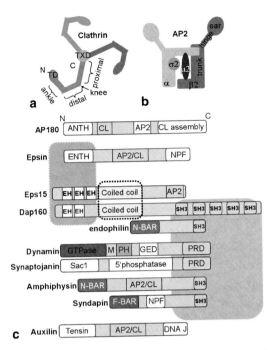

Fig. 11.2 Domain structure of major proteins thought to be involved in clathrin-mediated endocytosis. (A) Clathrin triskelion is formed by trimerization of three heavy chains (170 kDa) and three light chains (33 to 35 kDa) (not shown). The heavy chain consists of three main domains: an N-terminal domain (TD), a leg (harboring an ankle, distal, knee, and proximal portion), and a C-terminal trimerization domain (TXD). (B) Adaptor complex 2 (AP2) is a heterotetrameric complex of α, β_2, μ_2, and σ_2 subunits, which are also called "adaptins." (C) Domain structures of biochemically and genetically well-characterized endocytic proteins: AP180 (95 kDa), epsin (94 kDa), eps15 (100 kDa), DAP160/intersectin (145 kDa), endophilin (40 kDa), dynamin (100 kDa), synaptojanin (145 kDa), amphiphysin (76 kDa), syndapin (55 kDa), and auxilin (100 kDa). ANTH, AP180 amino-terminal homology; DNA-J, identified in the prokaryotic heat shock protein DnaJ and takes part in the chaperone system of protein folding; ENTH, epsin amino-terminal homology, and structurally related to ANTH; CL, clathrin binding domain; AP2, adaptor complex 2 binding domain; NPF, Asp-Pro-Phe motifs; EH, Eps15 homology; BAR, Bin1/Amphiphysin/Rvs domain; SH3, Src homology 3 domain; M, middle domain in dynamin; PH, pleckstrin homology domain; GED, GTPase effector domain; PRD, proline-rich domain; Sac1, suppressor of actin 1 domain

(CHCR0-7) forming the "proximal," "knee," "distal," and "ankle" portions of the leg of the subunit (21–24). CHC binds with its proximal leg domain to CLC while the distal leg domain is critical for trimerization (25). The N-terminal globular domain contains binding sites for numerous proteins that contain a "clathrin box" (26,27), and fine orchestration of multiple clathrin-protein interactions is believed to be critical for proper polymerization of clathrin triskelia during cage formation. Hence, the peculiar structure of clathrin molecules allows them to assemble into cage like structures while likely simultaneously serving as an organizing interaction scaffold stabilizing numerous endocytic proteins that regulate membrane internalization (3,28).

In most cell types, vesicles of variable diameter can be accommodated in different sized cages. Cryo-electron tomography indeed shows the ability of clathrin triskelia to self-assemble into cages of several designs. The sides of these structures are a combination of pentagonal, hexagonal, and occasionally heptagonal facets allowing clathrin to form cages of variable size (29,30). In contrast, electron micrographs of synaptic terminals indicate that synaptic vesicles are more uniform in size, ensuring the release of constant transmitter packages. As a result, vesicle formation and coat assembly are tightly regulated processes that involve numerous proteins.

Adaptor Proteins AP2 and AP180 Promote Clathrin Assembly During Synaptic Vesicle Endocytosis

Adaptor Proteins in Nerve Terminals

Several adaptor proteins are implicated in synaptic vesicle formation, among them the tetrameric AP2 complex and the monomeric AP180. Both proteins are enriched in nerve terminals and concentrate in endocytic zones (31,32). These adaptors not only bind clathrin but also interact with several other proteins implicated in synaptic vesicle retrieval, and loss-of-function analyses in several species show dramatic defects in synaptic vesicle recycling (31,33,34). Hence, AP2 and AP180 are crucial components of the endocytic machinery at the synapse.

AP2 Is an Interaction Hub

Adaptor proteins are organizing centers that link nascent vesicle membranes to the clathrin lattice while interacting with a cohort of endocytic proteins (35). The AP2 complex is a tetrameric complex that harbors two large, one medium, and one small subunit. The two large subunits, α-adaptin and β_2-adaptin, consist of an "appendage" (ear) domain, a "hinge" region, and a "trunk" region, joined by the medium and small subunits μ_2-adaptin (also called AP50) and σ_2-adaptin, respectively (Fig. 11.2B). The trunk region of AP2 recruits the complex to the membrane likely through the binding of membrane phosphoinositide lipids and cargo such as synaptotagmin, a transmembrane synaptic vesicle protein (36–38). While the trunk region is involved in mediating stable interactions, the appendage domains are held in the cytoplasm on top of flexible linkers (hinges) and are able to interact with a multitude of cytosolic endocytic proteins (35). Hence, AP2 links membrane cargo and cytosolic components.

Although some AP2-interacting proteins bind isolated appendages, others do so more effectively only when appendage domains are concentrated, forming so called "hubs." This happens when coated pits are formed and multiple AP2s interact with the membrane. Hub properties are then lost when clathrin is recruited and binds to the appendages, resulting in the displacement of endocytic components and the formation of stable coated vesicles. Hence, in this model, AP2 hubs exist transiently at the leading edge of coated pit formation and are key in organizing coated vesicle formation (3,18,36,39).

AP180 Is a Monomeric Adaptor Protein that Controls Vesicle Size

AP180 was originally isolated as a protein concentrated in nerve terminals and enriched on clathrin coated vesicles (40–42). AP180 harbors a conserved N-terminal phosphatidylinositol-4,5-bisphosphate (PtdIns(4,5)P2) and phosphatidylinositol-3,4,5-triphosphate (PtdIns(3,4,5)P3) binding region termed the ANTH domain (Fig. 11.2C). PtdIns(4,5)P2 and likely also PtdIns(3,4,5)P3 are critically involved in endocytosis and allow adaptors to bind the synaptic plasma membrane, initiating budding (43). The AP180 ANTH domain is followed by an unstructured region that binds clathrin as well as AP2 (44,45). Hence, similar to AP2, AP180 may be involved in endocytic pit formation through interactions with both the plasma membrane and clathrin.

In addition to binding clathrin, adaptor proteins also promote coat formation *in vitro*. While addition of AP2 to a coat formation assay stimulates the formation of uniform coats at physiologic pH, AP180 is approximately four times more effective (46,47). In addition, a more homogeneous population of cages is formed when AP180 is present (44), suggesting that AP180, assisted by AP2, controls the size of coated pits and new synaptic vesicles.

Loss of Adaptor Protein Function Blocks Clathrin-Mediated Endocytosis

Although in budding yeast adaptor-like proteins are dispensable for endocytosis (48), neurons are critically dependent on AP2 and AP180 to form new synaptic vesicles. Loss-of-function studies in *Drosophila* using *α-adaptin* mutations demonstrate the critical role for the AP2 complex in vesicle formation (31). Imaging of AP2 deficient neurons shows defects early in synaptic vesicle endocytosis. AP2 null mutants show almost no synaptic vesicles, and hypomorphic mutants fail to take up large amounts of FM 1–43, a fluorescent dye that is incorporated into newly formed vesicles. These data are consistent with a role for AP2 in budding, confirming biochemical studies.

While AP2 null mutant *Drosophila* die very early in life, AP180 mutants die much later, indicating that AP180, a synapse enriched protein, plays a more accessory role compared to AP2 that is also required in nonneuronal cells (30). Additional *in vivo* analyses confirm such a function. Mutant AP180 synapses show a general reduction in synaptic vesicle number and a concomitant decrease in the uptake of FM 1–43, indicating defects in vesicle recycling that are generally less severe than those observed in *α-adaptin* mutant animals. Interestingly, however, *AP180* fly mutants show synaptic vesicles with heterogeneous diameters as determined morphologically and electrophysiologically. Furthermore, injection of AP180 antibodies as well as genetic loss-of-function studies in *Caenorhabditis elegans* confirm these findings and indicate that AP180 is critical for the regulation of synaptic vesicle size in several organisms, as *in vitro* studies suggest (30,34,49).

Epsin Assists in Clathrin Lattice Formation

Epsin Is Present in Nerve Terminals and on Coated Vesicles

Epsin localizes to nerve terminals and is present on clathrin-coated vesicles, suggesting a role in recycling (50). In addition, epsin binds several endocytic proteins. Epsin harbors a central AP2 and clathrin-binding domain and three C-terminal NPF (asparagine, proline, and phenylalanine) motifs (Fig. 11.2C) that bind eps15 homology (EH) domain–containing proteins, including eps15 and dap160, which are involved in endocytosis (see next subsection) (51).

Epsin's N-terminal homology domain (ENTH) (52) further implicates the protein in vesicle formation. This domain is structurally similar to but functionally quite different from the ANTH domain of AP180 (53,54). Both ANTH and ENTH domains bind PtdIns(4,5)P2 (55); however, unlike ANTH domains, ENTH domains are also capable of deforming membranes. Indeed, *in vitro*, epsin and AP180 each can recruit clathrin and promote its polymerization on lipid monolayers; however, unlike AP180, epsin is also able to modify membrane curvature on binding to PtdIns(4,5)P2, suggesting epsin facilitates membrane budding (56,57).

In Vivo Studies of Epsin

The two epsin genes in *Saccharomyces cerevisae, ent1* and *ent2,* were shown to be essential for organismic viability and cells depleted of epsin showed reduced uptake of a fluorescent dye (FM 4-64), suggesting defects in vesicle endocytosis in these cells (58). However, in flies, loss of Liquid Facets, LQF (the *Drosophila* epsin homologue), shows only a slight reduction in evoked transmitter release and no abnormalities in FM 1-43 uptake at the synapse (59), suggesting that epsin does not play an important role in endocytosis. However, this analysis is complicated by potential redundant effects of another epsin homologue in the fly genome. Hence, careful *in vivo* analyses of the two epsins in flies or epsin in other species will be required to clarify the role of the protein at live synapses.

Stoned Proteins Act as Adaptor Proteins for Synaptotagmin in Endocytosis

Drosophila stoned (stn) mutants were identified more than 35 years ago in a behavioral screen for stress-sensitive mutants (60), and were shown to genetically interact with dynamin mutants (61). Meanwhile, a function for *stn* in endocytosis has been well established (62–64). Indeed, synapses of *stn* mutants show reduced FM 1-43 uptake upon stimulation, a hallmark of defects in recycling. In addition, electron microscopy of mutant nerve terminals shows that synaptic vesicles are reduced in number and heterogeneous in size, resembling phenotypes seen in other endocytic mutants (30,65–68). Combined, these data are reminiscent of those observed in *AP180* mutants and indicate a role of *stn* in endocytosis.

Mapping of the *stn* locus revealed it produces a bicistronic transcript encoding stnA and stnB proteins (69). Although both proteins are concentrated at nerve terminals (65,66), only the stnB protein is involved in endocytosis. While stnA does not show similarity to other endocytic proteins, stnB shows sequence similarity to the medium subunit of the AP2 complex, µ2 adaptin (69). In addition, stnB binds several endocytic proteins including eps15, dap160, and AP2 (70–72). Finally, genetic rescue experiments with stnB, but not stnA, alleviate the endocytic defects associated with the *stn* mutations (62), indicating that it is stnB that is critical for endocytosis.

Like stnB, its mammalian homologue stonin 2 is similar to µ2 adaptin in protein sequence. The similarity between stnB/stonin 2 and the medium subunit of the AP2 adaptor suggests that stnB and stonin 2 may function as specialized adaptors in synaptic endocytosis. Interestingly, *stn* binds the synaptic vesicle-associated protein synaptotagmin directly (63,71–73) and genes encoding these two proteins genetically interact. Furthermore, in *stn* mutants synaptotagmin is dramatically mislocalized (64,73), implying that *stn* may serve as a recycling adaptor for synaptotagmin. Corroborating this model, electrophysiologic analyses of neurotransmitter release in *stn* mutants phenocopy synaptotagmin mutants in *Drosophila,* suggesting that proper subcellular localization of synaptotagmin via stnB is essential to the function of synaptotagmin in neurotransmitter release (64). Together these data suggest that while AP2 is a general adaptor that links the endocytic machinery to cargo, stnB/stonin2 needs to function as a specialized sorting adaptor that cooperates with AP2 to ensure high-speed and high-fidelity recycling of synaptic membranes (63).

Synaptotagmin: A Synaptic Vesicle-Associated Protein Required for Synaptic Recycling

Synaptotagmin is generally known as a putative calcium sensor for fast synchronous neurotransmitter release, as described in Chapter 7. However, the interactions of synaptotagmin with AP2 and *stn* suggest that synaptotagmin also plays a role in the recycling of synaptic vesicle membranes (74–77). Consistent with this notion, injection of antibodies against the synaptotagmin C2B domain leads to vesicle depletion in squid synapses. In addition, synaptic vesicle number is reduced in *C. elegans* and specific fly synaptotagmin mutants (78–81). Finally, elegant acute perturbation studies using 4′,5′-bis(1,3,2-dithioarsolan-2-yl)fluorescein (FlAsH)-mediated fluorescein-assisted light inactivation (FALI) to inactivate synaptotagmin protein within seconds, combined with live imaging of exo- and endocytosis (using synaptopHluorin), further indicate the critical role of synaptotagmin in the synaptic recycling (82,83). Hence, the collaboration among AP2, *stn*, and synaptotagmin appears to form a high-fidelity endocytic cargo complex that initiates synaptic vesicle endocytosis via the clathrin-mediated pathway (84).

Early to Mid-Endocytosis: Bending Membranes to Form Deeply Invaginated Coated Pits

Membrane-Bending Domains

During assembly of clathrin and adaptor complexes, the membrane bends to accommodate the curved dome shape of the clathrin lattice. As this is not a trivial feat, several mechanisms likely act in concert to induce membrane curvature. While purified lipids do not spontaneously deform and take on the curves of synaptic vesicle membranes, concentrated fractions of specific lipid-types are capable of deforming liposomes into tubules, suggesting lipid composition is at least a permissive factor in inducing membrane curvature (85).

Another determinant of membrane deformation is the protein-lipid environment. Protein scaffolding surfaces that link membranes to curved templates have been suggested to sense, induce, and stabilize curvature. In addition, insertion of amphiphatic helices or other transmembrane segments that disrupt one leaflet of the flat plasma membrane have also been implicated in generating curvature (86). Interestingly, several proteins involved in synaptic vesicle endocytosis are thought to modify membrane curvature, including ENTH domain- and BAR (Bin1/Amphiphysin/Rvs) domain-containing proteins. Epsin, an ENTH domain protein that can induce curvature, was described in the previous section; in this section we highlight the role of the N-BAR domain of endophilin in inducing and stabilizing membrane curvature.

Endophilin Generates High-Curvature Membranes

Endophilin was isolated in a yeast-two-hydrid screen using the proline-rich domain (PRD) of synaptojanin as bait (87). Endophilin harbors a BAR domain and a C-terminal SH3 domain (Fig. 11.2C). The SH3 domain tightly interacts with synaptojanin and also binds dynamin and amphiphysin, three proteins implicated in CME (88–90). In addition, the protein is concentrated at synapses (87,91) and endocytic hotspots, colocalizes with clathrin in immunoelectron microscopy studies, and is present on internalizing vesicles (88,92–95). These data imply that endophilin is part of the endocytic interactome and plays an important role in CME in neurons. Indeed, cell free reconstitution assays and acute inhibition of endophilin function in lamprey neurons further implicate the protein in clathrin-mediated vesicle budding (88,96–98).

Additional analyses indicate that endophilin also induces membrane curvature to promote vesicle formation. Purified endophilin can bind and tubulate lipid bilayers with neck diameters very similar to those of deeply invaginated clathrin-coated pits, and this activity is contained in the N-terminal domain of the protein. The N-terminal portion of endophilin contains an N-BAR domain consisting of an N-terminal amphiphatic helix, a BAR domain, and an internal amphiphatic helix. Interestingly, these different sections of the N-BAR appear to cooperate to induce and stabilize curvature (99). First, the BAR domain forms a rigid positively charged

concave interaction surface that binds negatively charged membranes and dimer-
izes effectively, scaffolding curved membranes (100). In fact, endophilin binds
very strongly to membranes such that the binding energy of the BAR domain to the
membrane is close to that required to bend the membrane (101). This suggests that
endophilin would not only be able to bind to an already bent membrane but that the
protein actually would be able to induce and stabilize membrane curvature. Second,
the insertion of the N-terminal amphiphatic helix into the hydrophobic layer of the
bilayer has been implicated in inducing membrane curvature during membrane
budding, and this is believed to be a general feature of several curvature-inducing
domains (56,100,102). Finally, the internal amphipathic helix of endophilin appears
to stabilize N-BAR dimers. This helix also inserts into the membrane to further
promote the generation of membrane curvature (99). Hence, endophilin forms a
rigid curved charged interaction scaffold for binding the membrane while inducing
curvature by inserting amphiphatic helices in the plasma membrane.

   Loss-of-function analyses of endophilin in *C. elegans, Drosophila,* and lamprey
are consistent with a role for the protein in vesicle budding, but, interestingly, also
indicate that endophilin plays a more critical role at a later stage, following fission,
during vesicle-uncoating (91,94,103; also see below). Injection of inhibitory peptides
that block endophilin interactions in lamprey synapses leads to a block late in endocytosis at the uncoating stage (103). Similarly, in *C. elegans* and *Drosophila* endophilin null mutants, synaptic vesicle numbers are vastly reduced, stalled early
endocytic structures are not readily observed, and coated vesicles accumulate, a phenotype that is indistinguishable from *synaptojanin* mutants that block CME at the
uncoating stage (see Late Endocytosis, below) (43,90–92,94,104). Hence, these *in
vivo* studies indicate that endophilin plays a critical role during vesicle uncoating.

   While the *in vivo* data suggest endophilin acts late in endocytosis, they do not
exclude an earlier, nonessential function for endophilin (and synaptojanin). Indeed,
Drosophila hypomorphic *endophilin* mutants show an accumulation of budding
vesicles at the plasma membrane, not observed in controls (93). Although these
data are consistent with a block earlier in endocytosis, the data could also be the
result of a general slowing of the clathrin-mediated machinery. Nonetheless, injection of lamprey synapses with endophilin antibodies also shows stalled clathrin-
coated prefission intermediates (88), suggesting that aside from an essential role in
uncoating, endophilin may aid in vesicle budding, facilitating the transition from
early to late endocytic stages by sensing and inducing membrane curvature.

Mid-Late Endocytosis: Clathrin-Coated Pits are Disconnected from the Presynaptic Membrane by the Large Guanosine Triphosphatase Dynamin

Once deeply invaginated clathrin-coated pits are formed, they are pinched off from
the presynaptic membrane to become free clathrin-coated vesicles. While *in vitro*
as well as *in vivo* studies point to dynamin as being critical at the fission step (105),
its exact mode of action during fission remains an intensely studied topic.

A Multistep Model for Dynamin During Fission

Shibire Is Dynamin

The importance of dynamin in synaptic vesicle endocytosis was first highlighted with the identification of temperature-sensitive mutant alleles in *Drosophila melanogaster*. When such mutant flies are placed at high temperature, they paralyze, and this is reversible by bringing the animals back to room temperature (60). The locus responsible for this phenotype was named *"shibire,"* the Japanese word for "paralyzed." The *shibire (shi)* gene was subsequently identified and shown to encode the homologue of mammalian dynamin (105). While mammals express several dynamins (106,107), single isoforms of the classical dynamin in *D. melanogaster* and *C. elegans* are assumed to cover the functions of the multiple isoforms in mammals.

Dynamin is a large guanosine triphosphatase (GTPase) (100 kDa) harboring five well-defined domains (Fig. 11.2C): an N-terminal GTPase domain, a middle (M) domain, a pleckstrin homology (PH) domain, a GTPase effector (GED) domain, and a proline-rich domain (PRD). The GTPase domain contains four GTP-binding motifs, required for guanine nucleotide binding and GTP-hydrolysis. The middle domain consists of a coiled-coil region, shown to be involved in oligomerization (108). The GED also contains a coiled-coil region, which interacts with the GTPase and middle domain during oligomerization, mediating increased GTPase activity. Hence, while most GTPases require another protein to stimulate their activities, dynamin harbors an intrinsic GTPase-activating domain (GAD) (109). In addition, dynamin also contains two targeting domains: a PH and a PRD. The PH domain binds to PtdIns(4,5)P2, thereby inducing dynamin's GTPase activity (110), whereas the PRD binds to src-homology-3 (SH3) domain proteins, such as endophilin, amphiphysin, syndapin, and dynamin-associated protein (160 kDa) (dap160/intersectin) (87,111–114). Hence, during endocytosis, dynamin may interact with numerous partners to catalyze vesicle formation and fission.

Dynamin Is Essential for Endocytosis

Phenotypic analyses of *shi* mutants reveal the essential role of dynamin in synaptic vesicle endocytosis. When neurons of temperature-sensitive *shi^ts1* mutants are stimulated intensely at restrictive temperatures, they fail to maintain release and eventually run out of synaptic vesicles (94,115), a result also supported by experiments in hippocampal neurons where dynamin was acutely inhibited with a recently developed noncompetitive inhibitor of dynamin, dynasore (116). In line with these observations, morphologic analyses of *shi^ts1* mutant neurons show vesicle depletion and an accumulation of endocytic intermediates that fail to pinch off the synaptic membrane (117,118). These membrane structures often appear electron-dense and coated on the surface, resembling clathrin-coated pits (119). Interestingly, around the necks of these intermediates, electron-dense "collars," believed to contain dynamin, are visible (32,119). Hence, *in vivo* mutational analyses point to an essential role for dynamin in synaptic vesicle fission and recycling.

Dynamin Is a Mechanoenzyme Inducing Neck Constriction

How does dynamin mediate vesicle fission? *In vitro* experiments show that purified dynamin can self-assemble into rings and spirals when incubated in low salt buffers (120). Interestingly, these rings and spirals have the same dimensions as the collars observed in *shi*[ts1] flies and those seen on vesicle necks when rat brain synaptosomes are incubated with the nonhydrolyzable GTP-analogue GTPγS (121). Therefore, dynamin rings and spirals appear to be common intermediates in vesicle formation.

The role of dynamin during fission is further highlighted by tubulation assays. When purified dynamin is added to lipid bilayers, it initiates the formation of lipid tubules, and these are wrapped with dynamin helical rings. Interestingly, when GTP is added, the tubules twist and supercoil and are eventually disrupted to form vesicle-like structures (122,123). While these data suggest that dynamin can tubulate lipids, and mediate fission in a GTP-dependent fashion, recent evidence indicates that mechanoconstriction per se is not sufficient for fission. Only when the lipid tubules are under longitudinal tension can dynamin induce fission (123). Hence, at the short necks of synaptic vesicles, accessory factors may induce tension and cooperate with the constricting action of dynamin to induce vesicle fission.

Dynamin as Mechanoenzyme and Classical GTPase

The mechanoenzyme model for dynamin action during vesicle fission implicates GTP hydrolysis as a driving force. Consistent with this notion, addition of GTPγS, a nonhydrolyzable GTP analogue, or introduction of point-mutants into dynamin to prevent GTP binding, results in the disappearance of constrictive activity (124,125). It is well established that the GTPase activity of dynamin is stimulated by dynamin self-assembly. Surprisingly, dynamin mutants specifically defective in assembly-stimulated GTPase activity (GAD mutants) do not block but instead stimulate endocytosis. A GAD domain mutant of dynamin (K649A) inhibits self-assembly and therefore also assembly-stimulated GTPase activity. The same mutant, however, is mostly stuck in GTP bound form but still harbors basal GTPase activity (126,127). The data suggest that while basal GTPase activity of dynamin is essential for twisting and constricting membranes, dynamin's "active" state is the GTP-bound form, similar to other GTPases. In the GTP-bound state, dynamin could then recruit accessory proteins that mediate downstream endocytic events (39,126,128–131). Nonetheless, analyses with additional GED and GTPase domain mutants paint a more complicated picture where GTP-binding, interactions with downstream effectors, GTP hydrolysis, and conformational changes are all likely required for endocytosis and vesicle fission.

Such a multistep model is also supported by analyses of the *shi*[ts2] mutation in *Drosophila* (132). While *shi*[ts2] mutations show reduced GTP hydrolysis and GTP binding, addition of a mutation in the GAD domain of *shi*[ts2] can fully suppress the endocytic defects associated with *shi*[ts2]. Interestingly, these suppressors of *shibire* (abbreviated as *sushi*) mutants, do not restore the reduced GTPase activity of the *shi*[ts2] mutation but rather reduce it further, likely resulting in longer GTP binding times on the mutant protein. Hence, similar to the data obtained with overexpression of GAD domain mutants, these data suggest that GTP binding is essential for dynamin function during endocytosis, but do not exclude a role for self-assembled dynamin-stimulated GTP hydrolysis during later stages of endocytosis. Interestingly, acute pharmacologic inhibition of dynamin with dynasore reveals early as well as late endocytic intermediates at the plasma membrane, possibly indicating a role for GTP-bound dynamin and GTP hydrolysis by dynamin at different stages of vesicle formation (133). Hence, GTP-dynamin may be part of an endocytic scaffold that mediates membrane invagination, while during later steps its mechanoenzymatic properties and assembly-induced GTP hydrolysis are needed for fission.

Several SH3 Domain-Containing Proteins Interact with Dynamin

The list of dynamin-interacting proteins is ever expanding (134), and it is not our intention to list every one of these interactors here. Instead, we summarize the data for some and highlight their link with synaptic vesicle endocytosis. We discuss the roles of amphiphysin, dap160/intersectin, and syndapin here, while further highlighting the role of endophilin in synaptic vesicle retrieval in a later subsection.

Amphiphysin: A Regulator of Dynamin 1 Recruitment

Amphiphysin was originally identified by immunoscreening a complementary DNA (cDNA) expression library using antibodies directed against synaptic plasma membranes (135) and is arguably one of the best characterized binding partners of dynamin. This protein contains a number of "classical" features suggesting it plays a critical role in membrane endocytosis. Not only does amphiphysin harbor a central CLAP (clathrin and adaptor binding domain) (Fig. 11.2C) that binds the AP2 adaptor and clathrin, but it also contains a C-terminal SH3 domain that binds the proline-rich domains of dynamin and synaptojanin, both critical for synaptic vesicle endocytosis (35,111). In addition, amphiphysin is one of the founding members of the BAR domain-containing protein family, involved in membrane bending and curvature sensing (100). Indeed, *in vitro* studies have shown that purified amphiphysin, like dynamin, can tubulate spherical liposomes, suggesting the protein is involved in membrane bending during endocytosis (136,137). Combined, these studies implicate amphiphysin as an important multifunctional membrane-transforming adaptor, linking clathrin and adaptors to the endocytic machinery.

Additional studies point to a role for amphiphysin in regulating dynamin function. While dynamin can form vesicles from large liposomes *in vitro*, this activity is enhanced by addition of amphiphysin (136). Furthermore, the GTPase activity of dynamin increases when amphiphysin binds, and this interaction is regulated by activity. In addition, dynamin as well as amphiphysin are constitutively phosphorylated by cdk-5, attenuating the ability of amphiphysin to interact with the membrane (138). However, upon neuronal activity and calcium influx, the calcineurin phosphatase is activated, and both dynamin and amphiphysin are dephosphorylated, allowing them to assemble into ring-like structures that promote vesicle formation at the plasma membrane (139,140). Interestingly, these data are corroborated by ultrastructural studies in the lamprey giant synapse where amphiphysin immunore-activity redistributes from the vesicle cluster to endocytic zones in response to electrical stimulation of the nerve (141). Hence, in response to intense stimulation, amphiphysin may relocate and promote endocytosis by tubulating lipids and induc-ing dynamin-mediated vesicle fission.

To analyze the function of amphiphysin during neuronal vesicle recycling, several *in vivo* loss-of-function studies were undertaken. Interestingly, microinjection of inhibitory peptides or antibodies in the lamprey giant synapse causes severe endocytic defects. Stalled early endocytic intermediates and clathrin-coated vesicles accumulate upon acute blockage of amphiphysin function (141,142). However, gene knockout studies in mouse, flies, and nematodes fail to reveal a major role for the protein in synaptic vesicle recycling. In mice, loss of amphiphysin 1 leads to a parallel loss of the other isoform, amphiphysin 2, in the brain. Despite the lack of amphiphysin func-tion in these animals, the observed endocytic defects, compared to loss of other endo-cytic proteins, were rather mild (143), indicating a more accessory role of the protein in vesicle recycling. In line with this, RNA interference (RNAi) studies targeting the *amph-1* gene in *C. elegans* show no overt defects in the nervous system (www.wormbase.org), while null mutations in *Drosophila* also show no defects in synaptic vesicle recycling (144). The lack of obvious endocytic defects in these animals may be due to functional compensation by other BAR domain-containing proteins that operate in endocytosis. However, loss of other endocytic proteins, including BAR domain-con-taining ones, do show strong endocytic defects and hence fail to show such pheno-typic compensation, making this possibility unlikely. However, it is noteworthy that fly and nematode amphiphysins do not contain a CLAP domain and fly amphiphysin does not bind dynamin and is localized to muscle (145), thereby precluding a role for the protein in neurons of fruit flies. Instead, amphiphysin in flies and amphiphysin 2 in mice appear to play a critical role in muscles, during T-tubule biogenesis (144,146). The data may therefore indicate that amphiphysins play a critical role in remodeling muscle membranes, and that this function could have evolved to take on an accessory role during synaptic vesicle endocytosis in vertebrates.

Dap160 and eps15 Collaborate to Maintain High Dynamin Concentrations at the Endocytic Zone

Synapses harbor high dynamin concentrations to ensure reliable vesicle formation. As mentioned before, the dynamin GTPase activity is enhanced by the cooperative assembly of dynamin in oligomers. Hence, the efficiency of dynamin during endo-cytosis is positively correlated with its concentration, highlighting the importance of maintaining high dynamin levels at the synapse (129). Coincidentally, two endo-cytic scaffold molecules, dap160/intersectin and eps15, were recently shown to maintain high dynamin levels within endocytic zones, thereby promoting efficient synaptic vesicle endocytosis (69,114,147–149).

Eps15 is a 100-kDa multidomain protein that was originally discovered as a phosphorylation substrate of epidermal growth factor receptor (EGFR) kinase (149), but several lines of evidence from *in vitro* and cell culture studies clearly implicate the protein in endocytosis (150). Eps15 harbors three N-terminal eps15 homology (EH) domains (Fig. 11.2C), also found in other proteins of the EH-domain protein family (151), a central coiled-coil domain that serves as a binding site for dap160/intersectin (152) and eps15 itself (153), and 15 C-terminal DPF (Asp-Pro-Phe) protein–protein interaction motifs. While by virtue of these domains eps15 can interact with many endocytic proteins including epsin, AP180, synapto-janin, dap160, and AP2 (113,152,154), the functional implications of most of these interactions have not been investigated *in vivo*.

Eps15 is critical for synaptic vesicle formation. At the synapse, eps15 localizes to the edges of clathrin-coated pits (155) and is enriched in the clathrin-coated vesi-cle fraction (51). Injection of eps15 inhibitory peptides in squid giant synapses leads to defects in endocytosis (156). In addition, genetic loss-of-function studies in *C. elegans* and *Drosophila* provide strong evidence for a role of this protein in synaptic vesicle cycling (113,148,157). Eps15 mutant animals show characteristic synaptic vesicle depletion and behavioral defects. In flies, loss of eps15 also results in a defect to endocytose new vesicles as monitored with FM 1–43 dye and a failure to maintain release during intense stimulation, strongly implicating this protein in the recycling of synaptic vesicles. Interestingly, the levels of dynamin are severely reduced at eps15 mutant synapses, suggesting eps15 is responsible for maintaining high dynamin concentrations at endocytic sites.

The major binding partner of eps15 in neurons is dap160/intersectin (157,158). Like eps15, dap160 contains N-terminal EH domains, a central coiled-coil domain, and C-terminal SH3 domains (Fig. 11.2C). Dap160 localizes to endocytic zones and has also been shown to bind to a multitude of endocytic proteins including epsin, dynamin, stnB, and connecdenn, suggesting an important role in vesicle endocytosis (70,114,159). Interestingly, while fly dap160 holds four SH3 domains, vertebrate dap160 (intersectin 1L) harbors five such domains plus a GED, a PH, and a C2 domain (160), suggesting slightly divergent roles. Nonetheless, the particular domain structure of this protein indicates it may stabilize multiple protein–protein interactions during endocytosis (152).

Loss-of-function studies in lamprey and flies indeed strongly suggest dap160 is an endocytic scaffold molecule that cooperates with eps15. When lamprey giant synapses are injected with intersectin antibodies or inhibitory SH3 peptides, clathrin-coated pits and membrane invaginations reminiscent of a block in endocy-tosis are observed (161). In flies, complete loss of dap160 yields rather mild endocytic defects, but these are strongly exacerbated when the temperature is raised (68). Such a temperature-sensitive recycling defect in the absence of dap160 protein is consistent with a scaffolding function of the protein; while at low tem-perature sufficient interactions necessary for vesicle endocytosis can occur, the increased kinetic energy at high temperature prevents efficient formation of endo-cytic protein–protein and protein–lipid complexes, which are normally stabilized by dap160, thereby inhibiting endocytosis. Interestingly, mutations in the main binding partner of dap160, eps15, are also temperature-sensitive in *C. elegans*. In addition, numerous endocytic proteins are mislocalized at mutant fly synapses, including dynamin, synaptojanin, endophilin, and AP180, further supporting a scaffolding function for dap160 (68,147). Hence, loss-of-function analyses of both eps15 and dap160 are consistent with a model where these proteins stabilize transient protein–protein and protein–lipid interactions that need to occur during the formation of new vesicles. Furthermore, both dap160 and eps15 are responsible for maintaining high dynamin concentrations at the endocytic zone, and this was confirmed by localization studies in the lamprey (161).

Dap160 and eps15 both harbor a central coiled-coil domain allowing these two proteins to bind. These data suggest that the two proteins can join forces and create a large multidomain endocytic scaffold surface for endocytosis (151,152). This idea was supported by recent *in vivo* analyses of single and double mutants. Single mutants of *eps15* and *dap160* display nearly identical defects in vesicle formation, including reduced vesicle numbers, large membrane folds, stalled invaginated pits, severely reduced FM1–43 dye uptake into vesicles upon stimulation, and inability to maintain normal levels of neurotransmitter release during intense stimulation. Interestingly, *eps15; dap160* double mutants show almost identical defects in endocytosis. The lack of additive phenotypes is a strong indication that the two proteins act together at the same step in recycling (157).

Syndapin: A Link with the Actin Cytoskeleton

Actin dynamics have been strongly implicated in endocytosis (162). Actin is an abundant component of nerve terminals. Assembly of actin and myosin filaments may produce mechanical forces required for the different steps of endocytosis, including initiation of membrane invagination, scission of vesicles mediated by dynamin and propelling newly formed vesicles away from the plasma membrane (163). Indeed, as mentioned before, recent evidence indicates that vesicle fission is dependent both on dynamin function and the generation of tension (123), and this could possibly be mediated by the actin cytoskeleton. Furthermore, injection of compounds that interfere with actin function in lamprey giant synapses dramatically impairs synaptic vesicle recycling (164), and dynamic actin tails have been observed at the necks of clathrin-coated pits (165). These and several other observations suggest that actin serves structural and, perhaps, force-generating roles during vesicle recycling.

With the notion that the actin cytoskeleton plays a critical role in recycling came the discovery of numerous proteins that form a link between the actin network and the endocytic machinery. Here we highlight one of these proteins, syndapin (synaptic dynamin-associated protein), a conserved SH3 domain-containing protein originally identified as a binding partner of dynamin (112).

Several lines of evidence point to a role of syndapin in endocytosis. Syndapin not only competes with endophilin for dynamin binding in an activity-dependent manner (166,167) but also binds other proteins involved in vesicle cycling, including synaptojanin and synapsin (168). In addition, like amphiphysin and endophilin, syndapin harbors a BAR domain, allowing it to induce and sense membrane curvature. Indeed, recent evidence indicates that purified syndapin can tubulate lipids *in vitro* (169), suggesting it plays a central role in vesicle formation.

Syndapin links endocytosis to the actin cytoskeleton because it can bind N-WASP (neuronal Wiskott-Aldrich syndrome protein), an activator of the Arp2/3 complex that induces actin nucleation. Interestingly, evanescent wave studies colocalize actin, Arp2/3 as well as N-WASP at endocytic sites, and the presence of these components is coordinated with dynamin-induced vesicle scission (165). An attractive possibility is then that actin nucleation and dynamin-mediated fission coincide by using a common binding partner, syndapin (112). Although syndapin has been suggested to use the same SH3 domain (Fig. 11.2C) to interact both with dynamin and N-WASP, such a simultaneous interaction is theoretically possible as syndapin was recently shown to homodimerize (170). Hence, syndapin may coordinate dynamic interactions between the endocytic machine and the actin cytoskeleton network.

While *in vitro* and overexpression studies point to a role for syndapin in endocytosis, loss-of-function studies are limited and RNAi experiments in *C. elegans* and do not show any clear phenotype in recycling (www.wormbase.org). Moreover, *Drosophila* syndapin is not localized to endocytic zones where proteins such as dap160, esp15, or endophilin reside, but instead it colocalizes with amphiphysin in muscles (authors' unpublished observations). These results suggest that at least in worms and flies, syndapin may not mediate the retrieval of synaptic vesicles.

Late Endocytosis: Uncoating and Reformation of Functional Vesicles

Following fission, vesicles shed their clathrin and adaptor coats before refilling with neurotransmitters. In this section we describe the proteins that act on the synaptic vesicle membrane and coat components to promote the last step of synaptic vesicle formation: uncoating. Once they are uncoated, synaptic vesicles may immediately participate in a new round of release, can be stored in the "reserve pool" to be used at a later stage, or can fuse with intracellular compartments such as endosomes, allowing vesicles to redefine their lipid and membrane protein composition (171).

Hsc70 and Auxilin 1 Drive Clathrin Coat Disassembly

More than 20 years ago, uncoating of the clathrin coat was found to be mediated by a 70-kDa protein that shows clathrin-dependent adenosine triphosphatase (ATPase) activity: hsc70 (172,173). Hsc70 is constitutively expressed and is involved in many cellular processes that require the energy from ATP hydrolysis. Its specificity to the uncoating of endocytic vesicles appears to be conferred by auxilin (Fig. 11.2C), a J-domain–containing protein that binds hsc70 as well as clathrin, AP2, and dynamin

(130,174). Structural analyses of clathrin cages and auxilin suggest that auxilin may recruit hsc70 near a set of critical clathrin–clathrin interactions within the clathrin cage. Auxilin binding, in concert with the hsc70 ATPase activity, may then produce local structural changes in heavy-chain contacts, creating distortions of the clathrin coat leading to clathrin disassembly (17,175,176).

In addition to a role in uncoating, hsc70 and auxilin may be involved in other endocytosis-related clathrin rearrangements. They may catalyze rearrangements of clathrin during the invagination of coated pits at early endocytic steps (19,38,175). An interesting notion is that ATP hydrolysis by hsc70 may drive endocytosis, either by dissociation of the stable clathrin coat into more unstable monomers at the end of the endocytic cycle, or by facilitating the reorganization of the coat during membrane bending and vesicle formation.

Since hsc70 plays multiple roles in cellular biology, isolating a single role in endocytosis through classical loss-of-function studies may be difficult. Indeed, while some loss-of-function studies with *hsc70* mutants show defects in endocytosis of signaling components (177–179), others show normal endocytosis but defective vesicle fusion (180). In contrast, loss-of-function studies of auxilin suggest a role for the protein in CME. RNAi-mediated knockdown or mutational analyses of *auxilin* in yeast, nematodes, and flies all show endocytic defects. While in *auxilin* mutant flies, Notch signaling is defected due to reduced endocytosis of the Notch ligand Delta, in RNAi-treated nematodes, receptor-mediated endocytosis of yolk protein is significantly reduced. Hence, both studies suggest a role for auxilin in endocytosis. However, auxilin's role in synaptic vesicle recycling has not been investigated in *C. elegans* and *Drosophila* likely because early developmental defects preclude direct analysis of the nervous system of the mutants (177,181).

Nonetheless, a role of auxilin in synaptic vesicle endocytosis is supported by work with squid giant synapses. Acute inhibition of auxilin and hsc70 by microinjection of peptides that inhibit the ability of these proteins to uncoat CCVs *in vitro* does show dramatic effects on recycling (182). Synapses show an accumulation of coated vesicles and reduced neurotransmission, likely a result of less endocytosis. Hence, acute inhibition of hsc70 and auxilin function in squid supports a role for the proteins in clathrin uncoating, in line with *in vitro* studies.

Synaptojanin Is Essential for Synaptic Vesicle Uncoating

While auxilin and hsc70 partner to depolymerize clathrin coats, stripping the vesicle membrane of adaptor proteins is catalyzed by synaptojanin, a phosphatase whose activity and localization are tightly regulated by endophilin.

Synaptojanin Is a Synaptic Vesicle Cycle Protein

Synaptojanin is located at nerve terminals in all species tested and is associated with synaptic vesicles and coated endocytic intermediates (90,104,183,184), suggesting a role in synaptic vesicle cycling. Synaptojanin was also shown to inter-act with a variety of proteins and lipids involved in endocytosis. Synaptojanin con-tains two inositol phosphatase domains arranged in tandem (Fig. 11.2C). The N-terminal Sac1 domain acts upon phosphatidylinositol-3-phosphate, phosphati-dylinositol-4-phosphate and phosphatidylinositol-3,5-bisphosphate (185), whereas the central inositol 5-phosphatase domain dephosphorylates PtdIns(4,5)P2 and PtdIns(3,4,5)P3 at the 5-position of the inositol ring (43,184–186). The C-terminus contains a proline-rich domain allowing the protein to bind numerous endocytic proteins including AP2, clathrin, amphiphysin, endophilin, dap160, and syndapin, suggesting a central role in synaptic endocytosis (87,90,111,112,158,187).

Loss of Synaptojanin Inhibits Vesicle Uncoating

While a role for synaptojanin in synaptic vesicle endocytosis was proposed based on biochemical studies, this idea was conclusively demonstrated using loss-of-function analyses in a variety of organisms. *Synaptojanin 1* knockout mice die shortly after birth and exhibit strong neurologic phenotypes, consistent with defects in the synaptic vesicle cycle. In line with the enzymatic function of synaptojanin, these knockout mice show increased PtdIns(4,5)P2 levels accompanied by an accumulation of clathrin-coated ves-icles (43), suggesting a role in uncoating. Similarly, *synaptojanin* mutant *Drosophila* show increased synaptic PtdIns(4,5)P2 levels (Patrik Verstreken, Laura Swann, and Pietro De Camilli, unpublished observations), a vast reduction in the total number of synaptic vesicles, and an accumulation of coated vesicles (90). Lamprey synapses injected with synaptojanin inhibitory antibodies as well as synapses of zebrafish and nematode *synaptojanin* mutants also show defects in uncoating. Together, these studies clearly point to a role for synaptojanin in vesicle uncoating (104,183).

Interestingly, in fly photoreceptors, *synaptojanin* mutations lead to the accumula-tion of neatly ordered arrays of coated vesicles, as if the underlying cytoskeleton is defective (90). Confirming this notion, *C. elegans synaptojanin* mutants (104) as well as lamprey axons microinjected with antibodies against synaptojanin (103) show hypertrophy of the actin-rich matrix at endocytic zones, suggesting a role for synapto-janin and phosphoinositide lipids in maintenance of the cytoskeleton at the synapse.

Phosphoinositides and Vesicle Formation

Synaptojanin is an enzyme that mediates uncoating of synaptic vesicles. Adaptor proteins such as AP2 and AP180 bind the synaptic membrane through interactions with PtdIns(4,5)P2 and likely also $Ptd_{Ins(3,4,5)P3}$ (35,188,189). During vesicle forma-tion, the recruitment of adaptors to the synaptic membrane appears to be controlled by the phosphorylation state of phosphoinositides, which is regulated by the oppos-ing actions of synaptojanin phosphatase and phosphatidylinositol-4-phosphate 5-kinase (assisted by talin) (102,143) (Fig. 11.3). At a later stage following the fission, synaptojanin mediates the dissociation of adaptor complexes from the vesicle

Fig. 11.3 Phosphoinositides in synaptic vesicle endocytosis. Adaptors bind PtdIns(4,5)P2 and possibly Ptd$_{Ins(3,4,5)P3}$ in the plasma membrane. Current models suggest that a fine-tuned balance of phosphoinositide kinase and phosphatase activity drives vesicle formation. In a simplified model vesicle formation may initiate by phosphoinositide phosphorylation by phosphatidylinositol-4-phosphate 5-kinase creating membrane-adaptor interaction surfaces. Concentration of adaptors at the membrane forms hubs for yet other endocytic proteins to participate in membrane bending and vesicle formation. Following fission, dephosphorylation of phosphoinositides by synaptojanin then leads to dissociation of adaptors from the vesicle membrane (see text for details)

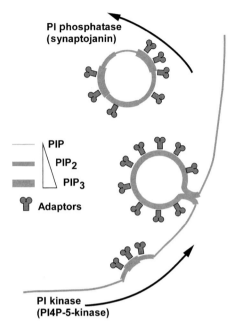

membrane by dephosphorylating polyphosphoinositides, thereby reducing the affinity of these clathrin adaptor proteins for the membrane (43). Therefore, phosphorylation and dephosphorylation cycles of phosphoinositides are critical for progression of vesicles through the vesicle cycle, and the tight regulation of kinases and phosphatases during early as well as late endocytic stages is critical for the formation of a new vesicle (Figs. 11.3 and 11.4).

Synaptojanin and Endophilin Are Partners During Vesicle Uncoating

Endophilin's main binding partner is synaptojanin (87,90,91,190), suggesting the proteins may function together, and this idea was confirmed by *in vivo* analyses. Detailed phenotypic studies on *synaptojanin* and *endophilin* mutant flies and worms revealed remarkably similar phenotypes, indicating the proteins function as partners in endocytosis. Both mutants show severe but similar amounts of vesicle depletion and dramatically increased numbers of coated vesicles. Interestingly, when stimulated at high frequency, both mutants fail to maintain normal neurotransmitter release, and the decline in transmission is nearly identical (90,91). The remarkable qualitative and quantitative phenotypic similarity between the two mutants suggests both proteins act together, at the same step in endocytosis. Indeed, the endocytic defects observed in *synaptojanin* or *endophilin* single mutants are not additive in their double mutants, suggesting that both endophilin and synaptojanin are essential for vesicle uncoating (90–92); however, the data do not exclude a

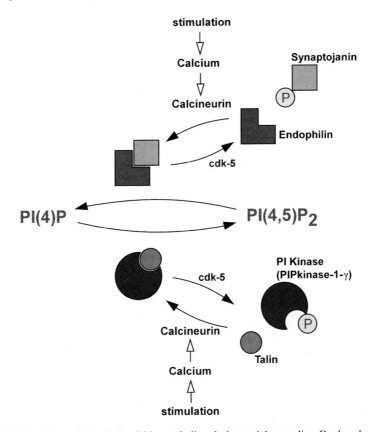

Fig. 11.4 Regulation of phosphoinositide metabolism during vesicle recycling. Dephosphorylation of synaptojanin and phosphatidylinositol-4-phosphate 5-kinase by calcineurin, activated by neuronal activity and calcium influx, allows downstream interactions to occur. Synaptojanin binds endophilin, stimulating phosphoinositide dephosphorylation, while phosphatidylinositol-4-phosphate 5-kinase binds talin, stimulating phosphoinositide phosphorylation

nonessential yet significant role during earlier stages when the adaptors are recruited and the membrane is bent.

Additional studies indicate endophilin serves as an adaptor for synaptojanin during vesicle endocytosis. While endophilin levels are mostly normal in *synaptojanin* mutants, synaptic synaptojanin levels are dramatically reduced in *endophilin* mutants. Hence, endophilin stabilizes synaptojanin at nerve terminals. Moreover, binding of endophilin to synaptojanin stimulates its phosphatase activity. It is noteworthy that the interaction between the two proteins is inhibited by phosphorylation of synaptojanin near its proline-rich domain (191). Interestingly, synaptojanin is dephosphorylated by calcineurin in response to nerve activity (192). Hence, dephosphorylation of phosphoinositide pools by synaptojanin appears to be regulated by activity through an interaction with endophilin (Fig. 11.4).

Conclusion

Synaptic vesicle recycling and sorting of vesicles in specific vesicle pools are critical components of the synaptic vesicle cycle as they are essential for sustained neurotransmission. Although different types of vesicle recycling mechanisms have been proposed to occur simultaneously (1,2), the molecular determinants of the clathrin-mediated pathway are studied the most. With the identification and, more importantly, characterization of the protein and lipid components of CME, we are arriving at a molecular description of the process. Our next challenge will not only be to complete the identification and characterization of molecular players involved through large-scale biochemical and genetic approaches, but also to understand the functional regulatory relations that exist among different proteins and lipids in CME as well as between CME and other mechanisms of recycling that operate at the synapse. Only this way we will arrive at a complete understanding of the mechanisms that regulate presynaptic function and plasticity.

Acknowledgments In writing this chapter and reviewing a large body of literature, we had to make difficult choices on what topics to include and which work to reference. We therefore would like to apologize to our colleagues whose work or opinions were not included or were overlooked. We are grateful to Hugo Bellen, Pietro De Camilli, and Oleg Shupliakov for stimulating discussions and to members of the Verstreken lab for comments on the manuscript. Patrik Verstreken's research is supported by a Marie Curie Excellence grant (MEXT-CT-2006-042267), the Research Fund of the K.U. Leuven and VIB.

References

1. Rizzoli SO, Jahn R. Kiss-and-run, collapse and "readily retrievable" vesicles. Traffic 2007;8(9):1137–1144.
2. Harata NC, Aravanis AM, Tsien RW. Kiss-and-run and full-collapse fusion as modes of exo-endocytosis in neurosecretion. J Neurochem 2006;97(6):1546–1570.
3. Schmid EM, Ford MG, Burtey A, et al. Role of the AP2 beta-appendage hub in recruiting partners for clathrin-coated vesicle assembly. PLoS Biol 2006;4(9):e262.
4. Pearse BM. Clathrin and coated vesicles. EMBO J 1987;6(9):2507–2512.
5. Kadota K, Kadota T. Isolation of coated vesicles, plain synaptic vesicles, and flocculent material from a crude synaptosome fraction of guinea pig whole brain. J Cell Biol 1973;58(1):135–151.
6. Crowther RA, Finch JT, Pearse BM. On the structure of coated vesicles. J Mol Biol 1976;103 (4):785–798.
7. Roth TF, Porter KR. Yolk protein uptake in the oocyte of the mosquito Aedes Aegypti. L. J Cell Biol 1964;20:313–332.
8. Lloyd TE, Verstreken P, Ostrin EJ, Phillippi A, Lichtarge O, Bellen HJ. A genome-wide search for synaptic vesicle cycle proteins in Drosophila. Neuron 2000;26(1):45–50.
9. Lemmon SK, Pellicena-Palle A, Conley K, Freund CL. Sequence of the clathrin heavy chain from Saccharomyces cerevisiae and requirement of the COOH terminus for clathrin function. J Cell Biol 1991;112(1):65–80.
10. Payne GS, Schekman R. A test of clathrin function in protein secretion and cell growth. Science 1985;230(4729):1009–1014.
11. Liu SH, Marks MS, Brodsky FM. A dominant-negative clathrin mutant differentially affects trafficking of molecules with distinct sorting motifs in the class II major histocompatibility complex (MHC) pathway. J Cell Biol 1998;140(5):1023–1037.

12. Baggett JJ, Wendland B. Clathrin function in yeast endocytosis. Traffic 2001;2(5):297–302.
13. Bazinet C, Katzen AL, Morgan M, Mahowald AP, Lemmon SK. The Drosophila clathrin heavy chain gene: clathrin function is essential in a multicellular organism. Genetics 1993;134 (4):1119–1134.
14. Granseth B, Odermatt B, Royle SJ, Lagnado L. Clathrin-mediated endocytosis is the dominant mechanism of vesicle retrieval at hippocampal synapses. Neuron 2006;51(6): 773–786.
15. Ungewickell E, Branton D. Assembly units of clathrin coats. Nature 1981;289(5796):420–422.
16. Kirchhausen T, Harrison SC. Structural domains of clathrin heavy chains. J Cell Biol 1984;99(5):1725–1734.
17. Fotin A, Cheng Y, Sliz P, et al. Molecular model for a complete clathrin lattice from electron cryomicroscopy. Nature 2004;432(7017):573–579.
18. Kirchhausen T. Clathrin. Annu Rev Biochem 2000;69:699–727.
19. Moskowitz HS, Yokoyama CT, Ryan TA. Highly cooperative control of endocytosis by clathrin. Mol Biol Cell 2005;16(4):1769–1776.
20. Ybe JA, Greene B, Liu SH, Pley U, Parham P, Brodsky FM. Clathrin self-assembly is regulated by three light-chain residues controlling the formation of critical salt bridges. EMBO J 1998;17(5):1297–1303.
21. ter Haar E, Musacchio A, Harrison SC, Kirchhausen T. Atomic structure of clathrin: a beta propeller terminal domain joins an alpha zigzag linker. Cell 1998;95(4):563–573.
22. Ungewickell E. Clathrin: a good view of a shapely leg. Curr Biol 1999;9(1):R32–35.
23. Kirchhausen T, Harrison SC, Chow EP, et al. Clathrin heavy chain: molecular cloning and complete primary structure. Proc Natl Acad Sci U S A 1987;84(24):8805–8809.
24. Brodsky FM. Cell biology: clathrin's Achilles' ankle. Nature 2004;432(7017):568–569.
25. Wilbur JD, Hwang PK, Brodsky FM. New faces of the familiar clathrin lattice. Traffic 2005;6 (4):346–350.
26. Dell' Angelica EC, Klumperman J, Stoorvogel W, Bonifacino JS. Association of the AP-3 adaptor complex with clathrin. Science 1998;280(5362):431–434.
27. ter Haar E, Harrison SC, Kirchhausen T. Peptide-in-groove interactions link target proteins to the beta-propeller of clathrin. Proc Natl Acad Sci U S A 2000;97(3):1096–1100.
28. Hinrichsen L, Meyerholz A, Groos S, Ungewickell EJ. Bending a membrane: how clathrin affects budding. Proc Natl Acad Sci U S A 2006;103(23):8715–8720.
29. Cheng Y, Boll W, Kirchhausen T, Harrison SC, Walz T. Cryo-electron tomography of clathrin-coated vesicles: structural implications for coat assembly. J Mol Biol 2007;365(3):892–899.
30. Zhang B, Koh YH, Beckstead RB, Budnik V, Ganetzky B, Bellen HJ. Synaptic vesicle size and number are regulated by a clathrin adaptor protein required for endocytosis. Neuron 1998;21(6):1465–1475.
31. Gonzalez-Gaitan M, Jackle H. Role of Drosophila alpha-adaptin in presynaptic vesicle recycling. Cell 1997;88(6):767–776.
32. Takei K, Haucke V, Slepnev V, et al. Generation of coated intermediates of clathrin-mediated endocytosis on protein-free liposomes. Cell 1998;94(1):131–141.
33. Boehm M, Bonifacino JS. Genetic analyses of adaptin function from yeast to mammals. Gene 2002;286(2):175–186.
34. Augustine GJ, Morgan JR, Villalba-Galea CA, Jin S, Prasad K, Lafer EM. Clathrin and synaptic vesicle endocytosis: studies at the squid giant synapse. Biochem Soc Trans 2006;34 (pt 1):68–72.
35. Slepnev VI, De Camilli P. Accessory factors in clathrin-dependent synaptic vesicle endocytosis. Nat Rev Neurosci 2000;1(3):161–172.
36. Owen DJ, Vallis Y, Pearse BM, McMahon HT, Evans PR. The structure and function of the beta 2-adaptin appendage domain. EMBO J 2000;19(16):4216–4227.
37. Rapoport I, Miyazaki M, Boll W, et al. Regulatory interactions in the recognition of endocytic sorting signals by AP2 complexes. EMBO J 1997;16(9):2240–2250.
38. Gaidarov I, Keen JH. Phosphoinositide-AP2 interactions required for targeting to plasma membrane clathrin-coated pits. J Cell Biol 1999;146(4):755–764.

39. Praefcke GJ, McMahon HT. The dynamin superfamily: universal membrane tubulation and fission molecules? Nat Rev Mol Cell Biol 2004;5(2):133–147.

40. Morris SA, Mann A, Ungewickell E. Analysis of 100–180-kDa phosphoproteins in clathrin-coated vesicles from bovine brain. J Biol Chem 1990;265(6):3354–3357.

41. Kohtz DS, Puszkin S. A neuronal protein (NP185) associated with clathrin-coated vesicles. Characterization of NP185 with monoclonal antibodies. J Biol Chem 1988;263(15):7418–7425.

42. Ahle S, Ungewickell E. Purification and properties of a new clathrin assembly protein. EMBO J 1986;5(12):3143–3149.

43. Cremona O, Di Paolo G, Wenk MR, et al. Essential role of phosphoinositide metabolism in synaptic vesicle recycling. Cell 1999;99(2):179–188.

44. Ye W, Lafer EM. Bacterially expressed F1–20/AP-3 assembles clathrin into cages with a narrow size distribution: implications for the regulation of quantal size during neurotransmission. J Neurosci Res 1995;41(1):15–26.

45. Mao Y, Chen J, Maynard JA, Zhang B, Quiocho FA. A novel all helix fold of the AP180 amino-terminal domain for phosphoinositide binding and clathrin assembly in synaptic vesicle endocytosis. Cell 2001;104(3):433–440.

46. Kirchhausen T, Harrison SC. Protein organization in clathrin trimers. Cell 1981;23(3):755–761.

47. Pearse BM, Robinson MS. Purification and properties of 100-kd proteins from coated vesicles and their reconstitution with clathrin. EMBO J 1984;3(9):1951–1957.

48. Huang KM, D'Hondt K, Riezman H, Lemmon SK. Clathrin functions in the absence of heterotetrameric adaptors and AP180-related proteins in yeast. EMBO J 1999;18(14):3897–3908.

49. Nonet ML, Holgado AM, Brewer F, et al. UNC-11, a Caenorhabditis elegans AP180 homologue, regulates the size and protein composition of synaptic vesicles. Mol Biol Cell 1999;10(7):2343–2360.

50. Chen H, Fre S, Slepnev VI, et al. Epsin is an EH-domain-binding protein implicated in clathrin-mediated endocytosis. Nature 1998;394(6695):793–797.

51. Rosenthal JA, Chen H, Slepnev VI, et al. The epsins define a family of proteins that interact with components of the clathrin coat and contain a new protein module. J Biol Chem 1999;274 (48):33959–33965.

52. Kay BK, Yamabhai M, Wendland B, Emr SD. Identification of a novel domain shared by putative components of the endocytic and cytoskeletal machinery. Protein Sci 1999;8(2):435–438.

53. Hyman J, Chen H, Di Fiore PP, De Camilli P, Brunger AT. Epsin 1 undergoes nucleocytosolic shuttling and its eps15 interactor NH(2)-terminal homology (ENTH) domain, structurally similar to Armadillo and HEAT repeats, interacts with the transcription factor promyelocytic leukemia Zn(2)+ finger protein (PLZF). J Cell Biol 2000;149(3):537–546.

54. De Camilli P, Chen H, Hyman J, Panepucci E, Bateman A, Brunger AT. The ENTH domain. FEBS Lett 2002;513(1):11–18.

55. Itoh T, Koshiba S, Kigawa T, Kikuchi A, Yokoyama S, Takenawa T. Role of the ENTH domain in phosphatidylinositol-4,5–bisphosphate binding and endocytosis. Science 2001;291(5506):1047–1051.

56. Ford MG, Mills IG, Peter BJ, et al. Curvature of clathrin-coated pits driven by epsin. Nature 2002;419(6905):361–366.

57. Kalthoff C, Alves J, Urbanke C, Knorr R, Ungewickell EJ. Unusual structural organization of the endocytic proteins AP180 and epsin 1. J Biol Chem 2002;277(10):8209–8216.

58. Wendland B, Steece KE, Emr SD. Yeast epsins contain an essential N-terminal ENTH domain, bind clathrin and are required for endocytosis. EMBO J 1999;18(16): 4383–4393.

59. Zhang B. Genetic and molecular analysis of synaptic vesicle recycling in Drosophila. J Neurocytol 2003;32(5–8):567–589.

60. Grigliatti TA, Hall L, Rosenbluth R, Suzuki DT. Temperature-sensitive mutations in Drosophila melanogaster. XIV. A selection of immobile adults. Mol Gen Genet 1973;120(2):107–114.

61. Petrovich TZ, Merakovsky J, Kelly LE. A genetic analysis of the stoned locus and its interaction with dunce, shibire and Suppressor of stoned variants of Drosophila melanogaster. Genetics 1993;133(4):955–965.

62. Estes PS, Jackson TC, Stimson DT, Sanyal S, Kelly LE, Ramaswami M. Functional dissection of a eukaryotic dicistronic gene: transgenic stonedB, but not stonedA, restores normal synaptic properties to Drosophila stoned mutants. Genetics 2003;165(1):185–196.
63. Diril MK, Wienisch M, Jung N, Klingauf J, Haucke V. Stonin 2 is an AP2-dependent endocytic sorting adaptor for synaptotagmin internalization and recycling. Dev Cell 2006;10 (2):233–244.
64. Fergestad T, Broadie K. Interaction of stoned and synaptotagmin in synaptic vesicle endocytosis. J Neurosci 2001;21(4):1218–1227.
65. Stimson DT, Estes PS, Rao S, Krishnan KS, Kelly LE, Ramaswami M. Drosophila stoned proteins regulate the rate and fidelity of synaptic vesicle internalization. J Neurosci 2001;21(9):3034–3044.
66. Fergestad T, Davis WS, Broadie K. The stoned proteins regulate synaptic vesicle recycling in the presynaptic terminal. J Neurosci 1999;19(14):5847–5860.
67. Ferguson SM, Brasnjo G, Hayashi M, et al. A selective activity-dependent requirement for dynamin 1 in synaptic vesicle endocytosis. Science 2007;316(5824):570–574.
68. Koh TW, Verstreken P, Bellen HJ. dap160/intersectin acts as a stabilizing scaffold required for synaptic development and vesicle endocytosis. Neuron 2004;43(2):193–205.
69. Andrews J, Smith M, Merakovsky J, Coulson M, Hannan F, Kelly LE. The stoned locus of Drosophila melanogaster produces a dicistronic transcript and encodes two distinct polypeptides. Genetics 1996;143(4):1699–1711.
70. Kelly LE, Phillips AM. Molecular and genetic characterization of the interactions between the Drosophila stoned-B protein and DAP-160 (intersectin). Biochem J 2005;388(pt 1):195–204.
71. Martina JA, Bonangelino CJ, Aguilar RC, Bonifacino JS. Stonin 2: an adaptor-like protein that interacts with components of the endocytic machinery. J Cell Biol 2001;153(5):1111–1120.
72. Walther K, Krauss M, Diril MK, et al. Human stoned B interacts with AP2 and synaptotagmin and facilitates clathrin-coated vesicle uncoating. EMBO Rep 2001;2(7):634–640.
73. Phillips AM, Smith M, Ramaswami M, Kelly LE. The products of the Drosophila stoned locus interact with synaptic vesicles via synaptotagmin. J Neurosci 2000;20(22):8254–8261.
74. Zhang JZ, Davletov BA, Sudhof TC, Anderson RG. Synaptotagmin I is a high affinity receptor for clathrin AP2: implications for membrane recycling. Cell 1994;78(5):751–760.
75. Littleton JT, Stern M, Schulze K, Perin M, Bellen HJ. Mutational analysis of Drosophila synaptotagmin demonstrates its essential role in Ca(2+)-activated neurotransmitter release. Cell 1993;74(6):1125–1134.
76. Perin MS, Johnston PA, Ozcelik T, Jahn R, Francke U, Sudhof TC. Structural and functional conservation of synaptotagmin (p65) in Drosophila and humans. J Biol Chem 1991; 266(1):615–622.
77. Han W, Rhee JS, Maximov A, et al. C-terminal ECFP fusion impairs synaptotagmin 1 function: crowding out synaptotagmin 1. J Biol Chem 2005;280(6):5089–5100.
78. Littleton JT, Bai J, Vyas B, et al. synaptotagmin mutants reveal essential functions for the C2B domain in Ca2+-triggered fusion and recycling of synaptic vesicles in vivo. J Neurosci 2001;21(5):1421–1433.
79. Jorgensen EM, Hartwieg E, Schuske K, Nonet ML, Jin Y, Horvitz HR. Defective recycling of synaptic vesicles in synaptotagmin mutants of Caenorhabditis elegans. Nature 1995;378 (6553):196–199.
80. Reist NE, Buchanan J, Li J, DiAntonio A, Buxton EM, Schwarz TL. Morphologically docked synaptic vesicles are reduced in synaptotagmin mutants of Drosophila. J Neurosci 1998;18(19):7662–7673.
81. Fukuda M, Moreira JE, Lewis FM, et al. Role of the C2B domain of synaptotagmin in vesicular release and recycling as determined by specific antibody injection into the squid giant synapse preterminal. Proc Natl Acad Sci U S A 1995;92(23):10708–10712.
82. Poskanzer KE, Marek KW, Sweeney ST, Davis GW. Synaptotagmin I is necessary for compensatory synaptic vesicle endocytosis in vivo. Nature 2003;426(6966):559–563.
83. Poskanzer KE, Fetter RD, Davis GW. Discrete residues in the c(2)b domain of synaptotagmin I independently specify endocytic rate and synaptic vesicle size. Neuron 2006;50(1):49–62.

84. De Camilli P, Takei K. Molecular mechanisms in synaptic vesicle endocytosis and recycling. Neuron 1996;16(3):481–486.

85. Bacia K, Schwille P, Kurzchalia T. Sterol structure determines the separation of phases and the curvature of the liquid-ordered phase in model membranes. Proc Natl Acad Sci U S A 2005;102(9):3272–3277.

86. McMahon HT, Gallop JL. Membrane curvature and mechanisms of dynamic cell membrane remodelling. Nature 2005;438(7068):590–596.

87. Ringstad N, Nemoto Y, De Camilli P. The SH3p4/Sh3p8/SH3p13 protein family: binding partners for synaptojanin and dynamin via a Grb2-like Src homology 3 domain. Proc Natl Acad Sci U S A 1997;94(16):8569–8574.

88. Ringstad N, Gad H, Low P, et al. Endophilin/SH3p4 is required for the transition from early to late stages in clathrin-mediated synaptic vesicle endocytosis. Neuron 1999;24(1):143–154.

89. Cestra G, Castagnoli L, Dente L, et al. The SH3 domains of endophilin and amphiphysin bind to the proline-rich region of synaptojanin 1 at distinct sites that display an unconventional binding specificity. J Biol Chem 1999;274(45):32001–32007.

90. Verstreken P, Koh TW, Schulze KL, et al. Synaptojanin is recruited by endophilin to promote synaptic vesicle uncoating. Neuron 2003;40(4):733–748.

91. Schuske KR, Richmond JE, Matthies DS, et al. Endophilin is required for synaptic vesicle endocytosis by localizing synaptojanin. Neuron 2003;40(4):749–762.

92. Fabian-Fine R, Verstreken P, Hiesinger PR, et al. Endophilin promotes a late step in endocytosis at glial invaginations in Drosophila photoreceptor terminals. J Neurosci 2003;23(33):10732–10744.

93. Guichet A, Wucherpfennig T, Dudu V, et al. Essential role of endophilin A in synaptic vesicle budding at the Drosophila neuromuscular junction. EMBO J 2002;21(7):1661–1672.

94. Verstreken P, Kjaerulff O, Lloyd TE, et al. Endophilin mutations block clathrin-mediated endocytosis but not neurotransmitter release. Cell 2002;109(1):101–112.

95. Rikhy R, Kumar V, Mittal R, Krishnan KS. Endophilin is critically required for synapse formation and function in Drosophila melanogaster. J Neurosci 2002;22(17):7478–7484.

96. Hill E, van Der Kaay J, Downes CP, Smythe E. The role of dynamin and its binding partners in coated pit invagination and scission. J Cell Biol 2001;152(2):309–323.

97. Schmidt A, Wolde M, Thiele C, et al. Endophilin I mediates synaptic vesicle formation by transfer of arachidonate to lysophosphatidic acid. Nature 1999;401(6749):133–141.

98. Simpson F, Hussain NK, Qualmann B, et al. SH3-domain-containing proteins function at distinct steps in clathrin-coated vesicle formation. Nat Cell Biol 1999;1(2):119–124.

99. Gallop JL, Jao CC, Kent HM, et al. Mechanism of endophilin N-BAR domain-mediated membrane curvature. EMBO J 2006;25(12):2898–2910.

100. Peter BJ, Kent HM, Mills IG, et al. BAR domains as sensors of membrane curvature: the amphiphysin BAR structure. Science 2004;303(5657):495–499.

101. Zimmerberg J, McLaughlin S. Membrane curvature: how BAR domains bend bilayers. Curr Biol 2004;14(6):R250–252.

102. Farsad K, Ringstad N, Takei K, Floyd SR, Rose K, De Camilli P. Generation of high curvature membranes mediated by direct endophilin bilayer interactions. J Cell Biol 2001;155(2):193–200.

103. Gad H, Ringstad N, Low P, et al. Fission and uncoating of synaptic clathrin-coated vesicles are perturbed by disruption of interactions with the SH3 domain of endophilin. Neuron 2000;27(2):301–312.

104. Harris TW, Hartwieg E, Horvitz HR, Jorgensen EM. Mutations in synaptojanin disrupt synaptic vesicle recycling. J Cell Biol 2000;150(3):589–600.

105. van der Bliek AM, Meyerowitz EM. Dynamin-like protein encoded by the Drosophila shibire gene associated with vesicular traffic. Nature 1991;351(6325):411–414.

106. Cao H, Garcia F, McNiven MA. Differential distribution of dynamin isoforms in mammalian cells. Mol Biol Cell 1998;9(9):2595–2609.

107. Cook T, Mesa K, Urrutia R. Three dynamin-encoding genes are differentially expressed in developing rat brain. J Neurochem 1996;67(3):927–931.

108. Smirnova E, Shurland DL, Newman-Smith ED, Pishvaee B, van der Bliek AM. A model for dynamin self-assembly based on binding between three different protein domains. J Biol Chem 1999;274(21):14942–14947.

109. Muhlberg AB, Warnock DE, Schmid SL. Domain structure and intramolecular regulation of dynamin GTPase. EMBO J 1997;16(22):6676–6683.

110. Salim K, Bottomley MJ, Querfurth E, et al. Distinct specificity in the recognition of phosphoinositides by the pleckstrin homology domains of dynamin and Bruton's tyrosine kinase. EMBO J 1996;15(22):6241–6250.

111. David C, McPherson PS, Mundigl O, de Camilli P. A role of amphiphysin in synaptic vesicle endocytosis suggested by its binding to dynamin in nerve terminals. Proc Natl Acad Sci U S A 1996;93(1):331–335.

112. Qualmann B, Roos J, DiGregorio PJ, Kelly RB. Syndapin I, a synaptic dynamin-binding protein that associates with the neural Wiskott-Aldrich syndrome protein. Mol Biol Cell 1999;10(2):501–513.

113. Salcini AE, Hilliard MA, Croce A, et al. The Eps15 C. elegans homologue EHS-1 is implicated in synaptic vesicle recycling. Nat Cell Biol 2001;3(8):755–760.

114. Yamabhai M, Hoffman NG, Hardison NL, et al. Intersectin, a novel adaptor protein with two Eps15 homology and five Src homology 3 domains. J Biol Chem 1998;273(47):31401–31407.

115. Delgado R, Maureira C, Oliva C, Kidokoro Y, Labarca P. Size of vesicle pools, rates of mobilization, and recycling at neuromuscular synapses of a Drosophila mutant, shibire. Neuron 2000;28(3):941–953.

116. Newton AJ, Kirchhausen T, Murthy VN. Inhibition of dynamin completely blocks compensatory synaptic vesicle endocytosis. Proc Natl Acad Sci U S A 2006;103(47):17955–17960.

117. Koenig JH, Ikeda K. Evidence for a presynaptic blockage of transmission in a temperature-sensitive mutant of Drosophila. J Neurobiol 1983;14(6):411–419.

118. Estes PS, Roos J, van der Bliek A, Kelly RB, Krishnan KS, Ramaswami M. Traffic of dynamin within individual Drosophila synaptic boutons relative to compartment-specific markers. J Neurosci 1996;16(17):5443–5456.

119. Kosaka T, Ikeda K. Reversible blockage of membrane retrieval and endocytosis in the garland cell of the temperature-sensitive mutant of Drosophila melanogaster, shibirets1. J Cell Biol 1983;97(2):499–507.

120. Hinshaw JE, Schmid SL. Dynamin self-assembles into rings suggesting a mechanism for coated vesicle budding. Nature 1995;374(6518):190–192.

121. Takei K, McPherson PS, Schmid SL, De Camilli P. Tubular membrane invaginations coated by dynamin rings are induced by GTP-gamma S in nerve terminals. Nature 1995;374 (6518):186–190.

122. Sweitzer SM, Hinshaw JE. Dynamin undergoes a GTP-dependent conformational change causing vesiculation. Cell 1998;93(6):1021–1029.

123. Roux A, Uyhazi K, Frost A, De Camilli P. GTP-dependent twisting of dynamin implicates constriction and tension in membrane fission. Nature 2006;441(7092):528–531.

124. Yamashita T, Hige T, Takahashi T. Vesicle endocytosis requires dynamin-dependent GTP hydrolysis at a fast CNS synapse. Science 2005;307(5706):124–127.

125. Warnock DE, Schmid SL. Dynamin GTPase, a force-generating molecular switch. Bioessays 1996;18(11):885–893.

126. Sever S, Damke H, Schmid SL. Dynamin:GTP controls the formation of constricted coated pits, the rate limiting step in clathrin-mediated endocytosis. J Cell Biol 2000;150(5):1137–1148.

127. Sever S, Muhlberg AB, Schmid SL. Impairment of dynamin's GAP domain stimulates receptor-mediated endocytosis. Nature 1999;398(6727):481–486.

128. Yoshida Y, Takei K. Stimulation of dynamin GTPase activity by amphiphysin. Methods Enzymol 2005;404:528–537.

129. Marks B, Stowell MH, Vallis Y, et al. GTPase activity of dynamin and resulting conformation change are essential for endocytosis. Nature 2001;410(6825):231–235.

130. Newmyer SL, Christensen A, Sever S. Auxilin-dynamin interactions link the uncoating ATPase chaperone machinery with vesicle formation. Dev Cell 2003;4(6):929–940.

131. Song BD, Yarar D, Schmid SL. An assembly-incompetent mutant establishes a requirement for dynamin self-assembly in clathrin-mediated endocytosis in vivo. Mol Biol Cell 2004;15(5):2243–2252.

132. Narayanan R, Leonard M, Song BD, Schmid SL, Ramaswami M. An internal GAP domain negatively regulates presynaptic dynamin in vivo: a two-step model for dynamin function. J Cell Biol 2005;169(1):117–126.

133. Macia E, Ehrlich M, Massol R, Boucrot E, Brunner C, Kirchhausen T. Dynasore, a cell-permeable inhibitor of dynamin. Dev Cell 2006;10(6):839–850.

134. Kim Y, Chang S. Ever-expanding network of dynamin-interacting proteins. Mol Neurobiol 2006;34(2):129–136.

135. Lichte B, Veh RW, Meyer HE, Kilimann MW. Amphiphysin, a novel protein associated with synaptic vesicles. EMBO J 1992;11(7):2521–2530.

136. Yoshida Y, Kinuta M, Abe T, et al. The stimulatory action of amphiphysin on dynamin function is dependent on lipid bilayer curvature. EMBO J 2004;23(17):3483–3491.

137. Takei K, Slepnev VI, Haucke V, De Camilli P. Functional partnership between amphiphysin and dynamin in clathrin-mediated endocytosis. Nat Cell Biol 1999;1(1):33–39.

138. Liang S, Wei FY, Wu YM, et al. Major Cdk5-dependent phosphorylation sites of amphiphysin 1 are implicated in the regulation of the membrane binding and endocytosis. J Neurochem 2007;102(5):1466–1476.

139. Bauerfeind R, Takei K, De Camilli P. Amphiphysin I is associated with coated endocytic intermediates and undergoes stimulation-dependent dephosphorylation in nerve terminals. J Biol Chem 1997;272(49):30984–30992.

140. Tomizawa K, Sunada S, Lu YF, et al. Cophosphorylation of amphiphysin I and dynamin I by Cdk5 regulates clathrin-mediated endocytosis of synaptic vesicles. J Cell Biol 2003;163(4):813–824.

141. Evergren E, Marcucci M, Tomilin N, et al. Amphiphysin is a component of clathrin coats formed during synaptic vesicle recycling at the lamprey giant synapse. Traffic 2004;5(7):514–528.

142. Shupliakov O, Low P, Grabs D, et al. Synaptic vesicle endocytosis impaired by disruption of dynamin-SH3 domain interactions. Science 1997;276(5310):259–263.

143. Di Paolo G, Pellegrini L, Letinic K, et al. Recruitment and regulation of phosphatidylinositol phosphate kinase type 1 gamma by the FERM domain of talin. Nature 2002;420(6911):85–89.

144. Razzaq A, Robinson IM, McMahon HT, et al. Amphiphysin is necessary for organization of the excitation-contraction coupling machinery of muscles, but not for synaptic vesicle endocytosis in Drosophila. Genes Dev 2001;15(22):2967–2979.

145. Zhang B, Zelhof AC. Amphiphysins: raising the BAR for synaptic vesicle recycling and membrane dynamics. Bin-Amphiphysin-Rvsp. Traffic 2002;3(7):452–460.

146. Lee E, Marcucci M, Daniell L, et al. Amphiphysin 2 (Bin1) and T-tubule biogenesis in muscle. Science 2002;297(5584):1193–1196.

147. Marie B, Sweeney ST, Poskanzer KE, Roos J, Kelly RB, Davis GW. dap160/intersectin scaffolds the periactive zone to achieve high-fidelity endocytosis and normal synaptic growth. Neuron 2004;43(2):207–219.

148. Majumdar A, Ramagiri S, Rikhy R. Drosophila homologue of Eps15 is essential for synaptic vesicle recycling. Exp Cell Res 2006;312(12):2288–2298.

149. Fazioli F, Minichiello L, Matoskova B, Wong WT, Di Fiore PP. eps15, a novel tyrosine kinase substrate, exhibits transforming activity. Mol Cell Biol 1993;13(9):5814–5828.

150. Salcini AE, Chen H, Iannolo G, De Camilli P, Di Fiore PP. Epidermal growth factor pathway substrate 15, Eps15. Int J Biochem Cell Biol 1999;31(8):805–809.

151. Santolini E, Salcini AE, Kay BK, Yamabhai M, Di Fiore PP. The EH network. Exp Cell Res 1999;253(1):186–209.

152. Sengar AS, Wang W, Bishay J, Cohen S, Egan SE. The EH and SH3 domain Ese proteins regulate endocytosis by linking to dynamin and Eps15. EMBO J 1999;18(5):1159–1171.

153. Tebar F, Confalonieri S, Carter RE, Di Fiore PP, Sorkin A. Eps15 is constitutively oligomerized due to homophilic interaction of its coiled-coil region. J Biol Chem 1997;272(24):15413–15418.

154. Benmerah A, Bayrou M, Cerf-Bensussan N, Dautry-Varsat A. Inhibition of clathrin-coated pit assembly by an Eps15 mutant. J Cell Sci 1999;112 (Pt 9):1303–1311.

155. Tebar F, Sorkina T, Sorkin A, Ericsson M, Kirchhausen T. Eps15 is a component of clathrin-coated pits and vesicles and is located at the rim of coated pits. J Biol Chem 1996;271 (46):28727–28730.

156. Morgan JR, Prasad K, Jin S, Augustine GJ, Lafer EM. Eps15 homology domain-NPF motif interactions regulate clathrin coat assembly during synaptic vesicle recycling. J Biol Chem 2003;278(35):33583–33592.

157. Koh TW, Korolchuk VI, Wairkar YP, et al. Eps15 and dap160 control synaptic vesicle membrane retrieval and synapse development. J Cell Biol 2007;178(2):309–322.

158. Roos J, Kelly RB. dap160, a neural-specific Eps15 homology and multiple SH3 domain-containing protein that interacts with Drosophila dynamin. J Biol Chem 1998;273 (30):19108–19119.

159. Allaire PD, Ritter B, Thomas S, et al. Connecdenn, a novel DENN domain-containing protein of neuronal clathrin-coated vesicles functioning in synaptic vesicle endocytosis. J Neurosci 2006;26(51):13202–13212.

160. Guipponi M, Scott HS, Hattori M, Ishii K, Sakaki Y, Antonarakis SE. Genomic structure, sequence, and refined mapping of the human intersectin gene (ITSN), which encompasses 250 kb on chromosome 21q22.1→q22.2. Cytogenet Cell Genet 1998;83(3–4):218–220.

161. Evergren E, Gad H, Walther K, Sundborger A, Tomilin N, Shupliakov O. Intersectin is a negative regulator of dynamin recruitment to the synaptic endocytic zone in the central synapse. J Neurosci 2007;27(2):379–390.

162. Schafer DA. Coupling actin dynamics and membrane dynamics during endocytosis. Curr Opin Cell Biol 2002;14(1):76–81.

163. Smythe E, Ayscough KR. Actin regulation in endocytosis. J Cell Sci 2006;119(pt 22):4589–4598.

164. Shupliakov O, Bloom O, Gustafsson JS, et al. Impaired recycling of synaptic vesicles after acute perturbation of the presynaptic actin cytoskeleton. Proc Natl Acad Sci U S A 2002;99(22):14476–14481.

165. Merrifield CJ, Feldman ME, Wan L, Almers W. Imaging actin and dynamin recruitment during invagination of single clathrin-coated pits. Nat Cell Biol 2002;4(9):691–698.

166. Anggono V, Robinson PJ. Syndapin I and endophilin I bind overlapping proline-rich regions of dynamin I: role in synaptic vesicle endocytosis. J Neurochem 2007;102(3):931–943.

167. Anggono V, Smillie KJ, Graham ME, Valova VA, Cousin MA, Robinson PJ. Syndapin I is the phosphorylation-regulated dynamin I partner in synaptic vesicle endocytosis. Nat Neurosci 2006;9(6):752–760.

168. Qualmann B, Kessels MM, Kelly RB. Molecular links between endocytosis and the actin cytoskeleton. J Cell Biol 2000;150(5):F111–116.

169. Itoh T, De Camilli P. BAR, F-BAR (EFC) and ENTH/ANTH domains in the regulation of membrane-cytosol interfaces and membrane curvature. Biochim Biophys Acta 2006;1761 (8):897–912.

170. Kessels MM, Qualmann B. Syndapin oligomers interconnect the machineries for endocytic vesicle formation and actin polymerization. J Biol Chem 2006;281(19):13285–13299.

171. Bonanomi D, Benfenati F, Valtorta F. Protein sorting in the synaptic vesicle life cycle. Prog Neurobiol 2006;80(4):177–217.

172. Braell WA, Schlossman DM, Schmid SL, Rothman JE. Dissociation of clathrin coats coupled to the hydrolysis of ATP: role of an uncoating ATPase. J Cell Biol 1984;99(2):734–741.

173. Schlossman DM, Schmid SL, Braell WA, Rothman JE. An enzyme that removes clathrin coats: purification of an uncoating ATPase. J Cell Biol 1984;99(2):723–733.

174. Prasad K, Barouch W, Greene L, Eisenberg E. A protein cofactor is required for uncoating of clathrin baskets by uncoating ATPase. J Biol Chem 1993;268(32):23758–23761.

175. Heymann JB, Iwasaki K, Yim YI, et al. Visualization of the binding of Hsc70 ATPase to clathrin baskets: implications for an uncoating mechanism. J Biol Chem 2005;280(8): 7156–7161.

176. Sousa R, Lafer EM. Keep the traffic moving: mechanism of the Hsp70 motor. Traffic 2006;7(12):1596–1603.

177. Hagedorn EJ, Bayraktar JL, Kandachar VR, Bai T, Englert DM, Chang HC. Drosophila melanogaster auxilin regulates the internalization of Delta to control activity of the Notch signaling pathway. J Cell Biol 2006;173(3):443–452.

178. Chang HC, Newmyer SL, Hull MJ, Ebersold M, Schmid SL, Mellman I. Hsc70 is required for endocytosis and clathrin function in Drosophila. J Cell Biol 2002;159(3):477–487.

179. Pishvaee B, Costaguta G, Yeung BG, et al. A yeast DNA J protein required for uncoating of clathrin-coated vesicles in vivo. Nat Cell Biol 2000;2(12):958–963.

180. Bronk P, Wenniger JJ, Dawson-Scully K, et al. Drosophila Hsc70-4 is critical for neurotransmitter exocytosis in vivo. Neuron 2001;30(2):475–488.

181. Greener T, Grant B, Zhang Y, et al. Caenorhabditis elegans auxilin: a J-domain protein essential for clathrin-mediated endocytosis in vivo. Nat Cell Biol 2001;3(2):215–219.

182. Morgan JR, Prasad K, Jin S, Augustine GJ, Lafer EM. Uncoating of clathrin-coated vesicles in presynaptic terminals: roles for Hsc70 and auxilin. Neuron 2001;32(2):289–300.

183. Van Epps HA, Hayashi M, Lucast L, et al. The zebrafish nrc mutant reveals a role for the polyphosphoinositide phosphatase synaptojanin 1 in cone photoreceptor ribbon anchoring. J Neurosci 2004;24(40):8641–8650.

184. McPherson PS, Garcia EP, Slepnev VI, et al. A presynaptic inositol-5-phosphatase. Nature 1996;379(6563):353–357.

185. Guo S, Stolz LE, Lemrow SM, York JD. SAC1-like domains of yeast SAC1, INP52, and INP53 and of human synaptojanin encode polyphosphoinositide phosphatases. J Biol Chem 1999;274(19):12990–12995.

186. Woscholski R, Finan PM, Radley E, et al. Synaptojanin is the major constitutively active phosphatidylinositol-3,4,5-trisphosphate 5-phosphatase in rodent brain. J Biol Chem 1997;272(15):9625–9658.

187. Haffner C, Di Paolo G, Rosenthal JA, de Camilli P. Direct interaction of the 170kDa isoform of synaptojanin 1 with clathrin and with the clathrin adaptor AP2. Curr Biol 2000; 10(8):471–474.

188. Jost M, Simpson F, Kavran JM, Lemmon MA, Schmid SL. Phosphatidylinositol-4,5–bisphosphate is required for endocytic coated vesicle formation. Curr Biol 1998;8(25):1399–1402.

189. Haucke V. Phosphoinositide regulation of clathrin-mediated endocytosis. Biochem Soc Trans 2005;33(pt 6):1285–1289.

190. Micheva KD, Kay BK, McPherson PS. Synaptojanin forms two separate complexes in the nerve terminal. Interactions with endophilin and amphiphysin. J Biol Chem 1997;272(43):27239–27245.

191. Lee SY, Wenk MR, Kim Y, Nairn AC, De Camilli P. Regulation of synaptojanin 1 by cyclin-dependent kinase 5 at synapses. Proc Natl Acad Sci U S A 2004;101(2):546–551.

192. Cousin MA, Tan TC, Robinson PJ. Protein phosphorylation is required for endocytosis in nerve terminals: potential role for the dephosphins dynamin I and synaptojanin, but not AP180 or amphiphysin. J Neurochem 2001;76(1):105–116.

193. Koenig JH, Ikeda K. Disappearance and reformation of synaptic vesicle membrane upon transmitter release observed under reversible blockage of membrane retrieval. J Neurosci 1989;9(11):3844–3860.

194. Clark SG, Shurland DL, Meyerowitz EM, Bargmann CI, van der Bliek AM. A dynamin GTPase mutation causes a rapid and reversible temperature-inducible locomotion defect in C. elegans. Proc Natl Acad Sci U S A 1997;94(19):10438–10443.

195. Moskowitz HS, Heuser J, McGraw TE, Ryan TA. Targeted chemical disruption of clathrin function in living cells. Mol Biol Cell 2003; 14:4437–4447.

Chapter 12
Lipids and Secretory Vesicle Exocytosis

Shona L. Osborne and Frederic A. Meunier

Contents

Abstract In recent years, the number of lipids implicated in the regulation of the synaptic vesicle exocytosis has risen dramatically. It is now clear that lipids such as the phosphoinositides, arachidonic acid, lysophospholipids, and cholesterol play a critical regulatory role in the processes leading up to exocytosis. Lipids may affect membrane fusion reactions by altering the physical properties of the membrane, recruiting key regulatory proteins, concentrating proteins into exocytic "hot spots,"

Frederic A. Meunier
Queensland Brain Institute and School of Biomedical Sciences, University of Queensland
St. Lucia, Queensland 4061, Australia
e-mail: f.meunier@uq.edu.au

or modulating protein function allosterically. This chapter discusses the different classes of lipids, the evidence linking them to secretory vesicle exocytosis, how they are thought to act to regulate key steps in the multistep process leading to exocytosis, and future directions.

Keywords Arachidonic acid, ceramide, cholesterol, lipid raft, phosphatidic acid, phosphoinositides, polyunsaturated fatty acids, sphingolipids.

While the role of proteins in neurosecretory vesicle cycling has been extensively investigated, the involvement of lipids has been slower to develop. However, a number of important findings have emerged from this growing field, which highlights the key role that membrane lipids play in coordinating the membrane trafficking and signaling events underlying neurotransmitter release. Multiple classes of lipids have been implicated and will be discussed in this chapter, including phosphoinositides, phosphatidic acid, lysophospholipids, cholesterol, sphingolipids, ceramide, and sphingophospholipids (Fig. 12.1A).

The synaptic vesicle cycle depends on co-ordinated membrane fusion and fission events. The favored model for membrane fusion to occur is via the formation of a lipidic hemifusion intermediate (Fig. 12.1B). According to this model, merging of the two proximal leaflets of the vesicle and plasma membrane bilayers to form the hemifusion intermediate would precede the merging of the two distal leaflets to form the fusion pore. Both fusion and fission require large deformations in membrane curvature. This deformation would be facilitated by the formation of high local concentrations of lipids with altered shapes (Fig. 12.1C). Certain lipids have a spontaneous curvature when in a monolayer, either positive (curvature in the direction of the polar head group) or negative (curvature in the direction of the hydrophobic tails). These lipids are classified as inverted-cone–shaped and cone-shaped, respectively. Examples that will be discussed include phosphatidic acid, a cone-shaped lipid, and lysophospholipids, which are inverted-cone shapes (Fig. 12.1C).

Fig. 12.1 Lipids and membrane fusion. (**a**) The structure of important classes of lipids is shown. Phospholipids (phosphatidylcholine, phosphatidylethanolamine, phosphatidylinositol, and phosphatidylserine) are the most abundant cellular lipids comprising the head group, which identifies the lipid, and two fatty acid chains linked by a glycerophosphate backbone. In addition to structural and other roles, they are precursors for signaling lipids such as phosphoinositides, phosphatidic acid, and lysophospholipids. Sphingomyelin, cholesterol, and ceramide are able to aggregate into lipidic microdomains that can target and localize certain classes of proteins into functional platforms. (**b**) The favored model for membrane fusion is via a lipidic hemifusion or stalk intermediate where lipid mixing of the two inner leaflets of the bilayer occurs prior to lipid mixing of the outer bilayers. (**c**) Certain classes of lipids are asymmetrical in shape and thus are unable to form planar structures. Such lipids can be classified into cone-shaped (e.g., phosphatidic acid) and inverted-cone–shaped (e.g., lysophosphatidic acid). Such lipids have a tendency to promote either negative or positive curvature as depicted for phosphatidic acid and lysophosphatidic acid. Aq, aqueous

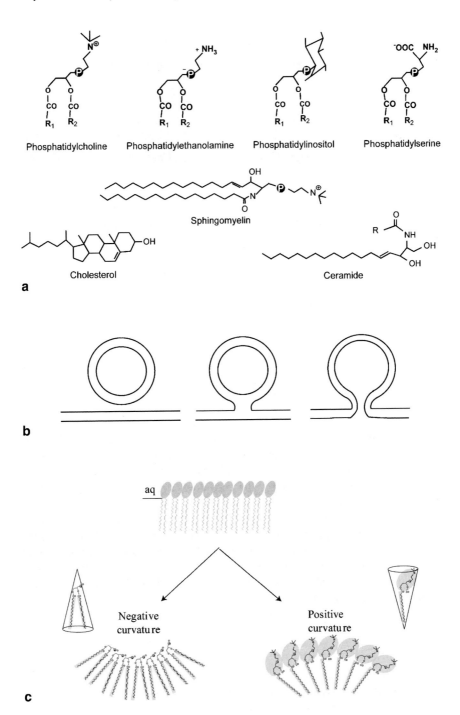

Phosphatidylcholine   Phosphatidylethanolamine   Phosphatidylinositol   Phosphatidylserine

Sphingomyelin

Cholesterol   Ceramide

a

b

aq

Negative curvature   Positive curvature

c

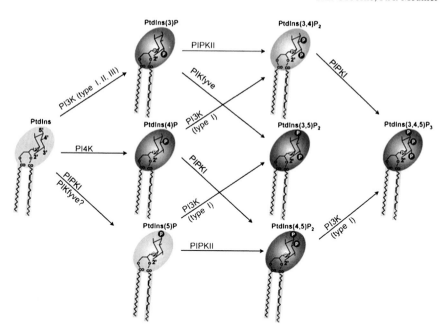

Fig. 12.2 Phosphoinositides. Phosphatidylinositol consists of two fatty acid side chains linked to the polar inositol head group via a glycerophosphate linkage and is mainly found on the cytosolic face of the membrane bilayer. The inositol head group can be reversibly phosphorylated by a series of kinases and phosphatases at three positions (3, 4, and 5) to form a family of seven phosphoinositides. PIKfyve-FYVE finger containing phosphoinositide kinase

In addition to their structural roles, it is increasingly becoming apparent that lipids can function as bona fide signaling molecules in many intracellular processes including membrane trafficking. One of the best studied classes of membrane lipids with signaling functions are the phosphoinositides (Fig. 12.2). Although phosphatidylinositol comprises only a minor proportion of total membrane lipids, its phosphorylated derivatives, the phosphoinositides (PIs), are important regulators of protein function. The generation of a high local concentration of phosphoinositides would serve as a signal for the site-specific recruitment of PI effectors or allosteric modulation of protein function. The rapid and reversible phosphorylation of phosphoinositides makes them ideal candidates for the tight spatiotemporal regulation of neurotransmitter release.

Phosphoinositides and the Synaptic Vesicle Cycle

Phospholipids (phosphatidylcholine, PtdCho; phosphatidylethanolamine, PtdEth; phosphatidylserine, PtdSer; and phosphatidylinositol, PtdIns) are the most abundant membrane lipids. Phospholipids consist of two fatty acid side chains whose composition can vary, linked to a polar head group via a glycerol molecule. In the case of PtdIns, the polar head group is the six-membered inositol ring linked to the glycerol backbone at the 1 position (Fig. 12.1A). PtdIns is unique among phospholipids in that the head group can be reversibly phosphorylated on the 3, 4, and 5 positions by a host of phosphatidylinositol kinases and phosphatases, producing a family of seven phosphoinositides (Fig. 12.2). Phosphoinositides phosphorylated at the 2 and 6 positions have not been described, and presumably cannot be synthesized due to steric hindrance. Phosphoinositides are key signaling molecules in many cellular processes and are the most studied lipid molecules in terms of their role in the synaptic vesicle cycle. The subcellular localization and regulated activity of phosphoinositide metabolic enzymes are key to understanding the role of phosphoinositides in exocytosis and will be discussed in detail below.

Phosphoinositide Metabolizing Enzymes at the Synapse

Much of our knowledge regarding the role of lipids has come from studies in model systems including bovine adrenal chromaffin cells and the rat pheochromocytoma (PC12) cell line. Earlier work focused on phosphatidylinositol-4,5-bisphosphate (PtdIns (4,5) P_2), and the role of PtdIns(4,5)P2 in exocytosis has begun to be extended from such model systems to neurons. More recently, evidence has been building in support of the involvement of other phosphoinositides including those synthesised by PI3-kinases. The contribution of enzymes involved in PtdIns(4,5)P2 metabolism will be discussed first since this is the best studied phosphoinositide with regard to the synaptic vesicle cycle, followed by PI3-kinases.

PtdIns(4,5)P2 and the Synaptic Vesicle Cycle

A number of enzymes involved in PtdIns(4,5)P2 production are found in neurons, including PI4 kinases, PtdIns(4)P-5 kinases, and phosphatases. The major pathways for PtdIns(4,5)P2 metabolism in neurons are illustrated in Figure 12.3. The first step is the phosphorylation of PtdIns by a PI4-kinase, generating PtdIns(4)P. The PtdIns(4)P then serves as a substrate for a PtdIns(4)P-5 kinase that adds a phosphate at the 5 position to generate PtdIns(4,5)P2. In neurons, there are two isoforms of PI4-kinase (PI4K) implicated in neurotransmitter release: PI4-kinase IIα and PI4-kinase IIIβ. The first, PI4-kinase IIα is present on synaptic vesicle (SV) and can produce PtdIns(4)P on immunoisolated SV *in vitro* (1), despite phosphatidylinositol comprising only a minor proportion of SV lipid composition (~1% lipid by mass) (2). However, whether PI4-kinase can generate PtdIns(4)P on synaptic vesicles *in vivo* is not clear, and furthermore the significance of a SV pool of PtdIns(4)P is also unclear given that the major PtdIns(4)P-5 kinase at the synapse, PIPKIγ, is cytosolic and PtdIns(4,5)P2 on the synaptic plasma membrane is required for exocytosis (3). One possibility is that PI4K IIα may be activated following fusion of the vesicle membrane with the plasma membrane and prior to endocytosis since PtdIns(4,5)P2 formation is also crucial for endocytosis.

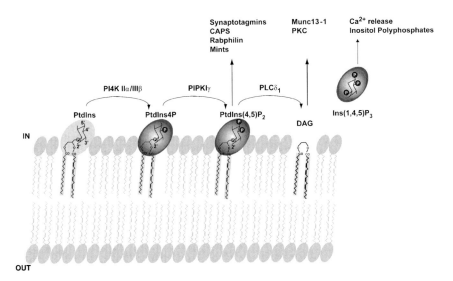

Fig. 12.3 Phosphoinositides and exocytosis. The major synaptic pathway for synthesis of PtdIns(4,5)P2 is depicted here since it is the best characterized phosphoinositide functioning in exocytosis and endocytosis. PtdIns(4,5)P2 functions as a signal to regulate the location and/or function of the synaptic proteins indicated and may also function as a substrate of phospholipase C δ1 (PLCδ1), which cleaves PtdIns(4,5)P2 generating soluble Ins(1,4,5)P_3 and diacylglycerol (DAG), which remains confined to the bilayer and regulates exocytosis through binding to Munc13-1 and protein kinase C (PKC)

The localization and activity of the second isoform, PI4K IIIβ, can be regulated potentially providing an extra control of exocytosis. PI4K IIIβ interacts with neuronal calcium sensor-1 (NCS-1, also known as frequenin). In PC12 cells, NCS-1 has been shown to regulate nucleotide-dependent exocytosis via PI4K IIIβ and both NCS-1 and PI4K IIIβ were shown to be transiently recruited to the plasma membrane upon stimulation of exocytosis (4), suggesting that PI4K IIIβ could synthesize the PtdIns(4)P used by cytosolic PIPKIγ to produce PtdIns(4,5)P2.

As mentioned above, the major PtdIns(4)P 5-kinase in neurons is PIPKIγ, which is a cytosolic protein. In PIPKIγ knockout mice, a loss of synaptic PtdIns(4,5)P2 correlated with a decrease in the size of the readily releasable pool of SV (5), consistent with a role for PtdIns(4,5)P2 in priming. PIPKIγ likely synthesizes the PtdIns(4,5)P2 required for both exocytosis and endocytosis since the knockout mouse shows endocytic defects in addition to the defects in priming (5). Many of the proteins required for clathrin-mediated endocytosis bind to PtdIns(4,5)P2 and since neurons in PIPKIγ knockout mice were shown to be lacking endocytic structures, PtdIns(4,5)P2 appears to be important for the recruitment of endocytic proteins and the process of clathrin-mediated endocytosis (5). Further evidence for the importance of PtdIns(4,5)P2 in clathrin-mediated synaptic vesicle endocytosis comes from mice lacking the protein synaptojanin. Synaptojanin is the major PtdIns(4,5)P2 phosphatase, and neurons from synaptojanin knockout mice exhibit a defect in vesicle uncoating (6).

Once synthesised, PtdIns(4,5)P2 can be removed either via the action of the PtdIns(4,5)P2 phosphatase synaptojanin, as is required for clathrin-coated vesicle uncoating, or through the action of a phospholipase C (PLC), producing the classical second messengers $Ins(1,4,5)P_3$ and diacylglycerol (DAG; see Phosphoinositide Metabolites and Exocytosis, below).

PI3-Kinases and the Synaptic Vesicle Cycle

PI3-kinases (PI3Ks) are a family of enzymes that phosphorylate PI on the 3 position. There are three classes of enzymes, I, II, and III, of which class I and class II enzymes have been implicated in the regulation of exocytosis. Class III enzymes are involved in constitutive trafficking through early endosomes and may be involved in synaptic vesicle recycling since recent evidence suggests that synaptic vesicle recycling occurs through PtdIns(3)P-positive presynaptic endosomes, a process tightly controlled by rab5 (7).

Type I PI3K predominantly phosphorylate PtdIns(4,5)P2, located on the plasma membrane, to form phosphatidylinositol-3,4,5-triphosphate (PtdIns(3,4,5)P3) and are the best studied class in all systems (8). However their involvement in synaptic processes is questionable. Classically, PI3Ks have been studied using the inhibitors wortmannin and LY294002 and an involvement of PI3K is inferred by sensitivity to these generic inhibitors. However, studies using these inhibitors at the synapse have yielded conflicting results. For example, little or no inhibition of exocytosis was observed from both synaptosomes and neurosecretory cells using wortmannin and LY294002 (1,3,9–11). However, wortmannin was shown to inhibit both spontaneous and evoked quantal neurotransmitter release at the neuromuscular junction (12), while high doses of LY294002 were shown both to inhibit synaptic vesicle recycling and to increase spontaneous acetylcholine release (13). These discrepancies may partly be due to the lack of specificity of LY294002, known to also block myosin light chain kinase activity, but may also be due to the involvement of other PI3 kinases such as PI3K-C2α (a class II PI3K), which is much less sensitive to both inhibitors. In this view, PI3K-C2α was recently shown to be necessary for the adenosine triphosphate (ATP)-dependent priming step of exocytosis in neurosecretory cells (14).

PI3K isoforms may also play other roles at different stages of the synaptic vesicle cycle. For example, the p85 subunit of type I PI3K interacts with synapsin and was shown to play an important role in regulating vesicle availability from the readily releasable pool (15) and a type I PI3K, PI3Kγ, has been implicated in the trafficking and insertion of neuronal calcium channels into the plasma membrane and the subsequent alterations in calcium influx could contribute to modulating exocytosis (16).

Phosphoinositide-Binding Proteins Involved in Exocytosis

PtdIns(4,5)P2 is mainly localized to the plasma membrane of neurons and neurosecretory cells. Plasma membrane PtdIns(4,5)P2 is likely to be important for exocytosis since modifying plasma membrane PtdIns(4,5)P2 levels in chromaffin cells alters secretion by regulating the number of vesicles available for fusion (3). A number of presynaptic proteins contain PI binding motifs and have been demonstrated to bind with varying degrees of selectivity to one or more phosphoinositides.

The best studied phosphoinositide-binding motif at the synapse is the C2B domain of synaptotagmin 1, the calcium-sensor for exocytosis (see Chapter 6). Synaptotagmin 1 binds both acidic phospholipids and phosphoinositides, particularly PtdIns(4,5)P2. There are two phosphoinositide-binding regions: a calcium-independent site discrete from the acidic phospholipid-binding sites being localized to a polybasic region on the C2B domain and a calcium-dependent site that is mediated through the calcium-binding loops. Other synaptotagmin isoforms including synaptotagmin 7 and the related synaptotagmin-like protein 4 (granuphilin) also bind PtdIns(4,5)P2 and may regulate large dense-core vesicle exocytosis (17).

While synaptotagmin isoforms are important for both large dense-core vesicle and synaptic vesicle exocytosis, calcium-activated protein for secretion (CAPS) is a cytosolic protein that was also found to bind to PtdIns(4,5)P2 and appears to regulate the exocytosis of large dense-core vesicles but not synaptic vesicles (18). Interestingly, a CAPS-1 knockout mouse primarily showed defects in vesicle filling and not in priming (19) so it is possible that CAPS-1 plays multiple roles in the vesicle cycle. Other PtdIns(4,5)P2-binding proteins include MINTS, annexin, and rabphilin; however, the importance of PtdIns(4,5)P2 binding for the function of these proteins is yet to be determined. What is clearer is the importance of PtdIns(4,5)P2 binding for the function of a number of key endocytic proteins such as the clathrin adaptor proteins AP-2 and AP-180, epsin, amphiphysin, and dynamin; disruption of PtdIns(4,5)P2-binding sites prevents their recruitment and inhibits endocytosis (20).

The identification of novel PtdIns(4,5)P2 effectors on secretory granules suggests that there may be further phosphoinositide binding proteins to be identified. Given the emerging significance of 3-phosphorylated phosphoinositides in exocytosis, it will be important to identify potential interacting proteins that may mediate the effects of these lipids on the synaptic vesicle cycle.

Phosphoinositide Metabolites and Exocytosis

PtdIns(4,5)P2 can be metabolized by the PLC that cleaves the glycerol side of the phosphoester bond, resulting in the production of DAG and myoinositol-1,4,5-triphosphate (Ins(1,4,5)P$_3$), both being important second messengers. DAG remains confined to the membrane bilayer where it can modulate the activity of proteins including protein kinase C (PKC) and Munc13, while Ins(1,4,5)P$_3$ is water soluble and can act to promote the release of Ca^{2+} from intracellular stores or can be further phosphorylated to inositol polyphosphates (Fig. 12.3).

DAG binding by both PKC and Munc13 is mediated by their C1 domains. Munc13 is a priming factor required for maintaining the readily releasable pool of SV (21,22). While the C1 domain is not essential for Munc13 function in priming, it is essential for the synaptic potentiation caused by phorbol ester treatment (23), suggesting it is the main target of DAG at the synapse. A recent study, however, has highlighted the importance of DAG action on both Munc13 and PKC for the potentiation of exocytosis through a coincidence detection mechanism (24). PKC has multiple targets at the synapse through which it may regulate exocytosis, including Munc18-1 (25), although recent work in *Caenorhabditis elegans* suggests that PKC-dependent phosphorylation of Munc18-1 functions in large dense-core vesicle but not synaptic vesicle exocytosis (26). A further, less well characterized target of DAG at the synapse is another protein kinase, protein kinase D (PKD). PKD contains a C1 domain, and consistent with a role for PKD in exocytosis, *C. elegans* lacking PKD displays movement defects (27).

Finally, DAG can be further metabolized by DAG lipase. In *Drosophila,* the protein rolling blackout (RBO) has homology to mammalian DAG lipases and is enriched presynaptically (28). Temperature-sensitive RBO mutants display a rapid paralysis that is restored upon return to the permissive temperature. In parallel to the loss of function, neurons were shown to become depleted of DAG and to accumulate PtdIns(4,5)P2 (28). In the mammalian system, there is no evidence to date of a similar role for a DAG lipase. However, in the striatum, DAG lipase α has been shown to be localized postsynaptically where it hydrolyses DAG to produce the endocannabinoid, 2-arachidonoyl-glycerol (2-AG). 2-AG has been shown to be the major endocannabinoid-mediating retrograde suppression in striatum (29). 2-AG is thought to act presynaptically via an action on either voltage-dependent calcium channels or the release machinery itself (29).

The $Ins(1,4,5)P_3$ released from PtdIns(4,5)P2 by PLC action is water soluble and its best characterized effect is to promote the release of Ca^{2+} from intracellular stores. However, $Ins(1,4,5)P_3$ can also be further phosphorylated at the 2, 3, and 6 positions by inositol polyphosphate kinases and then further phosphorylated to generate the inositol pyrophosphates. Inositol polyphosphates can act as signaling molecules in their own right, and several of the higher order inositol polyphosphates, in particular $InsP_6$, have been implicated in the regulation of exocytosis. $InsP_6$ was shown to be inhibitory for neurotransmission by affecting synaptotagmin 1 binding to PtdIns(4,5)P2 (30). Synaptotagmin 1 binds $InsP_6$ through the polybasic patch of the C2B domain, which suggests that $InsP_6$ could compete for binding with endogenous PtdIns(4,5)P2 or another effector of the C2B polybasic region such as the syntaxin/SNAP-25 heterodimer (31).

Discussion

Phosphoinositides, and in particular PtdIns(4,5)P2, have multiple functions at the synapse including the regulation of exocytosis, endocytosis, and calcium channels. To reconcile so many functions with one molecule, one can envisage that it is the localized production of PtdIns(4,5)P2 in microdomains that is critical to its pleiotropic function. Many phosphoinositide-binding proteins require simultaneous binding to a protein factor and phosphoinositide for correct and efficient localization and function. Such coincidence detection can explain how PtdIns(4,5)P2 might coordinate multiple pathways occurring in such a confined localization. While many questions remain to be addressed, it is clear that phosphoinositides occupy an important position in the hierarchy of factors regulating the synaptic vesicle cycle.

Phosphatidic Acid and Exocytosis

Phosphatidic Acid Metabolizing Enzymes

Phosphatidic acid is produced mainly from phosphatidylcholine through the action of phospholipase D (Fig. 12.4A). Phospholipase D cleaves phospholipids at the glycerophosphate linkage releasing the polar head group from the phosphatidic acid, which comprises the fatty acid side chains, the glycerol backbone, and a phosphate group. Phosphatidic acid can act either as a signaling molecule or by altering the biophysical properties of the membrane. Phosphatidic acid can also be further hydrolyzed by phosphatidic acid hydrolase, which removes the phosphate, producing diacylglycerol (see Phosphoinositide Metabolites and Exocytosis, above) or by phospholipase A_2 (PLA$_2$), which removes one fatty acid chain to produce lysophosphatidic acid (discussed further below).

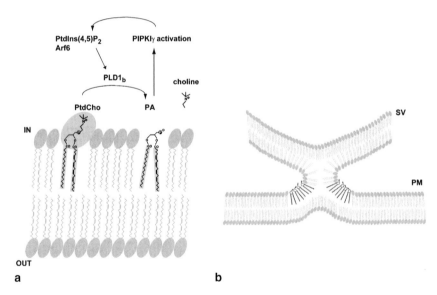

a   **b**

Fig. 12.4 Phosphatidic acid and exocytosis. (**a**) Phosphatidylcholine (PtdCho) is the major substrate for phospholipase D (PLD). During exocytosis, a PLD, likely PLD1$_b$, acts on PtdCho, liberating phosphatidic acid (PA) and free choline. While no role has been attributed to the soluble choline moiety, PA is known to activate type I phosphatidylinositol kinase, likely PIPKIγ. PtdIns(4,5)P2 produced by PIPKI is an essential cofactor for PLD1$_b$ activity and stimulates its activity together with the small GTPase Arf6, a possible positive feedback loop for the localized generation of PA. (**b**) PA may also act by promoting deformation of the membrane bilayer. PA is a cone-shaped lipid that promotes negative curvature of the bilayer as is required for formation of a fusion stalk intermediate prior to fusion pore formation and thus may act physically to promote exocytosis. SV, synaptic vesicle; PM, plasma membrane

There are two mammalian isoforms of PLD: PLD1 and PLD2. Both PLD1 and PLD2 require PtdIns(4,5)P2 as an essential cofactor for activation, while PLD1 activity is additionally regulated by small guanosine triphosphatase (GTPases) including Arf6. Work in chromaffin cells indicates that PLD1, and in particular PLD1$_b$, is the isoform that regulates exocytosis (32).

Phospholipase D Activity and Exocytosis

There is good evidence that PLD is required for exocytosis of secretory granules in chromaffin cells. Overexpression of PLD1 but not PLD2 potentiates exocytosis, while a catalytically inactive mutant inhibits exocytosis and knockdown of PLD1 by RNA interference inhibits exocytosis (33). PLD1$_b$ localizes to the plasma membrane and is thought to be the isoform responsible for this effect. PLD1 has been shown to act at a late stage of exocytosis, post docking (34).

There are two main hypotheses, not mutually exclusive, that could explain how phosphatidic acid affects exocytosis. The first is that phosphatidic acid has been shown to stimulate PIPKI activity. Thus, generation of phosphatidic acid by PLD would promote de novo synthesis of PtdIns(4,5)P2 by PIPKI known to promote exocytosis (3). In turn, PtdIns(4,5)P2 is an essential cofactor for PLD1, which would stimulate the production of phosphatidic acid in a positive feedback loop (Fig. 12.4A). This could act to rapidly form high local concentrations of PtdIns(4,5)P2 at sites of exocytosis. The second mechanism is via a biophysical effect of the phosphatidic acid (Fig. 12.4B). Phosphatidic acid is classified as a cone-shaped lipid that would promote negative curvature of a bilayer. When formed in the inner leaflet of the plasma membrane, phosphatidic acid would be predicted to increase the fusogenicity of the membrane at exocytic sites by promoting negative curvature and the formation of a hemifusion intermediate (33).

Future work will determine whether PLD1 plays an equivalent role in synaptic vesicle release, although work in Aplysia neurons has already pointed to the conservation of this pathway since microinjection of a catalytically inactive PLD1 inhibited ACh release (35). Another possibility that requires further investigation is that PLD activity may also play a role in the endocytic arm of the vesicle cycle since PLD activity is inhibited by several endocytic proteins including amphiphysins (36).

Lysophospholipids and Exocytosis

Lysophospholipid Metabolizing Enzymes

Lysophospholipids are generated by the action of PLA$_2$ activity on membrane phospholipids (Fig. 12.5A). There are multiple cellular forms of PLA$_2$, both intracellular and secretory. The actions of PLA$_2$ isoforms hydrolyze phospholipids at

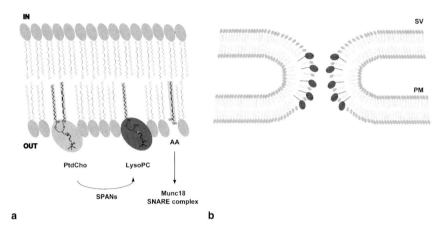

Fig. 12.5 Lysophosphatidic acid and exocytosis. (**a**) Phosphatidylcholine (PtdCho) is a major substrate for phospholipase A_2 and snake presynaptic phospholipase A_2 neurotoxins (SPANs), which cleave PtdCho asymmetrically, liberating a free fatty acid from the sn-2 position (frequently arachidonic acid (AA) as depicted or oleic acid) and lysophosphatidylcholine (LysoPC). (**b**) LysoPC is an inverted-cone–shaped lipid that promotes positive curvature of the bilayer. When formed in the outer leaflet of the plasma membrane (e.g., by SPANs), LysoPC would act to promote formation of the fusion pore. Arachidonic acid is a bioactive lipid and in particular may act on exocytosis through Munc18 and promotion of SNARE complex formation. SV, synaptic vesicle; PM, plasma membrane

the *sn*-2 ester bond to produce a free fatty acid and a lysophospholipid comprising a single fatty acid chain, the glycerol and phosphate group and the polar head group. Since the lysophospholipids retains the polar head group, they are named after the parent lipid (e.g., lysophosphatidylcholine, lysophosphatidic acid, etc.). Lysophospholipids are inverted cone shapes and generate positive curvature, while the free fatty acid (FA) promotes negative curvature (Fig. 12.5B). While the free FA can equilibrate itself between the two sides of the membrane bilayer, the lysophospholipid remains confined to the leaflet of the bilayer in which it was produced, which leads to an asymmetrical distribution of lipids with importance for membrane dynamics.

Phospholipase A_2 Activity and Exocytosis

The best evidence for the involvement of lysophospholipids during exocytosis has come from the study of the mechanism of action of snake presynaptic phospholipase A_2 neurotoxins (SPANs). SPANs cause progressive paralysis at the neuromuscular junction by stimulating exocytosis and blocking endocytosis. Originally, the stimulatory effect observed was believed to be promoted by the production of arachidonic acid (see Ceramide and Exocytosis, below). However, more recently, SPANs have been found to mainly act on PtdCho to produce LysoPtdCho and fatty acids (including arachidonic acid but mainly oleic acid [OA]) and as such, the paralytic effect can be mimicked by the addition of LysoPtdCho and OA (37). Ultrastructurally, the addition of LysoPtdCho and OA causes similar changes in the nerve terminal to SPANs, including a reduction in total number of vesicles and swelling of the nerve terminal. The effect is proposed to be due to effects on the membrane bilayer properties with the fatty acid in the inner leaflet promoting the negative curvature required for the formation of a hemifusion intermediate, and the inverted-cone shape lysophospholipids in the outer leaflet promoting the formation of the fusion pore (Fig. 12.5B). The same lipid distribution, on the other hand, would be predicted to destabilize structures requiring negative curvature including the invagination required for endocytosis and membrane fission, consistent with the block in endocytosis caused by SPANs. Further evidence in support of this biophysical hypothesis comes from the fact that microinjection of secretory PLA_2 into PC12 cells and hippocampal neurons blocks exocytosis, presumably because the presence of lysophospholipids on the inner leaflet of the bilayer would now be inhibitory for the formation of the hemifusion intermediate (38).

Phosphatidic acid is also a substrate for lysophosphatidic acid transferase (LPAAT) activity, which generates lysophosphatidic acid (LysoPA). LysoPA acts as a signaling molecule in many systems and, like lysoPtdCho and other lysophospholipids, has an inverted cone shape. Thus the action of a LPAAT would be predicted to switch a lipid from having cone-shaped to inverted cone-shape structure, thereby modifying the membrane bilayer properties. Endophilin, a protein involved in endocytosis, was shown to have LPAAT activity; however, this was subsequently demonstrated to be an artifact of the purification rather than an activity inherent to endophilin (39). The possibility remains, however, that such an activity could play a role in membrane dynamics during exo-endocytosis. What is clear from this work is that localized and asymmetric changes in the leaflets of the membrane bilayer can have important consequences on synaptic activity.

Cholesterol and Exocytosis

Cholesterol Metabolizing Enzymes

Cholesterol is a 27-carbon molecule that plays a major role in determining the lipid fluidity of the plasma membrane. In most organs, cholesterol is taken up by the cells as lipoprotein particles. Due to their size, lipoprotein particles are unable to pass the blood–brain barrier. Hence the brain is actually responsible for the biogenesis of cholesterol, which represents up to 30% of the total lipids of the brain since it is one of the major components of myelin. A number of metabolic enzymes are required for the de novo synthesis of cholesterol (40). Briefly, cholesterol synthesis from acetyl-CoA molecules consists of three majors steps: (1)

synthesis of mevalonate (C6) by the combined action of acetyl–coenzyme A (CoA) C-acetyltransferase, hydroxymethyglutaryl-CoA synthase, β-hydroxy-β-methyglytaryl-CoA reductase present in the endoplasmic reticulum; (2) mevalonate is then activated to produce isopentenyl-PP (C5) used as an elongation unit to synthesize a squalene (C30); (3) the latter is further cycled and demethylated to produce cholesterol (C27) (40). Although cholesterol can be synthesized by a number of embryonic neurons, adult neurons require additional cholesterol synthesized by glial cells as apolipoprotein (41,42). Glial cell–derived cholesterol is essential for synapse formation and maintenance as elegantly demonstrated (41,42), although the exact way cholesterol is involved in synapse formation is still unclear.

Cholesterol, Rafts, and Exocytosis

Due to the complex mechanism of cholesterol biosynthesis, transport, and delivery, genetic ablation of key metabolic enzymes would not be greatly informative. Much work however has been done on Niemann–Pick type C disease, characterized by an abnormal cholesterol accumulation in humans (43). In this disorder, cholesterol and sphingolipids accumulate in late endosomal compartments without reaching the endoplasmic reticulum, resulting in defective cholesterol esterification. Cholesterol has long been known to reduce the fluidity of the plasma membrane, which has major repercussions on the biophysical properties of ion channels and ligand-gated channels. In the last decade, an important body of work has ascribed a role for cholesterol as well as other lipids such as sphingolipids in plasma membrane microdomains called lipid rafts (44,45), which are noncaveolar microdomains enriched in cholesterol, soluble in Triton X100 and insoluble in Lubrol WX. Syntaxin and synaptosome-associated protein of 25 kDa (SNAP-25) have been found to be clustered on the plasma membrane of neurosecretory cells (46) and enriched in lipid rafts by flotation assays (44,46). Pharmacologic depletion of cholesterol inhibits exocytosis (44,46), suggesting that lipid rafts may be important to the functions of syntaxin and SNAP-25 (Fig. 12.6A).

SNAP-25 is believed to be a true raft protein partly via its palmitoylation (Fig. 12.6B) but the way syntaxin 1 is associated to lipid rafts is more enigmatic. Syntaxin 1 might be associated with lipid rafts by simple binding to SNAP-25 as suggested by perturbation of membrane clustering following botulinum type E treatment, which is known to prevent syntaxin/SNAP-25 interaction (31). Syntaxin could also be associated with lipid rafts via its binding to P/Q-type calcium channels, which have also been found in lipid rafts by flotation experiment (47). Importantly, another pool of syntaxin that is associated with Munc18a has been found not to be associated with lipid raft by flotation experiments (48). Considering the established role of Munc18 in maintaining syntaxin in a closed conformation, it is tempting to suggest that syntaxin can shuttle between raft and nonraft microdomains, and that lipid rafts are indeed necessary for exocytosis.

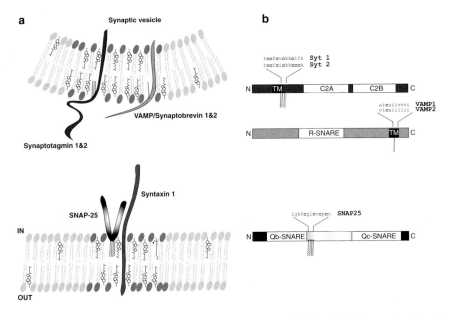

Fig. 12.6 Lipid microdomains, palmitoylation, and exocytosis. (**a**) Hypothetical representation of presynaptic lipid rafts and palmitoylated proteins involved in exocytosis. (**b**) Schematic of the structure of synaptotagmins (Syt) 1 and 2, vesicle-associated membrane protein (VAMP) 1 and 2, and synaptosome-associated protein of 25 kDa (SNAP-25) depicting the location of palmitoylated cysteines (highlighted in bold)

However, even though lipid rafts are undeniably important for exocytosis in neurosecretory cells and various other cells types (45), a clear model on how lipid rafts and cholesterol play a positive role in exocytosis is yet to emerge. The recent demonstration that cholesterol disrupts the balance between evoked and spontaneous release in hippocampal neurons adds to the complexity of the question, suggesting that it is the synchronization process of neurotransmitter release that is perturbed by cholesterol depletion (49). Moreover, the high cholesterol level found in synaptic vesicle suggests that lipid rafts could also be present in secretory vesicles. A recent study provided a detailed map of synaptic vesicle lipid composition, demonstrating a high percentage of cholesterol (~40 mol%) and low levels of phosphatidylinositol (2). Modeling of the protein component of vesicles assuming a homogeneous distribution indicated that the lipids might not be easily accessible. However, a high percentage of cholesterol may contribute to clustering of proteins of interest, allowing access to lipids such as phosphatidylinositol (see Phosphoinositides and the Synaptic Vesicle Cycle, above) and to the high curvature of the synaptic vesicle.

Clearly, more work needs to be done to clarify how cholesterol and rafts positively affect exocytosis. There is no doubt that the recent report highlighting a link between Alzheimer's disease and cholesterol will stir this exciting field of research (50).

Ceramide and Exocytosis

Ceramide and Sphingolipids Metabolism

Sphingolipids and their precursor ceramide (*N*-acylsphingosine) act as signaling molecules in a variety of cellular events (4). Upon various stimulation types, hydrolysis of sphingomyelin by endogenous sphingomyelinase promotes the formation of ceramide. A ceramidase converts ceramide to sphingosine, which can be further metabolized by sphingosine kinase to sphingosine 1-phosphate, an important regulator of apoptosis, mitosis, and motility. Ceramide was initially found to be phosphorylated in a Ca^{2+}-dependent manner through the action of ceramide-kinase located on synaptic vesicles.

Ceramide, Sphingolipids, and Exocytosis

The fact that ceramide-kinase co-purified with synaptic vesicles, and its activity was enhanced by micromolar concentrations of Ca^{2+} suggested, that it might play an important role in exocytosis (51). Interestingly, ceramide-1-phosphate was found to be a direct activator of cytosolic PLA_2, and is thereby involved in the production of arachidonic acid, an important lipid mentioned for its role in exocytosis (see next section). Recently, ceramide phosphatase activity was demonstrated to be necessary for mast cell degranulation and the Ca^{2+}-dependency of this enzyme was revealed to be mediated through its binding to the Ca^{2+} sensor calmodulin (52). Genetic evidence points to an important role of ceramide in synaptic transmission in *Drosophila* (53). In this study, genetic ablation of ceramidase leads to a severe phenotype. A presynaptic impairment of evoked synaptic currents was found, and a reduction of readily releasable vesicles was associated with fewer vesicles in reserve pool (53).

In PC12 cells ceramide was shown to be produced upon stimulation of exocytosis, and most importantly exogenous addition of cell-permeant ceramide was shown to stimulate dopamine release (54). Following the recent profiling of ceramides involved in excitotoxicity in the brain (55), various ceramide side chains were tested for their effect in exocytosis from PC12 cells, revealing that C2, C6, and C18 ceramide are capable of triggering exocytosis in PC12 cells (56). Sphingosine-1-phosphate was recently shown to act via an autocrine mechanism to promote glutamate exocytosis from hippocampal neurons (57). At this stage, it is not clear how ceramide or sphingosine are involved in exocytosis, but both have been associated with lipid rafts and could contribute to the negative curvature necessary to generate membrane fusion (53,58).

Fatty Acids Metabolism and Exocytosis

Fatty acids are an integral part of the hydrophobic lipid chain of phospholipids and are classically assigned a structural role in membranes. Investigating the role of lipids in exocytosis has revealed a more active role for fatty acids in exocytosis than previously anticipated. This section discusses palmitoylation, a process during which fatty acid is grafted as posttranslational modification on cysteine residues of certain proteins critically involved in exocytosis. Fatty acids and especially polyunsaturated fatty acids (PUFAs) released from the phospholipids of the plasma membrane through the action of various phospholipases also play an important role during exocytosis.

Palmitoylation and Exocytosis

Posttranslational lipid modifications such as the addition of fatty acid palmitoyl moieties (C16 chain) to proteins play an important role in exocytosis from yeast to neurons through the palmitoylation of proteins involved in exocytosis such as soluble N-ethylmaleimide–sensitive factor attachment receptor (SNARE) proteins. The enzymes catalyzing the transfer of palmitate, called palmitoyl transferases (PATs), were only recently described (59). However, the actual requirement of this enzyme to perform palmitoylation has been questioned, as palmitoylation can actually occur spontaneously on highly reactive cysteine residues (60).

In neurons and neuroendocrine cells, vesicle-associated membrane protein VAMP2, SNAP-25, and synaptotagmin can be palmitoylated (60–63) (Fig. 12.6B). Such lipid modification is known to increase the hydrophobicity of a protein, thereby facilitating its membrane insertion. However, in neurons, palmitoylation-deficient mutations in SNAP-25 did not affect plasma membrane targeting or its interaction with syntaxin 1 (64). Surprisingly, this study highlighted a clear inhibition of exocytosis and blockade of SNARE disassembly, suggesting that SNAP-25 palmitoylation could have a major functional role in exocytosis (64). This hypothesis is backed up by the observation that SNAP-25A, normally expressed during development and bearing a mutation in the sequence of cysteines, is much less efficient in mediating exocytosis (65). Clearly, not only palmitoylation but also the precise sequence of the palmitoylated cysteines in SNAP-25 are critical for optimal exocytosis. The possibility that palmitoylation could increase protein–protein interaction has been recently proposed (63).

PUFA Metabolizing Enzymes

Mammalian neurons are not capable of synthesizing endogenous omega-3 (n-3) fatty acids. This has fueled much research into how beneficial dietary precursors such as oleic acid are for brain function and development. The concentrations of long-chain polyunsaturated fatty acids of the n-6 and n-3 series in neurons are largely dependent on the food intakes of their precursors such as linoleic (18:2 n-6) and α-linolenic acids (18:3 n-3), and the preformed PUFA arachidonic acid (AA; 20:4 n-6), eicosapentaenoic acid (20:5 n-3), and docosahexaenoic acid (22:6 n-3).

Once in neurons, a variety of desaturase and elongase enzymes are capable of producing and maintaining a finely balanced concentration of various PUFA (66).

A number of early pharmacologic approaches have highlighted a positive role for AA, including studies by Piomelli *et al* (67,68), which identified a role for AA and its metabolites in modulating synaptic plasticity in Aplysia. Moreover, studies by Williams *et al* (69) demonstrated that AA played a role in mediating long-term plasticity in the hippocampus. In this early study, activity of AA was attributed to presynaptic sites, although the molecular mechanism was not defined. Numerous studies have shown that PLA$_2$ from various snake and insect venoms promotes fusion of secretory vesicles (70) (see also Phospholipase A$_2$ Activity and Exocytosis, above). PLA$_2$ is responsible for the cleavage of the *sn*-2 ester bond of 1,2-diacyl-3-*sn*-phosphoglycerides. Neurotoxins harboring PLA$_2$ activity release fatty acids such as AA from the phospholipids of the plasma membrane and promote extensive exocytosis accompanied with a blockade of endocytosis, leading to a complete depletion of synaptic vesicles in the presynaptic motor nerve terminals at the neuromuscular junction (70).

Morgan and Burgoyne (71) made a very interesting discovery that stimulation of exocytosis in neurosecretory cells increases concomitantly both endogenous AA production and catecholamine secretion. But pharmacologic dissection using the PKC inhibitor staurosporin allowed them to uncouple these two processes thereby completely preventing AA production with minimal effect on catecholamine secretion. This led to serious doubts about a direct role of AA in mediating exocytosis. However, more recently, in *Caenorhabditis elegans*, deletion of *fat-3*, a gene encoding a PUFA synthesizing enzyme, Δ6-desaturase, was found to result in an uncoordinated phenotype. Electrophysiologic examination of the neuromuscular junction in the *fat-3 C. elegans* mutant demonstrated a significant downregulation of phasic transmitter release (72). Importantly, this phenotype could be rescued by exogenous addition of AA, suggesting that AA could play a critical role in neurotransmitter release. These findings prompted more careful examinations of which PUFA is critically involved in exocytosis and by which mechanism.

Latham *et al* (73) screened a variety of PUFA molecules for their effects on secretion and found that only AA was capable of significantly potentiating catecholamine secretion from bovine chromaffin cells. Importantly, AA was found to dose-dependently increase SNARE complex formation, suggesting that AA could potentially act on the mechanism of exocytosis. Rickman and Davletov (74) found that various PUFA and detergents were capable of directly reverting the negative regulation of Munc18a. This was further substantiated with the demonstration that AA allows Munc18a to bind the SNARE complex, suggesting that Munc18a, like other related Munc/sec proteins, is capable of directly binding and promoting the formation of the SNARE complex. Clearly, SNARE binding to Munc18a is only revealed in the presence of AA, suggesting that AA is a critical component allowing a switch in Munc18a function (Fig. 12.7). AA can be found as free molecule or as a component of phospholipids. In this view, it is interesting to note that Munc18a binding to syntaxin 1 N-terminal peptide occurs on the plasma membrane, suggesting that the plasma membrane provides a component that favors the productive Munc18a mode versus the inhibitory mode (which occurs

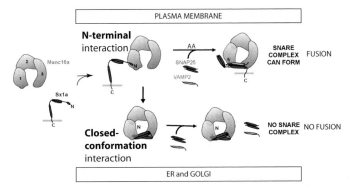

Fig. 12.7 Emerging hypothesis on how Munc18a controls soluble *N*-ethylmaleimide–sensitive factor attachment receptor (SNARE) complex formation. Munc18a can bind syntaxin 1 (Sx1) in either of two modes, depending on the lipidic environment: the classical inhibitory mode (preventing SNARE complex formation) occurring inside the cell, and the new productive mode (promoting SNARE complex assembly) occurring on or near the plasma membrane. ER, endoplasmic reticulum

inside the cell, presumably in the endoplasmic reticulum and the Golgi). Moreover, using fusion-competent membrane sheets, Jahn's group (75) has demonstrated that Munc18a allows the t-SNARE complex (syntaxin 1 and SNAP-25) to form as an acceptor intermediate for vesicle-bound VAMP2. Whether this effect is mediated by free AA itself or as side chain of plasma membrane phospholipids remains an open question. All these findings suggest that AA serves as a switch for Munc18a by acting as either a free molecule or a side chain of phospholipids (Fig. 12.7). Further research into this molecular switch could reveal how Munc18a tightly controls exocytosis both negatively (to avoid ectopic fusion events) and positively (to promote exocytosis of secretory vesicles with the plasma membrane).

Conclusion

Research into the molecular mechanisms of exocytosis and endocytosis has long focused on presynaptic proteins and has led to important discoveries as to how some proteins can locally control the lipid composition and fusogenicity. More recent work has revealed that certain lipids can actually orchestrate membrane fusion by providing microdomains both on the plasma membrane and on synaptic vesicles whose lipid and protein composition is critical for exocytosis and endocytosis. Some lipids, such as PtdIns(4,5)P2, have long been known to be intrinsically linked to the very late events in membrane fusion. But the focus on presynaptic lipids has recently shifted to the next level with reports that lipids present on or near the plasma membrane of neurosecretory cells have the ability to regulate the SNARE pathway to exocytosis by switching Munc18-1 function. No doubt this novel avenue will fuel much more research and continue to shed light onto the fascinating role played by lipids during neurotransmission.

References

1. Wiedemann C, Schafer T, Burger MM, Sihra TS. An essential role for a small synaptic vesicle-associated phosphatidylinositol 4-kinase in neurotransmitter release. J Neurosci 1998;18(15):5594–5602.
2. Takamori S, Holt M, Stenius K, et al. Molecular anatomy of a trafficking organelle. Cell 2006;127(4):831–846.
3. Milosevic I, Sorensen JB, Lang T, et al. Plasmalemmal phosphatidylinositol-4,5-bisphosphate level regulates the releasable vesicle pool size in chromaffin cells. J Neurosci 2005;25 (10):2557–2565.
4. de Barry J, Janoshazi A, Dupont JL, et al. Functional implication of neuronal calcium sensor-1 and phosphoinositol 4-kinase-beta interaction in regulated exocytosis of PC12 cells. J Biol Chem 2006;281(26):18098–18111.
5. Di Paolo G, Moskowitz HS, Gipson K, et al. Impaired PtdIns(4,5)P2 synthesis in nerve terminals produces defects in synaptic vesicle trafficking. Nature 2004;431(7007):415–422.
6. Cremona O, Di Paolo G, Wenk MR, et al. Essential role of phosphoinositide metabolism in synaptic vesicle recycling. Cell 1999;99(2):179–188.
7. Wucherpfennig T, Wilsch-Brauninger M, Gonzalez-Gaitan M. Role of Drosophila Rab5 during endosomal trafficking at the synapse and evoked neurotransmitter release. J Cell Biol 2003;161(3):609–624.
8. Hawkins PT, Anderson KE, Davidson K, Stephens LR. Signalling through Class I PI3Ks in mammalian cells. Biochem Soc Trans 2006;34(Pt 5):647–662.
9. Chasserot-Golaz S, Hubert P, Thierse D, et al. Possible involvement of phosphatidylinositol 3-kinase in regulated exocytosis: studies in chromaffin cells with inhibitor LY294002. J Neurochem 1998;70(6):2347–2356.
10. Martin TF. Phosphoinositides as spatial regulators of membrane traffic. Curr Opin Neurobiol 1997;7(3):331–338.
11. Wiedemann C, Schafer T, Burger MM. Chromaffin granule-associated phosphatidylinositol 4-kinase activity is required for stimulated secretion. EMBO J 1996;15(9):2094–2101.
12. Hong SJ, Chang CC. Inhibition of quantal release from motor nerve by wortmannin. Br J Pharmacol 1999;128(1):142–148.
13. Rizzoli SO, Betz WJ. Effects of 2-(4-morpholinyl)-8-phenyl-4H-1-benzopyran-4-one on synaptic vesicle cycling at the frog neuromuscular junction. J Neurosci 2002;22(24): 10680–10689.
14. Meunier FA, Osborne SL, Hammond GR, et al. Phosphatidylinositol 3-kinase C2alpha is essential for ATP-dependent priming of neurosecretory granule exocytosis. Mol Biol Cell 2005;16(10):4841–4851.
15. Cousin MA, Malladi CS, Tan TC, Raymond CR, Smillie KJ, Robinson PJ. Synapsin I-associated phosphatidylinositol 3-kinase mediates synaptic vesicle delivery to the readily releasable pool. J Biol Chem 2003;278(31):29065–29071.
16. Viard P, Butcher AJ, Halet G, et al. PI3K promotes voltage-dependent calcium channel trafficking to the plasma membrane. Nat Neurosci 2004;7(9):939–946.
17. Osborne SL, Wallis TP, Jimenez JL, Gorman JJ, Meunier FA. Identification of secretory granule phosphatidylinositol 4,5-bisphosphate-interacting proteins using an affinity pulldown strategy. Mol Cell Proteomics 2007;6(7):1158–1169.
18. Speese S, Petrie M, Schuske K, et al. UNC-31 (CAPS) is required for dense-core vesicle but not synaptic vesicle exocytosis in Caenorhabditis elegans. J Neurosci 2007;27(23):6150–6162.
19. Speidel D, Bruederle CE, Enk C, et al. CAPS1 regulates catecholamine loading of large dense-core vesicles. Neuron 2005;46(1):75–88.
20. Haucke V. Phosphoinositide regulation of clathrin-mediated endocytosis. Biochem Soc Trans 2005;33(Pt 6):1285–1289.
21. Basu J, Betz A, Brose N, Rosenmund C. Munc13-1 C1 domain activation lowers the energy barrier for synaptic vesicle fusion. J Neurosci 2007;27(5):1200–1210.

22. Bauer CS, Woolley RJ, Teschemacher AG, Seward EP. Potentiation of exocytosis by phospholipase C-coupled G-protein-coupled receptors requires the priming protein Munc13-1. J Neurosci 2007;27(1):212–219.

23. Rhee SG. Regulation of phosphoinositide-specific phospholipase C. Annu Rev Biochem 2001;70:281–312.

24. Wierda KDB, Toonen RFG, de Wit H, Brussaard AB, Verhage M. Interdependence of PKC-dependent and PKC-independent pathways for presynaptic plasticity. Neuron 2007;54 (2):275–290.

25. Nili U, de Wit H, Gulyas-Kovacs A, et al. Munc18-1 phosphorylation by protein kinase C potentiates vesicle pool replenishment in bovine chromaffin cells. Neuroscience 2006;143(2):487–500.

26. Sieburth D, Madison JM, Kaplan JM. PKC-1 regulates secretion of neuropeptides. Nat Neurosci 2007;10(1):49–57.

27. Feng H, Ren M, Wu SL, Hall DH, Rubin CS. Characterization of a novel protein kinase D: Caenorhabditis elegans DKF-1 is activated by translocation-phosphorylation and regulates movement and growth in vivo. J Biol Chem 2006;281(26):17801–17814.

28. Huang FD, Matthies HJ, Speese SD, Smith MA, Broadie K. Rolling blackout, a newly identified PIP2-DAG pathway lipase required for Drosophila phototransduction. Nat Neurosci 2004;7(10):1070–1078.

29. Uchigashima M, Narushima M, Fukaya M, Katona I, Kano M, Watanabe M. Subcellular arrangement of molecules for 2-arachidonoyl-glycerol-mediated retrograde signaling and its physiological contribution to synaptic modulation in the striatum. J Neurosci 2007;27 (14):3663–3676.

30. Llinas R, Sugimori M, Lang EJ, et al. The inositol high-polyphosphate series blocks synaptic transmission by preventing vesicular fusion: a squid giant synapse study. Proc Natl Acad Sci U S A 1994;91(26):12990–12993.

31. Rickman C, Archer DA, Meunier FA, et al. Synaptotagmin interaction with the syntaxin/SNAP-25 dimer is mediated by an evolutionarily conserved motif and is sensitive to inositol hexakisphosphate. J Biol Chem 2004;279(13):12574–12579.

32. Bader MF, Doussau F, Chasserot-Golaz S, Vitale N, Gasman S. Coupling actin and membrane dynamics during calcium-regulated exocytosis: a role for Rho and ARF GTPases. Biochim Biophys Acta 2004;1742(1–3):37–49.

33. Zeniou-Meyer M, Zabari N, Ashery U, et al. Phospholipase D1 production of phosphatidic acid at the plasma membrane promotes exocytosis of large dense-core granules at a late stage. J Biol Chem 2007;282(30):21746–21757.

34. Vitale N, Caumont AS, Chasserot-Golaz S, et al. Phospholipase D1: a key factor for the exocytotic machinery in neuroendocrine cells. EMBO J 2001;20(10):2424–2434.

35. Humeau Y, Vitale N, Chasserot-Golaz S, et al. A role for phospholipase D1 in neurotransmitter release. Proc Natl Acad Sci U S A 2001;98(26):15300–15305.

36. Lee C, Kim SR, Chung JK, Frohman MA, Kilimann MW, Rhee SG. Inhibition of phospholipase D by amphiphysins. J Biol Chem 2000;275(25):18751–18758.

37. Rigoni M, Caccin P, Gschmeissner S, et al. Equivalent effects of snake PLA2 neurotoxins and lysophospholipid-fatty acid mixtures. Science 2005;310(5754):1678–1680.

38. Wei S, Ong WY, Thwin MM, et al. Group IIA secretory phospholipase A2 stimulates exocytosis and neurotransmitter release in pheochromocytoma-12 cells and cultured rat hippocampal neurons. Neuroscience 2003;121(4):891–898.

39. Gallop JL, Butler PJ, McMahon HT. Endophilin and CtBP/BARS are not acyl transferases in endocytosis or Golgi fission. Nature 2005;438(7068):675–678.

40. Dietschy JM, Turley SD. Thematic review series: brain Lipids. Cholesterol metabolism in the central nervous system during early development and in the mature animal. J Lipid Res 2004;45(8):1375–1397.

41. Pfrieger FW. Cholesterol homeostasis and function in neurons of the central nervous system. Cell Mol Life Sci 2003;60(6):1158–1171.

42. Mauch DH, Nagler K, Schumacher S, et al. CNS synaptogenesis promoted by glia-derived cholesterol. Science 2001;294(5545):1354–1357.

43. Pentchev PG, Comly ME, Kruth HS, et al. A defect in cholesterol esterification in Niemann-Pick disease (type C) patients. Proc Natl Acad Sci 1985;82(23):8247–8251.
44. Chamberlain LH, Burgoyne RD, Gould GW. SNARE proteins are highly enriched in lipid rafts in PC12 cells: implications for the spatial control of exocytosis. Proc Natl Acad Sci U S A 2001;98(10):5619–5624.
45. Salaun C, James DJ, Chamberlain LH. Lipid rafts and the regulation of exocytosis. Traffic 2004;5(4):255–264.
46. Lang T, Bruns D, Wenzel D, et al. SNAREs are concentrated in cholesterol-dependent clusters that define docking and fusion sites for exocytosis. EMBO J 2001;20(9):2202–2213.
47. Taverna E, Saba E, Rowe J, Francolini M, Clementi F, Rosa P. Role of lipid microdomains in P/Q-type calcium channel (Cav2.1) clustering and function in presynaptic membranes. J Biol Chem 2004;279(7):5127–5134.
48. Chamberlain LH, Burgoyne RD, Gould GW. SNARE proteins are highly enriched in lipid rafts in PC12 cells: implications for the spatial control of exocytosis. Proc Natl Acad Sci U S A 2001;98(10):5619–5624.
49. Wasser CR, Ertunc M, Liu X, Kavalali ET. Cholesterol-dependent balance between evoked and spontaneous synaptic vesicle recycling. J Physiol 2007;579(2):413–429.
50. Gylys KH, Fein JA, Yang F, Miller CA, Cole GM. Increased cholesterol in Abeta-positive nerve terminals from Alzheimer's disease cortex. Neurobiol Aging 2007;28(1):8–17.
51. Bajjalieh SM, Martin TF, Floor E. Synaptic vesicle ceramide kinase. A calcium-stimulated lipid kinase that co-purifies with brain synaptic vesicles. J Biol Chem 1989;264(24):14354–14360.
52. Mitsutake S, Igarashi Y. Calmodulin is involved in the Ca2+-dependent activation of ceramide kinase as a calcium sensor. J Biol Chem 2005;280(49):40436–40441.
53. Rohrbough J, Rushton E, Palanker L, et al. Ceramidase regulates synaptic vesicle exocytosis and trafficking. J Neurosci 2004;24(36):7789–7803.
54. Jeon HJ, Lee DH, Kang MS, et al. Dopamine release in PC12 cells is mediated by Ca(2+)-dependent production of ceramide via sphingomyelin pathway. J Neurochem 2005;95 (3):811–820.
55. Guan XL, He X, Ong WY, Yeo WK, Shui G, Wenk MR. Non-targeted profiling of lipids during kainate-induced neuronal injury. FASEB J 2006;20(8):1152–1161.
56. Tang N, Ong WY, Zhang EM, Chen P, Yeo JF. Differential effects of ceramide species on exocytosis in rat PC12 cells. Exp Brain Res 2007;183(2):241–247.
57. Kajimoto T, Okada T, Yu H, Goparaju SK, Jahangeer S, Nakamura S. Involvement of sphingosine-1-phosphate in glutamate secretion in hippocampal neurons. Mol Cell Biol 2007;27(9):3429–3440.
58. Rogasevskaia T, Coorssen JR. Sphingomyelin-enriched microdomains define the efficiency of native Ca(2+)-triggered membrane fusion. J Cell Sci 2006;119(Pt 13):2688–2694.
59. Huang K, Yanai A, Kang R, et al. Huntingtin-interacting protein HIP14 is a palmitoyl transferase involved in palmitoylation and trafficking of multiple neuronal proteins. Neuron 2004;44(6):977–986.
60. Veit M. Palmitoylation of the 25–kDa synaptosomal protein (SNAP-25) in vitro occurs in the absence of an enzyme, but is stimulated by binding to syntaxin. Biochem J 2000;345 (pt 1):145–151.
61. Veit M, Becher A, Ahnert-Hilger G. Synaptobrevin 2 is palmitoylated in synaptic vesicles prepared from adult, but not from embryonic brain. Mol Cell Neurosci 2000;15(4):408–416.
62. Veit M, Sollner TH, Rothman JE. Multiple palmitoylation of synaptotagmin and the t-SNARE SNAP-25. FEBS Lett 1996;385(1–2):119–123.
63. Washbourne P. Greasing transmission: palmitoylation at the synapse. Neuron 2004;44(6):901–902.
64. Washbourne P, Cansino V, Mathews JR, Graham M, Burgoyne RD, Wilson MC. Cysteine residues of SNAP-25 are required for SNARE disassembly and exocytosis, but not for membrane targeting. Biochem J 2001;357(pt 3):625–634.

65. Sorensen JB, Nagy G, Varoqueaux F, et al. Differential control of the releasable vesicle pools by SNAP-25 splice variants and SNAP-23. Cell 2003;114(1):75–86.

66. Lauritzen L, Hansen HS, Jorgensen MH, Michaelsen KF. The essentiality of long chain n-3 fatty acids in relation to development and function of the brain and retina. Prog Lipid Res 2001;40(1–2):1–94.

67. Piomelli D, Shapiro E, Feinmark SJ, Schwartz JH. Metabolites of arachidonic acid in the nervous system of Aplysia: possible mediators of synaptic modulation. J Neurosci 1987;7(11):3675–3686.

68. Piomelli D, Volterra A, Dale N, et al. Lipoxygenase metabolites of arachidonic acid as second messengers for presynaptic inhibition of Aplysia sensory cells. Nature 1987;328 (6125):38–43.

69. Williams JH, Errington ML, Lynch MA, Bliss TV. Arachidonic acid induces a long-term activity-dependent enhancement of synaptic transmission in the hippocampus. Nature 1989;341(6244):739–742.

70. Schiavo G, Matteoli M, Montecucco C. Neurotoxins affecting neuroexocytosis. Physiol Rev 2000;80(2):717–766.

71. Morgan A, Burgoyne RD. Relationship between arachidonic acid release and Ca2(+)-dependent exocytosis in digitonin-permeabilized bovine adrenal chromaffin cells. Biochem J 1990;271(3):571–574.

72. Lesa GM, Palfreyman M, Hall DH, et al. Long chain polyunsaturated fatty acids are required for efficient neurotransmission in C. elegans. J Cell Sci 2003;116(pt 24):4965–4975.

73. Latham CF, Osborne SL, Cryle MJ, Meunier FA. Arachidonic acid potentiates exocytosis and allows neuronal SNARE complex to interact with Munc18a. J Neurochem 2007;100(6): 1543–1554.

74. Rickman C, Davletov B. Arachidonic acid allows SNARE complex formation in the presence of Munc18. Chem Biol 2005;12(5):545–553.

75. Zilly FE, Sorensen JB, Jahn R, Lang T. Munc18-bound syntaxin readily forms SNARE complexes with synaptobrevin in native plasma membranes. PLoS Biol 2006;4(10):e330.

Chapter 13
Neurotransmitter Reuptake and Synaptic Vesicle Refilling

Richard J. Reimer, Kimberly A. Zaia, and Hiroaki Tani

Contents

Richard J. Reimer
Department of Neurology and Neurological Sciences and Graduate Program in Neuroscience,
Stanford University School of Medicine, Stanford, CA 94305
e-mail: rjreimer@stanford.edu

Z.-W. Wang (ed.) *Molecular Mechanisms of Neurotransmitter Release,*
© Humana Press 2008 a part of Springer Science+Business Media, LLC

Abstract Intercellular information transfer in the nervous system is mediated by chemical neurotransmitters. The fidelity of this process requires the rapid release and clearance of the neurotransmitter from the synaptic cleft. In addition to metabolic pathways for synthesis of neurotransmitters, two specific mechanisms, vesicular storage and local reuptake, have evolved to facilitate neurotransmission. These processes are mediated by transporter proteins: vesicular neurotransmitter transporters to fill the vesicles and plasma membrane neurotransmitter transporters to clear the synaptic cleft. This chapter discusses the synthesis, packaging, and recycling of the classic neurotransmitters with an emphasis on the transporter proteins that are integral to these pathways.

Keywords Neurotransmitter, transporter, GABA, glutamate, glycine, acetylcholine, dopamine, serotonin, norepinephrine.

The complexity of vertebrate behavior relies on the spatially and temporally precise transfer of information between neurons. Synaptic transmission, the transfer of information through release of a chemical messenger at specialized sites of cell-cell apposition, is the primary mechanism for neuronal intercellular communication. The chemical messengers, referred to as neurotransmitters, are characterized by four widely accepted criteria: (1) accumulation in the presynaptic terminal; (2) release from the presynaptic neuron in response to stimulation; (3) direct application elicits a characteristic postsynaptic response; and (4) a mechanism exists for rapid removal from the synaptic cleft (1). In the vertebrate nervous system, substances that meet these criteria include acetylcholine, several monoamines (dopamine, norepinephrine, epinephrine, and serotonin), and the amino acids γ-aminobutyric acid (GABA), glycine, and glutamate (2).

Neurotransmitter Release and Reuptake Rely on Transporter Proteins

The rapid release and clearance of neurotransmitter from the intercellular junction are hallmarks of synaptic transmission. Two specific mechanisms that have evolved to facilitate these processes are vesicular storage and local reuptake. Vesicular storage allows for simultaneous release of thousands of neurotransmitter molecules into the synaptic cleft, while local reuptake facilitates clearance of the neurotransmitter from the synaptic cleft and allows for the recycling of the neurotransmitters. Both of these processes are dependent on transporter proteins—vesicular neurotransmitter transporters to fill the vesicles and plasma membrane neurotransmitter transporters to clear the synaptic cleft. Although a number of different neurotransmitters have been identified, basic aspects of molecular mechanisms for storage and reuptake are conserved.

Vesicular Neurotransmitter Transport is Necessary for Quantal Release

A little more than 50 years ago, Katz and colleagues demonstrated that the neurotransmitter acetylcholine is released at synapses in "packets" containing thousands of molecules (3). It is now accepted that release of these quanta occurs through exocytosis of small synaptic vesicles filled with neurotransmitter. Since neurotransmitters are typically synthesized in the cytoplasm, a mechanism is required for their uptake into synaptic vesicles. Indeed, biochemical studies have defined synaptic vesicle transport activities that mediate the uptake of each of the classic neurotransmitters. These transport processes are coupled to a large proton electrochemical gradient across the synaptic vesicle membrane that permits rapid filling of vesicles and generation of lumen-to-cytoplasm neurotransmitter concentration gradients of up to 10^4(4).

The synaptic vesicle proton electrochemical gradient ($\Delta\mu H^+$) is generated by a vacuolar-type H^+–adenosine triphosphatase (ATPase), a multimeric complex containing cytoplasmic (V1) and transmembrane (V0) domains each composed of several polypeptide subunits (5). Recent data suggest that each synaptic vesicle has a single H^+-ATPase (6). The H^+-ATPase couples hydrolysis of one adenosine triphosphate (ATP) molecule to the inward transmembrane movement of two protons and generation of a chemical (ΔpH) and an electrical ($\Delta\psi$) gradient. Under normal physiologic conditions, there is an estimated 1- to 2-pH unit gradient and a 40- to 80-mV potential (inside positive) across the synaptic vesicle membrane (4). Due to the small size of synaptic vesicles, inward proton transport rapidly generates a membrane potential. This membrane potential creates an energy barrier that hinders further proton influx and hence limits the maximal pH gradient that can be achieved. Anions such as Cl^- can permeate the synaptic vesicle membrane and reduce $\Delta\psi$, thus facilitating formation of a larger ΔpH (4). The flux of Cl^- through channels has been suggested as a major regulatory mechanism for acidification of intracellular vesicles including synaptic vesicles. The primary mediator of the Cl^- conductance in synaptic vesicles is believed to be ClC3, a member of the ClC family of Cl^- channels (7).

All vesicular neurotransmitter transport activities are dependent on $\Delta\mu H^+$. Bafilomycin, a specific inhibitor of the vacuolar H^+-ATPase, as well as the proton ionophores carbonyl cyanide m-chlorophenylhydrazone (CCCP) and carbonylcyanide p-(trifluoromethoxy) phenylhydrazone (FCCP), reduce vesicular storage of all neurotransmitters. The contribution of the chemical and electrical components of $\Delta\mu H^+$ in different transport systems has been studied *in vitro* by selectively reducing ΔpH and $\Delta\psi$ with weak bases and permeant anions, respectively (4). Such studies have shown that the vesicular monoamine and acetylcholine transport systems depend primarily on ΔpH, GABA transport relies on both ΔpH and $\Delta\psi$, and glutamate transport relies almost exclusively on $\Delta\psi$ (8). Bioenergetic differences between transport systems presumably reflect a combination of differences in substrate charge and the stoichiometry of coupling.

In addition to its role in proton translocation, the membranous V0 domain of the vacuolar H⁺-ATPase has also been implicated in formation of the exocytotic fusion pore. Biochemical studies had identified V0 as the mediatophore, a membrane protein complex that facilitates the release of acetylcholine at the synaptic cleft (9). This finding has been complemented by more recent genetic studies with *Saccharomyces cerevisiae* and *Drosophila melanogaster* that implicate the V0 domain in formation of membrane fusion pores (10,11).

Reuptake of Neurotransmitters Terminates Signaling and Facilitates Recycling

Control of the temporal and spatial patterns of neurotransmitter signaling is most readily achieved by removal of the neurotransmitter from the synaptic cleft. Two mechanisms by which this removal can occur are enzymatic inactivation and reuptake. Although mechanisms for enzymatic inactivation have only been described for some neurotransmitter systems, reuptake is utilized in some form by nearly all neurotransmitter systems. Reuptake of neurotransmitters was first proposed as a mechanism for signal termination in the 1960s. Shortly thereafter, biochemical studies demonstrated that transport activities for nearly all of the putative neurotransmitters share specific characteristics: a high affinity and relative specificity for the neurotransmitter and dependence on the Na⁺ gradient across the plasma membrane (12,13). In the early 1990s, a series of molecular biology studies characterized many of the proteins involved in such transport systems (14).

Rapid reuptake of neurotransmitter from the synaptic cleft is facilitated by the coupling of neurotransmitter transport activities to the large Na⁺ gradient at the plasma membrane generated by the Na⁺/K⁺-ATPase. The electrogenic nature of the transport processes leads to generation of large neurotransmitter gradients across the plasma membrane and thus low resting concentration of neurotransmitter in the synaptic cleft. The rate of clearance is enhanced by the high expression levels of the transporter on the membranes surrounding the synapse—some presynaptic, some postsynaptic, and some glial (15,16). These transport systems also allow for recycling of neurotransmitters—most directly in the case of the presynaptic transporters but also in the case of the glial transporters.

The Monoamines

The monoamines are a class of neurotransmitters derived from aromatic amino acids and defined by the presence of a single amine group attached to the aromatic ring. As a group, monoamines are modulators of central nervous system activity, with major roles in complex aspects of vertebrate brain function including initiation of voluntary movement and mood. They are the principal neurotransmitters in many neuroendocrine systems, and the monoamine norepinephrine is a primary neurotransmitter in the autonomic nervous system. In the central nervous system, monoaminergic neurons are predominantly localized to brainstem nuclei and the hypothalamus.

Monamines are Synthesized from Amino Acid Precursors

The catecholamines (dopamine, norepinephrine, and epinephrine) are a subclass of monoamines derived from tyrosine (Fig. 13.1). Catecholamine synthesis is carried out by a linear set of reactions starting with the addition of a hydroxyl group to the phenyl ring of tyrosine to produce dihydroxyphenylalanine (DOPA) (2). This reaction

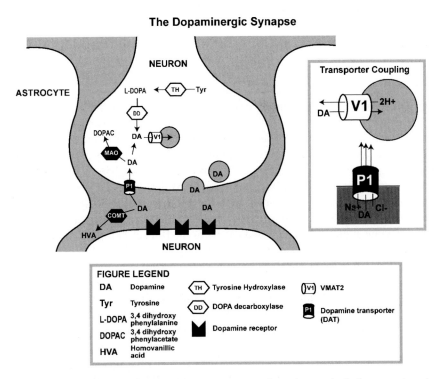

Fig. 13.1 The dopaminergic synapse. The first step in dopamine synthesis from tyrosine, the addition of a hydroxyl group to the phenyl ring of tyrosine to produce dihydroxyphenylalanine (DOPA), is catalyzed by tyrosine hydroxylase and is the rate-limiting step for the synthesis of all catecholamines. DOPA decarboxylase mediates the second step, synthesis of dopamine from DOPA. Dopamine is then packaged into secretory vesicles by the vesicular monoamine transporters (VMATs), which couple the transport of dopamine to the H^+ electrochemical gradient. Once released, the majority of dopamine is taken back up into the presynaptic neuron by perisynaptic Na^+- and Cl^--dependent dopamine transporter DAT. Degradation of dopamine by catechol-O-methyltransferase (COMT) and monoamine oxidase (MAO) A and B are minor mechanism in terminating dopamine signaling

is catalyzed by the cytosolic enzyme tyrosine hydroxylase and is the rate-limiting step for the synthesis of all catecholamines. In a subsequent reaction, DOPA decarboxylase mediates synthesis of dopamine from DOPA. Dopamine can then be converted into norepinephrine by dopamine β-hydroxylase, an enzyme restricted to the lumen of secretory vesicles. The intravesicular localization of dopamine β-hydroxylase suggests that dopamine must be transported into a secretory vesicle before it can be converted into norepinephrine (4). Interestingly, phenylethanolamine-*N*-methyltransferase (PMNT), the enzyme that metabolizes norepinephrine to epinephrine, is cytoplasmic, suggesting that newly synthesized norepinephrine is transported out of secretory vesicles before its conversion into epinephrine (4). For vesicular release, the epinephrine must then be transported back into secretory vesicles. The movement of catecholamines in and out of secretory vesicles throughout these synthetic steps is likely mediated by the vesicular monoamine transporters.

The enzymes involved in monoamine synthesis are restricted to the neurons that produce these neurotransmitters (17). PMNT is most prominently expressed in a small number of brainstem nuclei and the adrenal gland, but has also been detected in the amygdala. Dopamine β-hydroxylase is present in these PMNT-positive neurons as well as the locus ceruleus and additional brainstem nuclei. Finally, tyrosine hydroxylase is present in the epinephrinergic and norepinephrinergic neurons as well as the substantia nigra and ventral tegmentum and arcuate nucleus of the hypothalamus.

While catecholamines are derived from tyrosine, the monoamine serotonin is derived from tryptophan. Like the catecholamines, serotonin is synthesized through a multistep process that involves a rate-limiting enzymatic step mediated by an amino acid hydroxylase (tryptophan hydroxylase) followed by a decarboxylase reaction (mediated by aromatic L-amino-acid oxidase) (2). Expression of tryptophan hydroxylase, which is about 50% homologous to tyrosine hydroxylase, is restricted to cells that release serotonin, specifically the raphe nuclei in the brainstem, the pineal gland, platelets, and enterochromaffin cells (18).

Histamine is also a monoaminergic neurotransmitter. It is derived from histidine in a single-step process catalyzed by the enzyme histidine decarboxylase (2). As a signaling molecule histamine is best characterized in mast cells where it is stored in granules and released to mediate allergic reactions. Histamine is also stored in the enterochromaffin cells of the stomach and released to increase acid secretion from parietal cells. In the brain, histamine is secreted by neurons in the posterior hypothalamus that project to cortical neurons and is involved in wakefulness (19). No reuptake system has been identified for histamine, and it is believed that the primary mechanism for terminating histaminergic signaling is methylation in the extrasynaptic space.

Vesicular Monoamine Transport is Mediated by Two Unique Transporters

Two vesicular monoamine transporters, VMAT1 and VMAT2, have been cloned (20). They are predicted to have 12 transmembrane domains and are structurally related to the bacterial drug resistance transporters. Along with the closely related vesicular acetylcholine transporter (VAChT; see below), they comprise the solute carrier (SLC)18 family of proteins (21). VMAT1 transports dopamine, norepinephrine, epinephrine, and serotonin and is expressed by cells of the adrenal medulla, neurons in sympathetic ganglia, and other nonneural cells that release monoamines. VMAT2 is expressed by neuronal populations in the central nervous system. The substrate specificity for VMAT1 and VMAT2 is similar, and the apparent affinities for the monoamines are in the low micromolar range for both transporters; however, VMAT2 has a slightly higher apparent affinity for all monoamines (22). In addition, only VMAT2 appears able to transport histamine at physiologic concentrations. This is consistent with expression of VMAT2, but not VMAT1, by histamine-releasing mast cells and enterochromaffin cells (23).

Transport by the VMATs involves the exchange of two luminal protons for one singly protonated molecule of transmitter (24). Each cycle of transport thus yields outward movement of one net positive charge. For a vesicular pH gradient of ~1.5 pH units and membrane potential of ~60 mV the predicted intravesicular transmitter concentration is 10^4- to 10^5-fold greater than the cytoplasmic transmitter concentration. This approximation is consistent with the micromolar and near-molar catecholamine concentrations measured in cytosol and vesicles, respectively. Since osmotic forces limit free transmitter concentration to ~150 mM, a fraction of the measured concentration, it has been suggested that formation of macromolecular complexes consisting of a proteinaceous core, ATP, and the catecholamines reduces the effective osmolarity inside the vesicle (4).

Two well-characterized inhibitors act on the VMATs: reserpine and tetrabenazine. Both VMAT isoforms are irreversibly inhibited by reserpine, which appears to interact with the transporters near the site of substrate recognition (24). Reserpine initially showed clinical promise as an antihypertensive medication, but depression was a major side effect and limited its use. Tetrabenazine reversibly inhibits VMAT2 and is markedly less effective as an inhibitor of VMAT1. It has a limited clinical use in the treatment of some movement disorders. Amphetamines and 3,4-methylenedioxy-n-methylamphetamine (MDMA, exstacy) act as weak bases to reduce the vesicular ΔpH (25). Loss of this driving force for the vesicular transporters leads to efflux of the luminal contents into the cytoplasm and subsequent release of neurotransmitter from the neuron through reversal of the plasma membrane transporters. The specificity of their effects (amphetamines lead to dopamine and to a lesser extent norepinephrine release, while MDMA leads to serotonin release) is thought to be due to selective uptake by plasma membrane transporters (see below). The association of polymorphisms in the VMAT1 gene with an increased risk for bipolar disorder supports the link between vesicular monoamine transport and molecular psychopathology suggested by the neuropsychiatric effects of compounds that influence vesicular monoamine transport (26).

A major mechanism for regulation of vesicular monoamine transport appears to involve changes in protein trafficking. VMATs undergo phosphorylation by casein kinase, and this posttranslational modification influences their retrieval from maturing large dense-core vesicles (LDCVs) (27). Since sorting to LDCVs versus synaptic vesicles will determine the site and mode of transmitter release, the regulation of transporter trafficking has great potential to influence signaling. In particular, differential trafficking of VMAT2 in midbrain neurons can lead to release of dopamine from exocytosis at their cell bodies and dendrites if trafficked to LDCVs, or axon terminals if trafficked to synaptic vesicles (28). Regulation of VMAT activity by the heteromeric G protein $G\alpha_{o2}$ has also been demonstrated (29,30). It appears that intraluminal monoamines activate the G protein and downregulate uptake (31). This may be a mechanism to ensure consistency in quantal size and may also serve to limit efflux of neurotransmitter through reverse transport once a vesicle has been filled.

Monoamine Signaling is Terminated by Reuptake and Degradation

The primary mechanism for terminating monoamine signaling appears to be presynaptic reuptake by plasma membrane monoamine transporters, which, coupled with repackaging in secretory vesicles, serves as an efficient mechanism for recycling. In contrast to the vesicular transporters, which are broadly expressed in monoaminergic neurons, unique plasma membrane monoamine transporters are expressed selectively in dopaminergic neurons, noradrenergic neurons, and serotonergic neurons (17). The monoamine transporters are the primary site of action of pharmacologic agents used to depression and drugs of abuse (16). These transporters are part of SLC6, family of Na^+ and Cl^--dependent plasma membrane neurotransmitter transporters that also includes the plasma membrane GABA transporters (GATs) and glycine transporters (GlyTs). SLC6 proteins are predicted to have 12 transmembrane domains, with the amino and carboxy termini residing in the cytoplasm. While these proteins couple neurotransmitter transport to ionic gradients, they also mediate uncoupled conductances (32).

The dopamine transporter DAT and the norepinephrine transporter NET are homologous proteins of 618 and 617 amino acids, respectively (33). While selectively expressed in neurons that release their designated transmitters, both transporters readily recognize both dopamine and norepinephrine with high affinity. NET has submicromolar apparent affinities for both norepinephrine and dopamine, and DAT has low micromolar affinities for these catecholamines. Both transporters couple uptake of substrate with cotransport of Na^+ and Cl^- with a coupling of 1:1:1. Assuming that the monoamine carries a single positive charge, the process will be electrogenic (34).

The dopamine transporter DAT is present in nerve terminals and colocalizes with tyrosine hydroxylase and presynaptic D2 dopamine receptors (17). DAT appears to form a multimeric unit with intermolecular modulation of activity and is subject to regulation through a number of mechanisms. Protein kinase C (PKC) activation leads to downregulation of DAT through internalization. A number of proteins including LIM, PICK1, α-synuclein, Hic5, and the D2 dopamine receptor have been shown to interact with and regulate DAT (16). Alcohol also directly interacts with DAT and increases transport rate. The importance of DAT in clearance of synaptically released dopamine is demonstrated by the 300-fold reduction in rate at which dopamine is removed from the extracellular space in the DAT knockout compared to wild-type mice (35). Not surprisingly, these mice have a number of abnormal behavioral traits including hyperactivity, motor stereotypy, cognitive deficits, and dysregulation of sleep.

Like DAT, NET is regulated by PKC-induced internalization (16). Cell surface expression is also regulated by depolarization and by stimulation of muscarinic receptors and angiotensin II receptors. Direct interactions with the synaptic vesicle proteins syntaxin 1A and α-synuclein have also been implicated in the regulation of NET activity. Similar to findings in the DAT knockout mice, NET knockout mice exhibit elevated extracellular concentrations of norepinephrine (36). These mice also have reduced body weight, tachycardia, elevated blood pressure, and behavioral abnormalities including a blunted response to novel objects and altered responses to antidepressants. Orthostatic intolerance, a human disease characterized by an elevated heart rate without hypotension upon standing, is associated with a mutation leading to substitution of an alanine with a proline at residue 457 (A457P) (37).

The serotonin transporter SERT is a 630-amino-acid protein that is less closely related to DAT or NET than the catecholamine transporters are to each other (16). It is distributed widely in brain and peripheral tissues and is the target of the selective serotonin reuptake inhibitors (SSRIs) as well as other classes of antidepressants. In the brain, SERT is highly expressed on extrasynaptic axonal membranes arising from the raphe nuclei. Like DAT and NET, SERT has a very high apparent affinity (submicromolar) for its substrate. However, serotonin transport appears to require cotransport of 1 Na^+ and 1 Cl^- along with countertransport of 1 K^+ (38). Since serotonin is positively charged, transport is electroneutral. Studies indicate that SERT exists in complex with protein phosphatase 2A and that PKC activation leads to complex dissociation and SERT internalization. Interestingly the PKC effect is inhibited by transporter occupation. SERT interacts with a myristoylated alanine-rich C-kinase–related protein (MacMARCKS), and is also modulated by histamine, adenosine, and 5-hydroxytryptamine 1b (5-HT1b) receptors. As with the other high-affinity plasma membrane monoamine transporter knockout mice, SERT knockout mice have a sixfold higher concentration of extracellular serotonin and a greater than 50% reduction in intracellular levels (39). The mice exhibit signs of increased anxiety and abnormal gastric motility and have a reduced response to MDMA.

Recently a low-affinity plasma membrane monoamine transporter (PMAT) has been identified. The transporter is also known as equilibrative nucleoside transporter 4 (ENT4) and is a member of the SLC29 family of transporters (40). This protein is expressed throughout the brain in neurons (41). It mediates transport of both dopamine and serotonin with apparent affinities of ~0.3 mM and ~0.1 mM, respectively. Affinities for norepinephrine, epinephrine, and histamine are much lower. Organic cation transporter 3 (OCT3) also catalyzes monoamine uptake with similar low affinities, but with a preference for epinephrine and norepinephrine (42). The transport activities of both OCT3 and PMAT are Na^+ and Cl^- independent.

Although reuptake appears to be a predominant mechanism for the termination of monoaminergic signaling, enzymatic inactivation also occurs. The enzymes responsible for these activities, monoamine oxidase and catecholamine-O-methyl-transferase, are the targets for treatment of depression and Parkinson disease. Two isoforms of monoamine oxidase (MAO-A and MAO-B) are expressed in the nervous system (2). These enzymes are encoded by separate genes on the X-chromosome and share structural similarities, but the two isoforms display different preferences for substrates and inhibitors (43). MAO-A preferentially oxidizes serotonin and is inhibited by clorgyline, while MAO-B preferentially oxidizes phenylethanolamine and is specifically inhibited by selegiline. As for localization, MAO-A is expressed predominantly in catecholaminergic neurons with the highest levels in locus ceruleus. MAO-B is present in serotonergic neurons, histaminergic neurons and glia and is expressed at highest levels in the raphe nuclei. Deficiency of MAO-A in males of one family has been associated with aggressive behavior (44).

Catecholamines are also metabolized by catechol-O-methyltransferase (COMT). This enzyme exists in soluble and membrane anchored forms. Although not a primary mediator of catecholamine clearance, COMT may have a significant role in regions such as the prefrontal cortex where dopamine transporter expression is low (45). In humans, polymorphisms in COMT that lead to a reduction in enzymatic activity are associated with an increased sensitivity to pain (46).

Acetylcholine

Acetylcholine (ACh) was first described as a neurotransmitter in the 1920s. In a classic demonstration of chemical signaling between parasympathetic neurons and their target organs, Otto Loewi showed that electrical stimulation of the frog vagus nerve promotes the release of a soluble factor (originally termed "*vagusstoff*" and later identified as ACh) that reduces the heart rate. In recognition of their pioneering work on cholinergic neurotransmission, Loewi and his colleague Sir Henry Hallett Dale were awarded a Nobel Prize in 1936.

Characterized by the ability to synthesize, package, and release ACh, cholinergic neurons (Fig. 13.2) are distributed throughout the mammalian central and peripheral nervous systems. Immunoreactivity to the vesicular acetylcholine transporter (VAChT), a marker of cholinergic neurons, is found in the cerebral cortex, basal forebrain, brainstem, and spinal cord. VAChT immunoreactivity is also observed at presynaptic nerve terminals of motor neurons, preganglionic sympathetic and parasympathetic neurons, and postganglionic parasympathetic neurons (47).

Acetylcholine Synthesis is Mediated by Choline Acetyltransferase

ACh is synthesized in the cytoplasm of cholinergic neurons by choline acetyltransferase (ChAT), an enzyme that was first cloned from *Caenorhabditis elegans* as CHA-1 (48). ChAT generates ACh by catalyzing the transfer of an acetyl group from acetyl coenzyme A (acetyl CoA) to choline (49). Acetyl CoA is produced in cytosol and mitochondria by acetyl CoA synthetase (50), while choline is predominantly supplied by the blood and transported via membrane protein carriers across the blood–brain barrier and the neuronal plasma membrane (51).

The Cholinergic Synapse

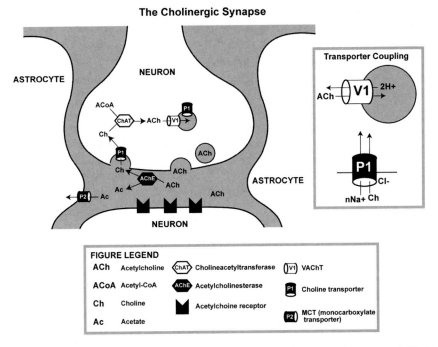

FIGURE LEGEND

ACh	Acetylcholine	ChAT	Cholineacetyltransferase	V1 VAChT
ACoA	Acetyl-CoA	AChE	Acetylcholinesterase	P1 Choline transporter
Ch	Choline		Acetylcholine receptor	
Ac	Acetate			P2 MCT (monocarboxylate transporter)

Fig. 13.2 The cholinergic synapse. Acetylcholine is synthesized from acetyl coenzyme A (CoA) and choline in a single-step reaction catalyzed by choline acetyltransferase. The neurotransmitter is packaged into vesicles by VAChT, the vesicular acetylcholine transporter through an H^+-coupled antiport mechanism. The primary mechanism for signal termination is hydrolysis of acetylcholine to choline and acetate by the synaptic enzyme acetylcholinesterase. Choline is taken up by the presynaptic Na^+-coupled Cl^--dependent choline transporter CHT, and acetate is likely removed from the synapse by glial monocarboxylate transporters. CHT is trafficked to synaptic vesicles and its localization to the plasma membrane is regulated by neuronal activity

The Vesicular Acetylcholine Transporter (VAChT) is Related to the VMATs

After synthesis, ACh is packaged into synaptic vesicles in the presynaptic nerve terminal. Early work indicated that vesicular storage of ACh at the neuromuscular junction (NMJ) is blocked by vesamicol, a compound that causes skeletal muscle paralysis (52). Subsequent studies on isolated synaptic vesicles from the *Torpedo californica* electric organ revealed that vesicular ACh accumulation is dependent on ATP and inhibited by vesamicol. The synaptic vesicle-localized protein that binds vesamicol and transports ACh from the cytoplasm into vesicles was first cloned from *C. elegans* as UNC-17 (53). The homologous vesicular acetylcholine transporter (VAChT) was later identified in the *Torpedo* and mammalian genomes (54).

VAChT is a 12-transmembrane domain protein that couples the influx of one ACh molecule to the efflux of two protons, using the proton electrochemical gradient generated by the vesicular proton ATPase to drive ACh accumulation (55,56). In mammals as in *C. elegans,* the coding sequence for VAChT (unc-17) is nested in the first intron of the ChAT (cha-1) transcript (57,58). Notably, the mature messenger RNA (mRNA) transcripts for both proteins can be generated by alternative splicing of a common precursor mRNA. This genetic organization enables the simultaneous regulation of synthetic and packaging components for cholinergic neurotransmission.

In vitro electrophysiologic studies have demonstrated that quantal size at the neuromuscular junction (NMJ), defined as the amount of ACh packaged and released per synaptic vesicle, may be regulated in several ways. For instance, over-expression of VAChT mRNA in developing *Xenopus* spinal neurons increases quantal size, an effect blocked by the VAChT inhibitor vesamicol (59). In addition, pretreatment with hypertonic solution increases quantal size at the *Xenopus* NMJ, while pretreatment with vesamicol decreases quantal size (60). Finally, Ca^{2+} influx through presynaptic ryanodine receptors at the *C. elegans* NMJ has also been shown to affect quantal size (61).

Hydrolysis of Acetylcholine in the Synaptic Cleft Terminates Signaling

Packaging of ACh into vesicles is followed by two final stages of neurotransmitter processing: release and recycling. Neuronal depolarization induces ACh release by promoting the Ca^{2+}-dependent fusion of ACh-filled synaptic vesicles with the presynaptic nerve terminal (see Chapter 4). ACh that is released into the synaptic cleft may exert downstream effects by binding to specific pre- and postsynaptic receptors. At the *C. elegans* NMJ, ACh signaling can be terminated by direct ACh uptake via the ACh transporter SNF-6 (62) as well as by acetylcholinesterase (AChE), an enzyme that hydrolyzes ACh to acetate and choline in the synaptic cleft. As there are no vertebrate homologues of SNF-6, ACh signaling in mammals is mostly terminated by AChE. The mammalian genome only has one AChE gene, but AChE exists in many different forms as a result of alternative C-terminal splicing, homomeric oligomerization, and heteromeric complex formation (63). The predominant isoform of AChE expressed in the brain and muscle is the "S" or "tailed" subunit, which features a distinct C-terminal peptide capable of tetramerization. At the NMJ, tetramers of AChE-S are anchored to the basal lamina through association with the extracellular matrix protein collagen Q (ColQ) (64). Meanwhile, at both the NMJ and in the brain, tetramers of AChE-S are anchored to pre- and postsynaptic membranes through association with the proline-rich membrane anchor (PRiMA) (65).

After ACh is hydrolyzed in the synaptic cleft, about half of the choline generated through ACh degradation is transported back into the presynaptic terminal and mostly recycled into new ACh. Choline reuptake is mediated by the Na^+/Cl^--dependent, hemicholinium-3-sensitive, high-affinity choline transporter (CHT), a 13-transmembrane-domain protein expressed specifically in cholinergic neurons (66). By protein sequence homology, CHT belongs to the SLC5 family that includes sodium-glucose cotransporters SGLT1-6 (67). Similar to solute transport mediated by other SLC5 proteins, CHT couples the transport of choline to the symport of sodium across the synaptic plasma membrane.

The choline transporter predominantly localizes to cholinergic synaptic vesicle membranes under basal conditions (68). Neuronal stimulation promotes the fusion of synaptic vesicles with the plasma membrane, allowing delivery of CHT to the cell surface (69). Since CHT-mediated choline uptake is the rate-limiting step of ACh synthesis (70), the activity-dependent increase in CHT surface expression provides a mechanism for regulating intracellular ACh levels. Biochemical studies on human CHT expressed in *Xenopus laevis* oocytes show that choline transport and choline-induced currents are pH-dependent with a pKa of 7.4. This finding suggests that CHT is inactive when localized to synaptic vesicles due to the acidic vesicle lumen (pH ~5.5), but becomes activated upon fusion with the plasma membrane and exposure to the extracellular space (pH ~7.5) (71).

At the NMJ, acetate produced from ACh degradation can be taken up and metabolized by muscle (72). In the brain, acetate is primarily transported into astrocytes where it is converted into CO_2 or intermediate metabolites (73). Although a specific acetate transporter has not been described, astrocytic acetate uptake *in vitro* is blocked by α-cyano-4-hydroxycinnamate (CHC), a competitive inhibitor of some proton-coupled monocarboxylate transporters (MCT family) (50). Both MCT1 and MCT4 are expressed by muscle and astrocytes and thus may contribute to acetate uptake.

γ–Aminobutyric Acid (GABA)

Originally isolated from brain as a factor that could inhibit spontaneous discharges at the crayfish stretch receptor, GABA is known to be the primary inhibitory neurotransmitter in the mammalian brain. Like the monoamines, GABA is uniquely expressed in cells that release it as a signaling molecule (74). It is estimated that about 15% of cortical neurons are GABAergic.

GABA is Synthesized from Glutamate

γ–aminobutyric acid is derived from glutamate and present only in cells expressing glutamic acid decarboxylase (GAD), the enzyme that carries out this reaction (Fig. 13.3). The two mammalian isoforms of GAD, GAD-65 and GAD-67, are

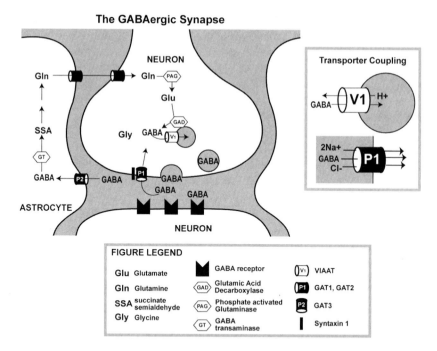

Fig. 13.3 The GABAergic synapse. Glutamic acid decarboxylase GAD mediates the synthesis of γ–aminobutyric acid (GABA) from glutamate. GABA uptake into vesicles occurs by VIAAT, the vesicular inhibitory amino acid transporter. Once released, GABA is taken up by one of the Na^+/Cl^--dependent GABA transporters (GATs). GAT1 is expressed in the presynaptic neuron and is the primary mediator of GABA clearance. It is estimated that one fifth of synaptically released GABA is taken up by the astrocytic GAT3. GABA taken up presynaptically can be repackaged, while GABA transported into astrocytes can be recycled through a glutamine-glutamate shuttle. In mixed GABAergic/glycinergic neurons GABA competes with glycine for transport into vesicles through VIAAT

encoded by separate genes, but typically are coexpressed in GABAergic cells. The isoforms differ in their binding of pyridoxal phosphate (PLP), a cofactor required by both isoforms. GAD67 appears to have one PLP site, while GAD65 appears to have two binding sites with faster association and dissociation rates than the GAD67 binding sites (75). More strikingly, the isoforms have markedly different localizations: GAD67 is localized predominantly in cell bodies, while GAD65 is more closely associated with synaptic vesicles (76). The relative contributions to GABA synthesis are suggested by the phenotypes of GAD65 and GAD67 knockouts; the GAD65 knockout mice have mild behavioral phenotypes and little change in GABA levels, while the GAD67 knockout mice have severe cleft palates leading to early postnatal death and markedly reduced GABA levels in the brain (77,78).

Vesicular GABA and Vesicular Glycine Transport are Mediated by a Single Protein, VIAAT

Early biochemical studies defining vesicular transport systems for GABA were carried out on mixed synaptic vesicles purified from either bovine or rodent brain (79). The molecular identity of the vesicular GABA transporter was determined from a screen for *C. elegans* genes involved in GABAergic synaptic transmission (80). Functional characterization of a vertebrate orthologue of the protein encoded by *unc-47,* a gene identified in the screen, confirmed that the multitransmembrane domain protein mediated vesicular GABA transport. The transporter shows no sequence similarity to VMATs or VAChT. Rather, it belongs to a large family of transporters that includes H^+-coupled amino acid transporters. As predicted from studies with purified synaptic vesicles, the transporter mediates uptake of GABA with an apparent affinity in the low millimolar range and can be driven by ΔpH or $\Delta\Psi$. The transporter also recognizes glycine as a substrate, but with a lower affinity and is thus referred to as the vesicular inhibitory amino acid transporter (VIAAT) (81). VIAAT is expressed in GABAergic and glycinergic neurons as well as islet cells in the pancreas and glial cells of the pineal gland (82). Transport mediated by VIAAT can be competitively inhibited by γ-vinyl GABA, a derivative of GABA used in the clinical treatment of epilepsy.

Recent studies indicate that proper localization of the unc-47 encoded protein in *C. elegans* requires expression of another gene, *unc-46* (83). The protein encoded by *unc-46* is related to LAMPs (lysosomal-associated membrane proteins). A vertebrate homologue is expressed in the developing mouse brain, but its role in targeting VIAAT to synaptic vesicles is unclear. Targeted disruption of the VIAAT gene in mice leads to a marked reduction in synaptic release of GABA and glycine (84). Loss of the transporter leads to embryonic lethality, failure of proper gut development, and formation of a cleft palate. It has been suggested that these defects are secondary to the paralysis that results from loss of inhibitory neurotransmission.

Clearance of GABA from the Synaptic Space is Mediated by a Family of Related Proteins

Once released into the synaptic cleft, GABA is rapidly cleared through the activity of a family of plasma membrane GABA transporters (GATs). The GATs are members of the SLC6 family of transporters that also includes the high-affinity monoamine transporters (16). GAT1 was the first neurotransmitter transporter to be identified on a molecular level and since then three closely related proteins have been identified (85). The rat and human isoforms of these proteins have been designated GAT2, GAT3, and BGT1 with the corresponding mouse isoforms designated mGAT3, mGAT4, and mGAT2. All of the transporters are Na^+ and Cl^- dependent and have a high affinity for GABA with apparent affinities in the low to submicro-molar range with the exception of BGT1.

GAT1 is the predominant GABA transporter in the mammalian central nervous system and is expressed in axons and presynaptic terminals of GABA releasing neurons throughout the brain, spinal cord, and retina (16). There is some suggestion of GAT1 expression in astrocytes surrounding GABAergic synapses as well. The Na^+:Cl^-:GABA stoichiometry for GAT1 transport is 2:1:1, with all ions moving in the same direction. Since GABA is zwitterionic, the process is electrogenic with each transport cycle moving a single net positive charge (86). About half of the protein is on the plasma membrane with the remainder in an intracellular vesicular compartment. Surface GAT1 expression can approach 1000 transporters/μm^2 in some brain regions. Similar to the other SLC6 neurotransmitter transporters, GAT1 plasma membrane expression is downregulated by PKC (16). A number of G-protein–coupled receptors can activate PKC and thus regulate GAT1 surface expression. Conversely, phosphorylation of GAT1 increases surface expression. GAT1 also appears to be regulated through protein–protein interactions. The amino-terminus of GAT1 directly interacts with syntaxin 1A (87). This interaction leads to a reduction in GAT1 transporter activity. Reverse transport through GAT1 has also been implicated in depolarization-dependent nonvesicular release of GABA. Electrophysiologic studies employing GAT1 inhibitors demonstrate that GAT1 activity regulates signaling mediated by both $GABA_A$ and $GABA_B$ receptors. This finding is supported by detailed electrophysiologic studies of GAT1 knockout mice that have determined that extracellular GABA levels are increased leading to altered $GABA_A$ and $GABA_B$ signaling (88).

GAT2 has 52% identity with GAT1. It is expressed in the brain, retina, liver, and kidney. Within the brain, expression is highest in meninges, ependyma, and choroid plexus (16). Faint expression is seen in neurons and glial cells as well. GAT3 shares 52% homology with GAT1 and appears to be expressed exclusively in astrocytes, specifically in distal processes located near GABAergic synapses (89). GAT2 and GAT3 are also downregulated by PKC activation (16). BGT1 shares 54% identity with GAT1. It is expressed pre-dominantly in the kidney and brain, and to a lesser extent in other tissues. BGT1 recognizes both betaine and GABA as substrates and transports with a Na^+:Cl^-:betaine/GABA stoichiometry of 3:2:1 (90). Although BGT has a higher apparent affinity for GABA (20 to 100 µM) than for betaine (200 to 400 µM), the lack of colocalization with GABAergic synapse markers suggests that its primary role may be in betaine transport and associated osmoregulation rather than in GABA reuptake (91).

Once removed from the synapse by the GATs, GABA can undergo degrada-tion through the activity of GABA transaminase. This enzyme is found in glial cells, and to a lesser extent neurons (2,92). In GABAergic neurons the fate of GABA taken up from the synapse is therefore mixed with either repackaging or catabolism as potential paths. GABA taken up into glial cells through the activity of GAT3 is catabolized by GABA transaminase to succinate semialde-hyde, which is further catabolized by succinate semialdehyde dehydrogenase to succinate. The latter in turn can enter the tricarboxylic acid (TCA) cycle and eventually form glutamate (see discussion below on *de novo* synthesis of glutamate in astrocytes) (93).

Glycine

The ubiquitous amino acid glycine is a primary inhibitory neurotransmitter in the vertebrate brainstem and spinal cord and can be co-released with GABA (2,82). Although glycine receptors are not present in the forebrain, *N*-methyl-D-aspartate (NMDA) receptors contain glycine-binding sites that regulate receptor activation, suggesting that release and clearance mechanisms for glycine in the forebrain may regulate excitability in the vertebrate neocortex.

Glycine Synthesis Occurs Ubiquitously, but Vesicular Storage Requires Expression of VIAAT

In the nervous system glycine appears to be synthesized primarily from serine through the activity of serine transhydroxymethylase (Fig. 13.4), a ubiquitously expressed enzyme (2). Similar to GAD, this enzyme requires PLP. Other synthetic pathways for glycine synthesis exist and may contribute, but their relative contributions to synaptically released glycine remain unknown. As mentioned above, glycine is a substrate for VIAAT, which is expressed in glycinergic neurons of the brainstem and spinal cord (82). As an amino acid used in protein synthesis, glycine is present in all cells including GABAergic neurons. Since the affinity of VIAAT for GABA is about 10-fold higher than for glycine, the amount of glycine released from these cells is far less than the amount of GABA. Nonetheless, glycine release from GABAergic cells may provide the glycine that interacts with NMDA receptors in the forebrain.

The Glycine Transporters GlyT1 and GlyT2 Mediate Uptake and Recycling of Glycine

Removal of synaptically released glycine appears to be mediated by GlyT1 and GlyT2 transporters (16). These proteins are structurally related to the monoamine and GABA plasma membrane transporters and are members of the SLC6 family. GlyT1 is expressed throughout the brain, but restricted to glial cells, not neurons. Variable splicing leads to five different isoforms of GlyT1. GlyT1a is expressed in several tissues, while GlyT1b and GlyT1c are nervous system–specific and GlyT1e and GlyT1f are expressed in the retina. The GlyT1 isoforms likely play a role in

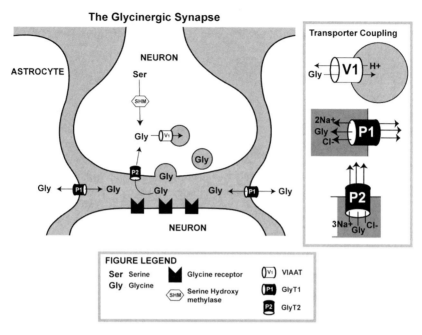

Fig. 13.4 The glycinergic synapse. The inhibitory amino acid glycine is derived primarily from serine through the activity of serine hydroxymethyltransferase, but recycling of released glycine through reuptake by GlyT2 is necessary for sustained release of glycine. VIAAT transports glycine into synaptic vesicles through a process driven by the H^+ electrochemical gradient. Termination of glycine signaling relies primarily on GlyT1, the astrocytic Na^+/Cl^--dependent high-affinity glycine transporter. GlyT1 cotransports glycine with 2 Na^+ and is reversible, while GlyT2 couples glycine transport to 3 Na^+ and is irreversible

uptake of synaptically released glycine, but their role in the forebrain, which lacks glycinergic synapses, is less clear. It has been suggested that it may function to control levels of glycine at glutamatergic synapses containing NMDA receptors. GlyT2 is ~50% homologous to GlyT1 and expressed presynaptically on glycinergic neurons and GABAergic Golgi cells of the cerebellum. There are two GlyT2 isoforms: a functional GlyT2a and a nonfunctional GlyT2b that differ by five amino acids in the N-terminal tail.

Although GlyT1 and GlyT2 have similar apparent affinities for glycine (~25 μM), they differ in their $Na^+:Cl^-:Gly$ stoichiometry; GlyT1 stoichiometry is 2:1:1 and GlyT2 is 3:1:1 (94). Because of the differences in coupling, GlyT2 has a greater driving force from the Na^+ electrochemical gradient and is capable of generating a much larger transmembrane glycine gradient than GlyT1. In addition, GlyT1 is also capable of reverse transport, whereas GlyT2 is not. Similar to the other SLC6 family members, GlyT1 and GlyT2 are downregulated by activators of PKC through reduction in surface expression, and also directly interact with syntaxin 1A, similar to GAT1 (16).

Targeted disruption of the GlyT1 and GlyT2 genes has revealed the relative contributions of the two proteins to glycinergic transmission and NMDA-mediated glutamatergic transmission (95). The GlyT1 knockout is neonatal lethal, but appears to have normal development of glycinergic synapses. Recordings at glycinergic synapses of tissue preparations from these animals demonstrate an increased Cl⁻ conductance at rest, suggesting enhanced glycine receptor activation. Inhibitory postsynaptic potentials also have a prolonged decay in these preparations. These findings suggest that GlyT1 has a major role in removing released glycine from glycinergic synapses. The effect of GlyT1 on glutamate transmission has also been analyzed through studies with the heterozygous mice. Glutamatergic synapses from GlyT1−/+ mice have enhanced NMDA:AMPA (α-amino-3-hydroxy-5-methyl-4-isoxazole propionic acid) ratios compared to wild-type mice, suggesting that GlyT1 normally attenuates NMDA-mediated transmission by clearing glycine from excitatory synapses. The GlyT1−/+ mice also faired better than wild-type littermates in the Morris water maze, indicating that this effect was marked enough to influence NMDA dependent behavior.

GlyT2−/− mice live longer than the GlyT1−/− mice, but are dead by the end of the second postnatal week. Physiologic studies have demonstrated that glycine-dependent inhibitory postsynaptic currents (IPSCs) are reduced in GlyT2−/− mice. This suggests that rather than playing a crucial role in clearing the synapse of glycine, the primary role for GlyT2 is to maintain a readily available supply of glycine in the presynaptic terminal. The GlyT2−/− mice display a phenotype characteristic of severe hyperexplexia (a disease defined by an enhanced startle response). This correlation is strengthened by genetic studies in humans with the disease, which have demonstrated an association between mutations in GlyT2 and hereditary hyperexplexia (96).

Glutamate

The amino acid glutamate was first implicated as a neuroactive substance in the 1950s when Takashi Hayashi described seizures resulting from administration of glutamate directly on exposed cortex in animals, and Curtis, Phillis, and Watkins demonstrated that L-glutamate depolarized and excited neurons in the spinal cord (97,98). It is now clear that glutamate is the primary excitatory neurotransmitter in the vertebrate nervous system (99).

Synaptically Released Glutamate is Derived from Glutamine

Glutamate is present in all cells and can be synthesized from α-ketoglutarate, an intermediate in the TCA cycle (Fig. 13.5). Since neurons lack pyruvate carboxylase, an enzyme that feeds oxaoloacetate into the TCA cycle and permits siphoning off intermediates, they have a relatively low capacity for synthesis of glutamate

The Glutamatergic Synapse

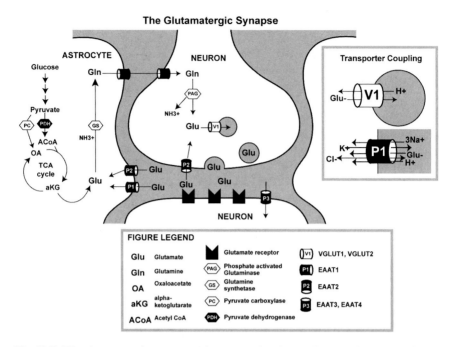

Fig. 13.5 The glutamatergic synapse. After exocytotic release, glutamate in the synaptic cleft is removed predominantly by astrocytic plasma membrane transporters EAAT1 and EAAT2. Postsynaptic uptake via EAAT3 and EAAT4 (in the cerebellum) also occurs to a lesser extent. EAAT2 is expressed on presynaptic membranes, but at low levels. Within astrocytes, glutamate is metabolized to glutamine (gln) by glutamine synthetase (GS). Glutamine is then released from astrocytes, presumably by the astrocytic glutamine transporters SNAT3 and SNAT5 and then taken up by neurons, possibly the SNAT1 and SNAT2. Neuronal glutamine is rapidly metabolized to glutamate by phosphate-activated glutaminase (PAG) and repackaged by the vesicular glutamate transporter. It is estimated that about half of the released glutamate is recycled through this pathway. Glutamate is also synthesized *de novo* in astrocytes from α-ketoglutarate, an intermediate in the tricarboxylic acid (TCA) cycle. The expression of pyruvate carboxylase, which allows for anaplerosis, is restricted to astrocytes in the central nervous system

from this pathway (100). Instead excitatory neurons appear to synthesize glutamate from glutamine, which is readily taken up from the extracellular space where it is present in high concentrations (~0.5 mM) (101). The conversion of glutamine to glutamate is carried out by the enzyme glutaminase. Two isoforms of glutaminase have been characterized—a liver isoform and a renal isoform (102). The glutaminase expressed in the brain is the renal isoform. It is associated with mitochondria and is regulated by phosphate levels. This regulation has led to its designation as phosphate-activated glutaminase (PAG). In addition to regulation by phosphate, brain glutaminase is also inhibited by ammonia, a product of the reaction that the enzyme catalyzes. The role of this enzyme in the synthesis of glutamate in neurons is demonstrated by the marked reduction in glutamate release caused by pharmacologic inhibition of PAG with 6-diazo-5-oxo-L-norleucine (DON).

Vesicular Glutamate Transporters Define Glutamatergic Neurons

Three unique vesicular glutamate transporters (VGLUT1-3) have been identified (103). VGLUT1 was initially isolated in a screen for mRNA transcripts upregulated in cultured neurons by subtoxic doses of NMDA. Structural similarity of this protein to a class of proteins characterized as inorganic phosphate transporters led to an initial impression that the protein was an Na^+-dependent phosphate transporter and to a temporary designation of the protein as brain-specific Na^+-dependent inorganic phosphate transporter (BNPi) (104). Subsequent studies have demonstrated that the primary function of the protein is synaptic vesicle glutamate transport leading to a new name, VGLUT1 (105,106). The role of the protein in phosphate transport remains unclear.

The expression of VGLUT1 is limited to a subset of glutamatergic neurons in the brain. A highly homologous protein (VGLUT2), also initially characterized as a phosphate transporter and named differentiation-associated Na^+-dependent phosphate transporter (DNPi), has a nearly complementary pattern of expression with one of the two proteins present in all established glutamatergic neurons (107,108). In general, VGLUT1 predominates in the neocortex and cerebellar cortex, while VGLUT2 predominates in the brainstem nuclei, thalamic nuclei, and cerebellar deep nuclei. The septal nuclei, nuclei of the diagonal band, and hypothalamus, also express VGLUT2. Although all cortical layers express VGLUT1, layer IV of frontal and parietal cortex and layers IV and VI of temporal cortex also express VGLUT2. Conversely, VGLUT2 predominates in the thalamus, but certain thalamic nuclei such as the medial habenula express VGLUT1. In the hippocampus, dentate gyrus granule cells express only VGLUT1 while pyramidal neurons from CA1 through CA3 express VGLUT1 as well as lower levels of VGLUT2. In the amygdala, the medial and central nuclei express VGLUT2, and the lateral and basolateral nuclei express VGLUT1.

A third vesicular glutamate transporter, VGLUT3 is expressed in neurons not classically considered glutamatergic (109–111). Immunohistochemical and in situ studies indicate VGLUT3 is expressed in GABAergic, serotonergic, dopaminergic, and cholinergic neurons as well as astrocytes. VGLUT1 and VGLUT2 also appear to be expressed in astrocytes but at low levels (112,113).

Although the VGLUTs exhibit similar transport activities, they are expressed in cells with very different properties. For example, compared to VGLUT1-containing neurons, VGLUT2 neurons, in general, have a lower firing rate and a higher probability of release (108). The three isoforms also appear to have different subcellular localizations that could influence glutamate release characteristics. Most notably VGLUT3 is expressed in vesicular structures within dendrites of some neurons in the hippocampus and striatum, suggesting a role in retrograde signaling (109). Further, two polyproline domains, which are present in the C-terminal cytoplasmic tail of VGLUT1 but not VGLUT2 or VGLUT3, mediate interactions with the endocytic protein endophilin. This interaction may regulate synaptic vesicle recycling and the mode of VGLUT1 internalization after synaptic vesicle exocytosis (114).

Recent studies indicate that VGLUT1 and VGLUT2 are present in multiple copies on synaptic vesicles. Correcting for the number of vesicles containing the transporters, it is estimated that there are ~9 and ~14 copies of VGLUT1 and VGLUT2, respectively, in synaptic vesicles in which they are expressed (6). However, in *D. melanogaster* a single copy of the vesicular glutamate transporter per vesicle is sufficient for maintaining synaptic function (115).

Glutamate uptake by the VGLUTs depends primarily on $\Delta\psi$ rather than ΔpH with apparent affinities in the low millimolar range. Interestingly, the VGLUTs do not appear to recognize aspartate (103). This is consistent with studies of synaptic vesicles and suggests that aspartate is not readily accumulated in synaptic vesicles through an active transport system (116). Vesicular glutamate transport shows a biphasic dependence on Cl⁻ with an optimum at 2 to 10 mM, and studies with purified VGLUT2 suggest that glutamate transport requires Cl⁻ (117,118). Like VMAT transport, VGLUT transport also appears to be regulated by $G\alpha_{o2}$. Specifically, $G\alpha_{o2}$ reduces the chloride dependence of transport (31). The role of Cl⁻ in vesicular glutamate transport is further complicated by the finding that expression of VGLUT1 appears to increase the vesicular Cl⁻ conductance (105).

Several compounds that inhibit vesicular glutamate transport have been identified; they include the dyes Evans Blue and Rose Bengal, and the stilbene derivative 4,4′-diisothiocyanatostilbene-2,2′-disulfonic acid (DIDS), a compound commonly used as an inhibitor of anion channels (103). With the exception of Rose Bengal, which is membrane permeant, most known inhibitors have a limited utility as they do not readily cross lipid membranes. No inhibitors unique for specific VGLUT isoforms have been identified.

Clearance of Glutamate is Primarily Mediated by Astrocytic Transporters

The transporters that clear synaptically released glutamate, the EAATs (excitatory amino acid transporters), comprise a group of structurally related proteins, with five different members (EAAT1–5) identified in the mammalian nervous system (15,119). These proteins all couple glutamate uptake to symport of 3 Na⁺ and 1 H⁺ and antiport of 1 K⁺. EAAT1, EAAT2, and EAAT3 are often referred to by the names of the rat isoforms GLAST (*gl*utamate *a*spartate *t*ransporter), GLT (*glu*tamate *t*ransporter), and EAAC1 (excitatory amino acid carrier 1), respectively. The majority of glutamate appears to be cleared by the two astroglial EAATs: EAAT1 and EAAT2. Throughout the forebrain, including the hippocampus, EAAT2 is the major glutamate transporter. Although expressed predominantly on astrocytes, one isoform of EAAT2 (EAAT2a) is also on neuronal presynaptic membranes (120). The relative contribution of the presynaptically localized EAAT2a to clearance of synaptically released glutamate, however, is unclear. EAAT3 is also expressed in the forebrain, but is expressed in neurons and on the cell bodies and dendrites, not on axon terminals. One exception to this is EAAT3 expression in GABAergic presynaptic terminals (15). Reduction in EAAT3 expression leads to a reduction in GABA derived from extracellular glutamate, suggesting that the presynaptic EAAT3 on GABAergic neurons provides glutamate for GABA synthesis. EAAT4 is expressed at highest levels in the postsynaptic dendritic spines of cerebellar Purkinje cells near glutamatergic synapses, but is also expressed at very low levels in the forebrain (15). EAAT5 is expressed exclusively in photoreceptors and bipolar cells of the retina (121).

In addition to mediating glutamate uptake, the EAATs display a glutamate gated anion conductance. This is most prominent in EAAT4 and EAAT5 (122). Although the physiologic significance of the anion conductance is unclear in most cases, the anion conductance appears to be a major mechanism for signaling in the retina. In retinal bipolar cells, activation of the anion conductance of the presynaptic EAAT5 transporters hyperpolarizes the cell (123). The glutamate concentration from spillover to nearby synapses is also high enough to inhibit neighboring bipolar cells, providing a form of lateral inhibition.

Similar to the other reuptake transporters, the EAATs are subjected to regulation. It has been demonstrated that the trafficking and activities of the EAATs can be modulated through posttranslational modifications and interactions with other proteins (124). Signaling through CNTF (ciliary neurotrophic factor) and PDGF (platelet-derived growth factor) appears to increase glycosylation and enhance delivery of EAAT1 and EAAT2 to lipid rafts on the plasma membrane. The proteins GTRAP41 and GTRAP48 have been shown to interact with the carboxy terminal tail of EAAT4 and increase its expression on the cell surface; meanwhile, GTRAP3-18 has been shown to interact with the carboxy terminus of EAAT3 and lower its affinity for glutamate (125,126).

An Intercellular Glutamate-Glutamine Shuttle Facilitates Recycling of Synaptically Released Glutamate

Since the majority of released glutamate is taken up from the synapse by the astroglial EAAT1 and EAAT2, recycling of glutamate is more complex than for other neurotransmitters. It appears that recycling relies on a series of enzymes and transporters that form a glial-neuronal glutamate-glutamine shuttle. The shuttle requires the conversion of glutamate to glutamine in glia and glutamine to glutamate in neurons (102). This is accomplished by the relatively restricted expression of glutamine synthetase (GS) in glia and phosphate activated glutaminase (PAG) in neurons. GS, which amidates glutamate to form glutamine, is expressed at highest levels in the brain, but is also present in the kidney and liver (127). Within the brain, GS is expressed in glial cells and is not present in neurons. Glia are also capable of de novo synthesis of glutamate from glucose. Pyruvate carboxylase, an enzyme expressed in glia, but not neurons, metabolizes pyruvate to oxaloacetate, a TCA cycle intermediate. Entry of this four-carbon intermediate into the TCA cycle leads to an increase in the production of other TCA cycle intermediates, including α-ketoglutarate. Glutamate can be derived from α-ketoglutarate through an amino acid transaminase reaction, converted into glutamine through the activity of GS, and then enter the glutamate-glutamine shuttle. It has been estimated that this *de novo* pathway contributes about half of the glutamate that is released as a neurotransmitter.

The shuttle also requires transfer of glutamine from glia to neurons. A family of transporters that mediate glutamine transport have been implicated in this process (128). These proteins—the system N/A transporters (SNATs)—consist of structurally related transporters that mediate the classically described transport activities designated as system N and system A. Both activities are Na^+ dependent and recognize glutamine as a substrate. The system N proteins (SNAT3 and SNAT5) and the system A transporters (SNAT1, SNAT2, and SNAT4) are related to VGAT, the vesicular GABA transporter. Both the system N and system A transporters are pH sensitive, but the system N transporters also couple glutamine transport to exchange for H^+ (129). Because glutamine has no net charge and the Na^+ and H^+ move in opposite directions, the transporter readily reverses under normal physiologic conditions. The system A transporters, on the other hand, couple amino acid transport only to Na^+ cotransport and are not reversible, but interestingly retain a sensitivity to pH (130–133). The expression of SNAT3 and SNAT5 in glia and the reversibility of these transporters suggest that they have a role in the efflux of glutamine from glia. SNAT1 and SNAT2, which appear to only mediate uptake, are expressed exclusively on glutamatergic and GABAergic neurons. The complementary expression of the system N and system A transporters suggests that they are capable of mediating the directional flow of glutamine from glia to neurons. While the system N transporters are expressed at the perisynaptic spaces (129,134), there is no direct evidence that implicates these proteins in the shuttle. Studies with the system A transporter-specific blocker methylamino isobutyric acid (MeAIB) provide some evidence for SNAT1 or SNAT2 in neuronal glutamine uptake. MeAIB inhibits glutamate-dependent epileptiform activity and the activity-dependent release of GABA, suggesting that system A–dependent glutamine uptake contributes to synthesis of both glutamate and GABA (135–137). However, SNAT1 and SNAT2 are expressed predominantly at the cell body and dendrites (138). This subcellular localization of the SNAT1 and SNAT2 indicates that if there is a perisynaptic glutamate-glutamine shuttle, another transport system may be involved in neuronal uptake of glutamine.

Neuromodulators are Also Stored in Vesicles and Released Through Exocytosis

Synaptic vesicles mediate the release of neuropeptides and small molecules other than classic neurotransmitters. Neuropeptides enter the lumen of the endoplasmic reticulum through cotranslational translocation and are sorted to the secretory vesicle pathway where they undergo processing to form the biologically active species (2). After release, it is believed that neuropeptides are degraded and not repackaged. Of the synaptically released small molecule neuromodulators, zinc and ATP are the best characterized. NMDA and GABA receptors contain binding sites for zinc, and zinc exerts a direct effect on excitatory and inhibitory neurotransmission

(139). ATP activates both ionotropic and G-protein–coupled receptors (140). As with the classic neurotransmitters, the exocytotic release of these compounds requires transport into synaptic vesicles.

The multitransmembrane domain protein ZnT3 has been implicated in zinc uptake by synaptic vesicles. ZnT3 belongs to a family of zinc transporters and localizes to synaptic vesicles (141). Mice deficient in ZnT3 show a loss of zinc staining from hippocampal neurons, and expression of ZnT3 in PC12 cells increases vesicular zinc staining (142,143). Although ZnT3 transport has not been directly demonstrated, these findings strongly support a role for ZnT3 in synaptic vesicle zinc transport. The phenotype of ZnT3-deficient mice is mild, with the most striking abnormality being an increased susceptibility to seizures.

Chromaffin granules, platelet dense-core vesicles, and synaptic vesicles contain concentrations of ATP manyfold higher than cytosolic concentrations, suggesting active vesicular uptake (144). ATP transport has been demonstrated in chromaffin granules and synaptic vesicles, and the process appears to depend on the H^+ electrochemical gradient. It has generally been assumed that ATP is co-stored only with monoamines and acetylcholine, as an anion to balance to the cationic charge of those transmitters. However, the extent of ATP storage and release by different neuronal populations remains unknown, and the proteins responsible for ATP uptake by secretory vesicles have not been identified.

One of the first synaptic vesicle membrane proteins to be identified was SV2. This protein is a multitransmembrane domain protein with limited structural similarity to the VMATs and VAChT. The protein was first identified in *T. californica,* and three isoforms (A, B, and C) have been identified in mammals (145). The expression patterns of the vertebrate proteins show partial overlap and together cover essentially all neurons. Targeted disruption of isoform A and both isoforms A and B demonstrate that these proteins are crucial for normal brain function (146,147). Although a specific biochemical function has not been defined by these studies, it was suggested that SV2 might be involved in regulating the size of the readily releasable pool of vesicles or calcium homeostasis at the nerve terminal. SV2 is thought to be the binding site for botulinum A toxin entry into neurons and to be a binding site for the antiseizure medication levetiracetam (148,149). It has also been suggested that the long sugar chains on SV2 serve as a "smart gel" that regulates the release of neurotransmitters for the fused vesicle by limiting diffusion (150).

Structure of Proteins

Recent work has led to the crystallization of bacterial transmembrane proteins that bear homology to two families of neurotransmitter transporters: the SLC6 family that includes DAT, NET, SERT, the GATs, and GlyT1 and GlyT2; and the EAAT family (Fig. 13.6). Structures derived for these bacterial transporters have confirmed biochemical studies on the mammalian neurotransmitter transporters and advanced our understanding of the structure and function of these proteins.

EXTRACELLULAR

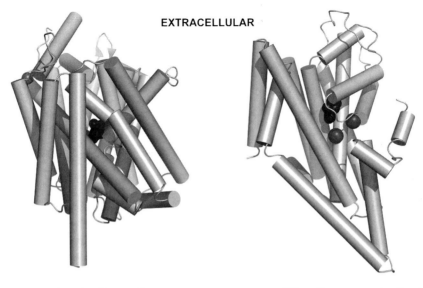

LeuT$_{Aa}$, *Aquifex aeolicus*   Glt$_{Ph}$, *Pyrococcus horikoshii*

Fig. 13.6 High-resolution structures of two bacterial transporters with structural homology to the neurotransmitter transporters. The x-ray crystal structure of the Na$^+$ and Cl$^-$-dependent leucine transporter protein LeuT$_{Aa}$ (left) demonstrates a 12 transmembrane domain structure with a pseudo-twofold symmetry such that the first five transmembrane domains (TM1 to TM5) correspond to TM6 to TM10 with inverted topology. The leucine substrate and two Na$^+$ are directly interacting with nonhelical segments of TM1 and TM6 and a Cl$^-$ ion is present near the extracellular surface of the protein. LeuT$_{Aa}$ has structural similarities to the monoamine, GABA, and glycine plasma membrane transporters. The x-ray crystal structure of Glt$_{Ph}$ (right) demonstrates an extracellular bowl formed by eight transmembrane domains with two hairpin structures that are predicted to partially span the lipid bilayer. Two Na$^+$ and amino acid substrate are evident at the base of the bowl. Glt$_{Ph}$ has structural and functional similarities to the EAAT family of glutamate/aspartate transporters. The structures were obtained from the Research Collaboratory for Structural Bioinformatics (RCSB) Protein Data Bank and rendered with PyMOL software (DeLano Scientific). Helical segments are represented by cylinders and ions and substrate atoms as spheres

The Na$^+$ and Cl$^-$ dependent leucine transporter protein LeuT$_{Aa}$ expressed by the bacterial species *Aquifex aeolicus* has structural similarity to the members of the SLC6 family of transporters. The x-ray crystal structure of LeuT$_{Aa}$ was recently solved to 1.65 Å with a substrate molecule (leucine) and 2 Na$^+$ and 1 Cl$^-$ bound (151). The repeating structure in the crystal is a dimer of a 12-transmembrane domain structure. A pseudo-twofold symmetry was found within the protein structure with the first five transmembrane domains (TM1 to TM5) corresponding to TM6 to TM10 with inverted topology. TM1 and TM6 run antiparallel, and each consists of two α-helices separated by a short segment in the middle of the membranous segment. In the solved structure the leucine substrate and two Na$^+$ are directly interacting with these nonhelical segments.

Glt$_{Ph}$, a bacterial homologue of the EAATs expressed in the bacterial species *Pyrococcus horikoshii,* has also been crystallized and the structure has been solved to 3.5 Å (152). As with LeuT$_{Aa}$, the structure was solved with ions (2 Na$^+$), and substrate (aspartate) present. Consistent with biochemical studies on higher order structures in the EAATs, the repeating structure of Glt$_{Ph}$ is a trimer. The crystal structure demonstrates an extracellular bowl formed by eight transmembrane domains with two hairpin structures that are predicted to partially span the lipid bilayer. These hairpin segments have nonhelical loops that form the binding site for the 2 Na$^+$ and amino acid substrate in a position equivalent to the middle of the membrane. Transport and flux studies have demonstrated that Glt$_{Ph}$ is capable of mediating glutamate and aspartate transport. The parallel to the EAATs extends beyond substrate specificity; DL-threo-É¿-benzyloxy-aspartate (TBOA), a non-transportable blocker of the glutamate transporters, binds to and locks the Glt$_{Ph}$ in a nonfunctioning conformation, and a Glt$_{Ph}$-mediated Cl$^-$ conductance has been identified (153). These similarities indicate that further structure-function analysis of Glt$_{Ph}$ will likely uncover characteristics of the EAATs that will be important in understanding their function and regulation at glutamatergic synapses.

Conclusion

The quantal release of neurotransmitters underlies information transfer in nervous systems in all organisms from invertebrates to humans. This process requires carefully coordinated systems for packaging neurotransmitters into vesicles and for rapidly removing neurotransmitters from the synaptic space to terminate signaling and prevent spillover to neighboring synapses. Transport proteins play crucial roles in regulating neurotransmitter release, reuptake, and recycling, and their regulation is a primary mechanism for modulating signaling. As more information is gathered on the structure and function of these proteins and the mechanisms that regulate them, a more refined understanding of nervous system function and regulation is emerging.

References

1. Fonnum F. Glutamate: a neurotransmitter in mammalian brain. J Neurochem 1984;42:1–11.
2. Cooper J, Bloom F, Roth R. The biochemical basis of neuropharmacology. New York: Oxford University Press, 2003.
3. Katz B. Neural transmitter release: from quantal secretion to exocytosis and beyond. The Fenn Lecture. J Neurocytol 1996;25:677–686.
4. Johnson RG. Accumulation of biological amines into chromaffin granules: a model for hormone and neurotransmitter transport. Physiol Rev 1988;68:232–307.
5. Nishi T, Forgac M. The vacuolar (H+)-ATPases—nature's most versatile proton pumps. Nat Rev Mol Cell Biol 2002;3:94–103.
6. Takamori S, Holt M, Stenius K, et al. Molecular anatomy of a trafficking organelle. Cell 2006;127:831–846.
7. Stobrawa SM, Breiderhoff T, Takamori S, et al. Disruption of ClC-3, a chloride channel expressed on synaptic vesicles, leads to a loss of the hippocampus. Neuron 2001;29:185–196.

8. Maycox PR, Hell JW, Jahn R. Amino acid neurotransmission: spotlight on synaptic vesicles. Trends Neurosci 1990;13:83–87.

9. Israel M, Morel N, Lesbats B, Birman S, Manaranche R. Purification of a presynaptic membrane protein that mediates a calcium-dependent translocation of acetylcholine. Proc Natl Acad Sci U S A 1986;83:9226–9230.

10. Peters C, Bayer MJ, Buhler S, Andersen JS, Mann M, Mayer A. Trans-complex formation by proteolipid channels in the terminal phase of membrane fusion. Nature 2001;409:581–588.

11. Hiesinger PR, Fayyazuddin A, Mehta SQ, et al. The v-ATPase V0 subunit a1 is required for a late step in synaptic vesicle exocytosis in Drosophila. Cell 2005;121:607–620.

12. Logan WJ, Snyder SH. Unique high affinity uptake systems for glycine, glutamic and aspartic acids in central nervous tissue of the rat. Nature 1971;234:297–299.

13. Weil-Malherbe H, Whitby LG, Axelrod J. The uptake of circulating [3H]norepinephrine by the pituitary gland and various areas of the brain. J Neurochem 1961;8:55–64.

14. Amara SG, Arriza JL. Neurotransmitter transporters: three distinct gene families. Curr Biol 1993;3:337–344.

15. Danbolt NC. Glutamate uptake. Prog Neurobiol 2001;65:1–105.

16. Chen NH, Reith ME, Quick MW. Synaptic uptake and beyond: the sodium- and chloride-dependent neurotransmitter transporter family SLC6. Pflugers Arch 2004;447:519–531.

17. Lorang D, Amara SG, Simerly RB. Cell-type-specific expression of catecholamine transporters in the rat brain. J Neurosci 1994;14:4903–4914.

18. Iijima K, Sato M. An immunocytochemical study using the PAP method for tyrosine hydroxylase and serotonin in alternate sections, and in situ hybridization to detect tryptophan hydroxylase mRNA in the rat's locus ceruleus. Acta Histochem 1991;90:159–172.

19. Takahashi K, Lin JS, Sakai K. Neuronal activity of histaminergic tuberomammillary neurons during wake-sleep states in the mouse. J Neurosci 2006;26:10292–10298.

20. Peter D, Liu Y, Sternini C, de Giorgio R, Brecha N, Edwards RH. Differential expression of two vesicular monoamine transporters. J Neurosci 1995;15:6179–6188.

21. Eiden LE, Schafer MK, Weihe E, Schutz B. The vesicular amine transporter family (SLC18): amine/proton antiporters required for vesicular accumulation and regulated exocytotic secretion of monoamines and acetylcholine. Pflugers Arch 2004;447:636–640.

22. Finn JP, Edwards RH. Individual residues contribute to multiple differences in ligand recognition between vesicular monoamine transporters 1 and 2. J Biol Chem 1997;272:16301–16307.

23. Merickel A, Edwards RH. Transport of histamine by vesicular monoamine transporter-2. Neuropharmacology 1995;34:1543–1547.

24. Schuldiner S, Shirvan A, Linial M. Vesicular neurotransmitter transporters: from bacteria to humans. Physiol Rev 1995;75:369–392.

25. Sulzer D, Chen T-K, Lau YY, Kristensen H, Rayport S, Ewing A. Amphetamine redistributes dopamine from synaptic vesicles to the cytosol and promotes reverse transport. J Neurosci 1995;15:4102–4108.

26. Lohoff FW, Dahl JP, Ferraro TN, et al. Variations in the vesicular monoamine transporter 1 gene (VMAT1/SLC18A1) are associated with bipolar i disorder. Neuropsychopharmacology 2006;31:2739–4277.

27. Krantz DE, Peter D, Liu Y, Edwards RH. Phosphorylation of a vesicular monoamine transporter by casein kinase II. J Biol Chem 1997;272:6752–6759.

28. Li H, Waites CL, Staal RG, et al. Sorting of vesicular monoamine transporter 2 to the regulated secretory pathway confers the somatodendritic exocytosis of monoamines. Neuron 2005; 48:619–633.

29. Ahnert-Hilger G, Nurnberg B, Exner T, Schafer T, Jahn R. The heterotrimeric G protein G02 regulates catecholamine uptake by secretory vesicles. EMBO J 1998;17:406–413.

30. Höltje M, von Jagow B, Pahner I, et al. The neuronal monoamine transporter VMAT2 is regulated by the trimeric GTPase Go(2). J Neurosci 2000;20:2131–2141.

31. Brunk I, Holtje M, von Jagow B, et al. Regulation of vesicular monoamine and glutamate transporters by vesicle-associated trimeric G proteins: new jobs for long-known signal transduction molecules. Handb Exp Pharmacol 2006:305–325.

32. DeFelice LJ, Goswami T. Transporters as channels. Annu Rev Physiol 2007;69:87–112.
33. Buck KJ, Amara SG. Chimeric dopamine-norepinephrine transporters delineate structural domains influencing selectivity for catecholamines and 1-methyl-4-phenylpyridinium. Proc Natl Acad Sci U S A 1994;91:12584–12588.
34. Gu H, Wall S, Rudnick G. Ion coupling stoichiometry for the norepinephrine transporter in membrane vesicles from stably transfected cells. J Biol Chem 1996;271:6911–6916.
35. Jones SR, Gainetdinov RR, Hu XT, et al. Loss of autoreceptor functions in mice lacking the dopamine transporter. Nat Neurosci 1999;2:649–655.
36. Xu F, Gainetdinov RR, Wetsel WC, et al. Mice lacking the norepinephrine transporter are supersensitive to psychostimulants. Nat Neurosci 2000;3:465–471.
37. Garland EM, Hahn MK, Ketch TP, et al. Genetic basis of clinical catecholamine disorders. Ann N Y Acad Sci 2002;971:506–514.
38. Mager S, Min C, Henry DJ, et al. Conducting states of a mammalian serotonin transporter. Neuron 1994;12:845–859.
39. Kalueff AV, Fox MA, Gallagher PS, Murphy DL. Hypolocomotion, anxiety and serotonin syndrome-like behavior contribute to the complex phenotype of serotonin transporter knock-out mice. Genes Brain Behav 2007;6:389–400.
40. Engel K, Zhou M, Wang J. Identification and characterization of a novel monoamine transporter in the human brain. J Biol Chem 2004;279:50042–10049.
41. Dahlin A, Xia L, Kong W, Hevner R, Wang J. Expression and immunolocalization of the plasma membrane monoamine transporter in the brain. Neuroscience 2007;146:1193–1211.
42. Amphoux A, Vialou V, Drescher E, et al. Differential pharmacological in vitro properties of organic cation transporters and regional distribution in rat brain. Neuropharmacology 2006;50:941–952.
43. Shih JC, Chen K, Ridd MJ. Monoamine oxidase: from genes to behavior. Annu Rev Neurosci 1999;22:197–217.
44. Vishnivetskaya GB, Skrinskaya JA, Seif I, Popova NK. Effect of MAO A deficiency on different kinds of aggression and social investigation in mice. Aggress Behav 2007;33:1–6.
45. Meyer-Lindenberg A, Kohn PD, Kolachana B, et al. Midbrain dopamine and prefrontal function in humans: interaction and modulation by COMT genotype. Nat Neurosci 2005;8:594–596.
46. Nackley AG, Shabalina SA, Tchivileva IE, et al. Human catechol-O-methyltransferase haplotypes modulate protein expression by altering mRNA secondary structure. Science 2006;314:1930–1933.
47. Weihe E, Tao-Cheng J-H, Schafer MK-H, Erickson JD, Eiden LE. Visualization of the vesicular acetylcholine transporter in cholinergic nerve terminals and its targeting to a specific population of small synaptic vesicles. Proc Natl Acad Sci U S A 1996;93:3547–3552.
48. Alfonso A, Grundahl K, McManus JR, Rand JB. Cloning and characterization of the choline acetyltransferase structural gene (cha-1) from C. elegans. J Neurosci 1994;14:2290–2300.
49. Wu D, Hersch LB. Choline acetyltransferase: celebrating its fiftieth year. J Neurochem 1994;62:1653–1663.
50. Waniewski RA, Martin DL. Astrocytes and synaptosomes transport and metabolize lactate and acetate differently. Neurochem Res 2004;29:209–217.
51. Lockman PR, Allen DD. The transport of choline. Drug Dev Ind Pharm 2002;28:749–771.
52. Parsons SM, Prior C, Marshall IG. Acetylcholine transport, storage and release. Int Rev Neurobiol 1993;35:279–390.
53. Alfonso A, Grundahl K, Duerr JS, Han H-P, Rand JB. The Caenorhabditis elegans unc-17 gene: a putative vesicular acetylcholine transporter. Science 1993;261:617–619.
54. Roghani A, Feldman J, Kohan SA, et al. Molecular cloning of a putative vesicular transporter for acetylcholine. Proc Natl Acad Sci U S A 1994;91:10620–10624.
55. Nguyen ML, Cox GD, Parsons SM. Kinetic parameters for the vesicular acetylcholine transporter: two protons are exchanged for one acetylcholine. Biochemistry 1998;37:13400–13410.

56. Erickson JD, Varoqui H, Schafer MD, et al. Functional identification of a vesicular acetyl-choline transporter and its expression from a "cholinergic" gene locus. J Biol Chem 1994;269:21929–21932.

57. Alfonso A, Grundahl K, McManus JR, Asbury JM, Rand JB. Alternative splicing leads to two cholinergic proteins in Caenorhabditis elegans. J Mol Biol 1994;241:627–630.

58. Bejanin S, Cervini R, Mallet J, Berrard S. A unique gene organization for two cholinergic markers, choline acetyltransferase and a putative vesicular transporter of acetylcholine. J Biol Chem 1994;269:21944–21947.

59. Song H-j, Ming G-l, Fon E, Bellocchio E, Edwards RH, Poo M-m. Expression of a putative vesicular acetylcholine transporter facilitates quantal transmitter packaging. Neuron 1997;18:815–826.

60. Van der Kloot W, Molgo J, Cameron R, Colasante C. Vesicle size and transmitter release at the frog neuromuscular junction when quantal acetylcholine content is increased or decreased. J Physiol 2002;541:385–393.

61. Liu Q, Chen B, Yankova M, et al. Presynaptic ryanodine receptors are required for normal quantal size at the Caenorhabditis elegans neuromuscular junction. J Neurosci 2005;25: 6745–6754.

62. Kim H, Rogers MJ, Richmond JE, McIntire SL. SNF-6 is an acetylcholine transporter interacting with the dystrophin complex in Caenorhabditis elegans. Nature 2004;430:891–896.

63. Massoulie J. The origin of the molecular diversity and functional anchoring of cholineste-rases. Neurosignals 2002;11:130–143.

64. Krejci E, Thomine S, Boschetti N, Legay C, Sketelj J, Massoulie J. The mammalian gene of acetylcholinesterase-associated collagen. J Biol Chem 1997;272:22840–22847.

65. Perrier AL, Massoulie J, Krejci E. PRiMA: the membrane anchor of acetylcholinesterase in the brain. Neuron 2002;33:275–285.

66. Okuda T, Haga T, Kanai Y, Endou H, Ishihara T, Katsura I. Identification and characteriza-tion of the high-affinity choline transporter. Nat Neurosci 2000;3:120–125.

67. Wright EM, Turk E. The sodium/glucose cotransport family SLC5. Pflugers Arch 2004;447:510–518.

68. Ferguson SM, Savchenko V, Apparsundaram S, et al. Vesicular localization and activity-dependent trafficking of presynaptic choline transporters. J Neurosci 2003;23: 9697–9709.

69. Simon JR, Kuhar MG. Impulse-flow regulation of high affinity choline uptake in brain cholinergic nerve terminals. Nature 1975;255:162–163.

70. Haga T. Synthesis and release of (14 C)acetylcholine in synaptosomes. J Neurochem 1971;18:781–798.

71. Iwamoto H, Blakely RD, De Felice LJ. Na+, Cl-, and pH dependence of the human choline transporter (hCHT) in Xenopus oocytes: the proton inactivation hypothesis of hCHT in syn-aptic vesicles. J Neurosci 2006;26:9851–9859.

72. Bertocci LA, Jones JG, Malloy CR, Victor RG, Thomas GD. Oxidation of lactate and acetate in rat skeletal muscle: analysis by 13C-nuclear magnetic resonance spectroscopy. J Appl Physiol 1997;83:32–39.

73. Waniewski RA, Martin DL. Preferential utilization of acetate by astrocytes is attributable to transport. J Neurosci 1998;18:5225–5233.

74. Watanabe M, Maemura K, Kanbara K, Tamayama T, Hayasaki H. GABA and GABA recep-tors in the central nervous system and other organs. Int Rev Cytol 2002;213:1–47.

75. Chen CH, Battaglioli G, Martin DL, Hobart SA, Colon W. Distinctive interactions in the holoenzyme formation for two isoforms of glutamate decarboxylase. Biochim Biophys Acta 2003;1645:63–71.

76. Soghomonian JJ, Martin DL. Two isoforms of glutamate decarboxylase: why? Trends Pharmacol Sci 1998;19:500–505.

77. Kash SF, Johnson RS, Tecott LH, et al. Epilepsy in mice deficient in the 65–kDa isoform of glutamic acid decarboxylase. Proc Natl Acad Sci U S A 1997;94:14060–14065.

78. Condie BG, Bain G, Gottlieb DI, Capecchi MR. Cleft palate in mice with a targeted mutation in the gamma-aminobutyric acid-producing enzyme glutamic acid decarboxylase 67. Proc Natl Acad Sci U S A 1997;94:11451–11455.
79. Hell JW, Maycox PR, Stadler H, Jahn R. Uptake of GABA by rat brain synaptic vesicles isolated by a new procedure. EMBO J 1988;7:3023–3029.
80. McIntire SL, Reimer RJ, Schuske K, Edwards RH, Jorgensen EM. Identification and characterization of the vesicular GABA transporter. Nature 1997;389:870–876.
81. Sagne C, El Mestikawy S, Isambert M-F, et al. Cloning of a functional vesicular GABA and glycine transporter by screening of genome databases. FEBS Lett 1997;417:177–183.
82. Chaudhry FA, Reimer RJ, Bellocchio EE, et al. The vesicular GABA transporter VGAT localizes to synaptic vesicles in sets of glycinergic as well as GABAergic neurons. J Neurosci 1998;18:9733–9750.
83. Schuske K, Palfreyman MT, Watanabe S, Jorgensen EM. UNC-46 is required for trafficking of the vesicular GABA transporter. Nat Neurosci 2007;10:846–853.
84. Wojcik SM, Katsurabayashi S, Guillemin I, et al. A shared vesicular carrier allows synaptic corelease of GABA and glycine. Neuron 2006;50:575–587.
85. Guastella J, Nelson N, Nelson H, et al. Cloning and expression of a rat brain GABA transporter. Science 1990;249:1303–1306.
86. Mager S, Kleinberger-Doron N, Keshet GI, Davidson N, Kanner BI, Lester HA. Ion binding and permeation at the GABA transporter GAT-1. J Neurosci 1996;16:5405–5414.
87. Quick MW. The role of SNARE proteins in trafficking and function of neurotransmitter transporters. Handb Exp Pharmacol 2006:181–196.
88. Jensen K, Chiu CS, Sokolova I, Lester HA, Mody I. GABA transporter-1 (GAT1)-deficient mice: differential tonic activation of GABAA versus GABAB receptors in the hippocampus. J Neurophysiol 2003;90:2690–2701.
89. Itouji A, Sakai N, Tanaka C, Saito N. Neuronal and glial localization of two GABA transporters (GAT1 and GAT3) in the rat cerebellum. Brain Res Mol Brain Res 1996;37:309–316.
90. Matskevitch I, Wagner CA, Stegen C, et al. Functional characterization of the Betaine/gamma-aminobutyric acid transporter BGT-1 expressed in Xenopus oocytes. J Biol Chem 1999;274:16709–16716.
91. Conti F, Minelli A, Melone M. GABA transporters in the mammalian cerebral cortex: localization, development and pathological implications. Brain Res Brain Res Rev 2004;45:196–212.
92. Chan-Palay V, Wu JY, Palay SL. Immunocytochemical localization of gamma-aminobutyric acid transaminase at cellular and ultrastructural levels. Proc Natl Acad Sci U S A 1979;76:2067–2071.
93. Schousboe A. Pharmacological and functional characterization of astrocytic GABA transport: a short review. Neurochem Res 2000;25:1241–1244.
94. Supplisson S, Roux MJ. Why glycine transporters have different stoichiometries. FEBS Lett 2002;529:93–101.
95. Gomeza J, Armsen W, Betz H, Eulenburg V. Lessons from the knocked-out glycine transporters. Handb Exp Pharmacol 2006:457–483.
96. Eulenburg V, Becker K, Gomeza J, Schmitt B, Becker CM, Betz H. Mutations within the human GLYT2 (SLC6A5) gene associated with hyperekplexia. Biochem Biophys Res Commun 2006;348:400–405.
97. Curtis DR, Phillis JW, Watkins JC. The chemical excitation of spinal neurones by certain acidic amino acids. J Physiol 1960;150:656–682.
98. Hayashi T. Effects of sodium glutamate on the nervous system. Keio J Med 1954;3:183–192.
99. Ottersen OP, Storm-Mathisen J. Glutamate. In: Bjorklund A, Hokfelt T, eds. Handbook of chemical neuroanatomy, vol 18. Amsterdam: Elsevier, 2000.
100. Shank RP, Bennett GS, Freytag SO, Campbell GL. Pyruvate carboxylase: an astrocyte-specific enzyme implicated in the replenishment of amino acid neurotransmitter pools. Brain Res 1985;329:364–367.
101. Fishman RA. Cerebrospinal fluid in diseases of the nervous system. Philadelphia: WB Saunders, 1992.

102. Kvamme E. Glutamine and glutamate in mammals. Boca Raton, FL: CRC Press, 1988.
103. Reimer RJ, Edwards RH. Organic anion transport is the primary function of the SLC17/type I phosphate transporter family. Pflugers Arch 2004;447:629–635.
104. Ni B, Rosteck PR, Nadi NS, Paul SM. Cloning and expression of a cDNA encoding a brain-specific Na+-dependent inorganic phosphate cotransporter. Proc Natl Acad Sci U S A 1994;91:5607–5611.
105. Bellocchio EE, Reimer RJ, Fremeau RT, Jr., Edwards RH. Uptake of glutamate into synaptic vesicles by an inorganic phosphate transporter. Science 2000;289:957–960.
106. Takamori S, Rhee JS, Rosenmund C, Jahn R. Identification of a vesicular glutamate transporter that defines a glutamatergic phenotype in neurons. Nature 2000;407:189–194.
107. Takamori S, Rhee JS, Rosenmund C, Jahn R. Identification of differentiation-associated brain-specific phosphate transporter as a second vesicular glutamate transporter (VGLUT2). J Neurosci 2001;21:RC182.
108. Fremeau RT, Troyer MD, Pahner I, et al. The expression of vesicular glutamate transporters defines two classes of excitatory synapse. Neuron 2001;31:247–260.
109. Fremeau RT, Jr., Burman J, Qureshi T, et al. The identification of vesicular glutamate transporter 3 suggests novel modes of signaling by glutamate. Proc Natl Acad Sci U S A 2002;99:14488–14493.
110. Gras C, Herzog E, Bellenchi GC, et al. A third vesicular glutamate transporter expressed by cholinergic and serotoninergic neurons. J Neurosci 2002;22:5442–5451.
111. Schafer MK, Varoqui H, Defamie N, Weihe E, Erickson JD. Molecular cloning and functional identification of mouse vesicular glutamate transporter 3 and its expression in subsets of novel excitatory neurons. J Biol Chem 2002;277:50734–50748.
112. Bezzi P, Gundersen V, Galbete JL, et al. Astrocytes contain a vesicular compartment that is competent for regulated exocytosis of glutamate. Nat Neurosci 2004;7:613–620.
113. Jourdain P, Bergersen LH, Bhaukaurally K, et al. Glutamate exocytosis from astrocytes controls synaptic strength. Nat Neurosci 2007;10:331–339.
114. Voglmaier SM, Kam K, Yang H, et al. Distinct endocytic pathways control the rate and extent of synaptic vesicle protein recycling. Neuron 2006;51:71–84.
115. Daniels RW, Collins CA, Chen K, Gelfand MV, Featherstone DE, DiAntonio A. A single vesicular glutamate transporter is sufficient to fill a synaptic vesicle. Neuron 2006;49:11–16.
116. Maycox PR, Deckwerth T, Hell JW, Jahn R. Glutamate uptake by brain synaptic vesicles. Energy dependence of transport and functional reconstitution in proteoliposomes. J Biol Chem 1988;263:15423–15428.
117. Jahn R, Hell J, Maycox PR. Synaptic vesicles: key organelles involved in neurotransmission. J Physiol (Paris) 1990;84:128–133.
118. Juge N, Yoshida Y, Yatsushiro S, Omote H, Moriyama Y. Vesicular glutamate transporter contains two independent transport machineries. J Biol Chem 2006;281:39499–39506.
119. Krantz DE, Chaudhry FA, Edwards RH. Neurotransmitter transporters. In: Bellen HJ, ed. Neurotransmitter release. Oxford: Oxford Press, 1999:145–207.
120. Chen W, Mahadomrongkul V, Berger UV, et al. The glutamate transporter GLT1a is expressed in excitatory axon terminals of mature hippocampal neurons. J Neurosci 2004; 24:1136–1148.
121. Fairman WA, Vandenberg RJ, Arriza JL, Kavanaugh MP, Amara SG. An excitatory amino-acid transporter with properties of a ligand-gated chloride channel. Nature 1995;375:599–603.
122. Wadiche JI, Amara SG, Kavanaugh MP. Ion fluxes associated with excitatory amino acid transport. Neuron 1995;15:721–728.
123. Veruki ML, Morkve SH, Hartveit E. Activation of a presynaptic glutamate transporter regulates synaptic transmission through electrical signaling. Nat Neurosci 2006;9:1388–1396.
124. Torres GE, Amara SG. Glutamate and monoamine transporters: new visions of form and function. Curr Opin Neurobiol 2007;17:304–312.
125. Jackson M, Song W, Liu MY, et al. Modulation of the neuronal glutamate transporter EAAT4 by two interacting proteins. Nature 2001;410:89–93.
126. Lin CI, Orlov I, Ruggiero AM, et al. Modulation of the neuronal glutamate transporter EAAC1 by the interacting protein GTRAP3-18. Nature 2001;410:84–88.

127. Mearow KM, Mill JF, Vitkovic L. The ontogeny and localization of glutamine synthetase gene expression in rat brain. Brain Res Mol Brain Res 1989;6:223–232.

128. Chaudhry FA, Reimer RJ, Edwards RH. The glutamine commute: take the N line and transfer to the A. J Cell Biol 2002;157:349–355.

129. Chaudhry FA, Reimer RJ, Krizaj D, et al. Molecular analysis of system N suggests novel physiological roles in nitrogen metabolism and synaptic transmission. Cell 1999;99:769–780.

130. Reimer RJ, Chaudhry FA, Gray AT, Edwards RH. Amino acid transport System A resembles System N in sequence but differs in mechanism. Proc Natl Acad Sci U S A 2000;97:7715–7720.

131. Chaudhry FA, Krizaj D, Larsson P, et al. Coupled and uncoupled proton movement by amino acid transport system N. EMBO J 2001;20:7041–7051.

132. Chaudhry FA, Schmitz D, Reimer RJ, et al. Glutamine uptake by neurons: interaction of protons with system a transporters. J Neurosci 2002;22:62–72.

133. Albers A, Broer A, Wagner CA, et al. Na+ transport by the neural glutamine transporter ATA1. Pflugers Arch 2001;443:92–101.

134. Cubelos B, Gonzalez-Gonzalez IM, Gimenez C, Zafra F. Amino acid transporter SNAT5 localizes to glial cells in the rat brain. Glia 2005;49:230–244.

135. Tani H, Bandrowski A, Parada I, et al. Modulation of epileptiform activity by glutamine and system A transport in a model of post-traumatic epilepsy. Neurobiol Dis 2007;25(2):230–238.

136. Liang SL, Carlson GC, Coulter DA. Dynamic regulation of synaptic GABA release by the glutamate-glutamine cycle in hippocampal area CA1. J Neurosci 2006;26:8537–8548.

137. Fricke MN, Jones-Davis DM, Mathews GC. Glutamine uptake by System A transporters maintains neurotransmitter GABA synthesis and inhibitory synaptic transmission. J Neurochem 2007;102(6):1895–1904.

138. Conti F, Melone M. The glutamine commute: lost in the tube? Neurochem Int 2006; 48:459–464.

139. Li YV, Hough CJ, Sarvey JM. Do we need zinc to think? Sci STKE 2003;2003:pe19.

140. Burnstock G. Purinergic signalling. Br J Pharmacol 2006;147(suppl 1):S172–181.

141. Palmiter RD, Cole TB, Quaife CJ, Findley SD. ZnT-3, a putative transporter of zinc into synaptic vesicles. Proc Natl Acad Sci U S A 1996;93:14934–14939.

142. Cole TB, Wenzel HJ, Kafer KE, Schwartzkroin PA, Palmiter RD. Elimination of zinc from synaptic vesicles in the intact mouse brain by disruption of the ZnT3 gene. Proc Natl Acad Sci U S A 1999;96:1716–1721.

143. Salazar G, Craige B, Love R, Kalman D, Faundez V. Vglut1 and ZnT3 co-targeting mechanisms regulate vesicular zinc stores in PC12 cells. J Cell Sci 2005;118:1911–1921.

144. Zimmermann H. Signalling via ATP in the nervous system. Trends Neurosci 1994; 17:420–426.

145. Bajjalieh SM, Frantz GD, Weimann JM, McConnell SK, Scheller RH. Differential expression of synaptic vesicle protein 2 (SV2) isoforms. J Neurosci 1994;14:5223–5235.

146. Crowder KM, Gunther JM, Jones TA, et al. Abnormal neurotransmission in mice lacking synaptic vesicle protein 2A (SV2A). Proc Natl Acad Sci U S A 1999;96:15268–15273.

147. Janz R, Goda Y, Geppert M, Missler M, Sudhof TC. SV2A and SV2B function as redundant Ca2+ regulators in neurotransmitter release. Neuron 1999;24:1003–1016.

148. Lynch BA, Lambeng N, Nocka K, et al. The synaptic vesicle protein SV2A is the binding site for the antiepileptic drug levetiracetam. Proc Natl Acad Sci U S A 2004;101:9861–9866.

149. Dong M, Yeh F, Tepp WH, et al. SV2 is the protein receptor for botulinum neurotoxin A. Science 2006;312:592–596.

150. Reigada D, Diez-Perez I, Gorostiza P, et al. Control of neurotransmitter release by an internal gel matrix in synaptic vesicles. Proc Natl Acad Sci U S A 2003;100:3485–3490.

151. Yamashita A, Singh SK, Kawate T, Jin Y, Gouaux E. Crystal structure of a bacterial homologue of Na+/Cl—dependent neurotransmitter transporters. Nature 2005;437:215–223.

152. Boudker O, Ryan RM, Yernool D, Shimamoto K, Gouaux E. Coupling substrate and ion binding to extracellular gate of a sodium-dependent aspartate transporter. Nature 2007;445: 387–393.

153. Ryan RM, Mindell JA. The uncoupled chloride conductance of a bacterial glutamate transporter homolog. Nat Struct Mol Biol 2007;14:365–371.

Chapter 14
Regulation of Neurotransmitter Release by Presynaptic Receptors

Matthew Frerking and Joyce Wondolowski

Contents

Abstract The release of neurotransmitter is subject to powerful modulatory control by receptors located in or near the presynaptic terminal. These presynaptic receptors are a diverse group of proteins, but they can be broadly divided into two classes: metabotropic receptors and ionotropic receptors. Most metabotropic receptors are coupled to G proteins and inhibit release by an interaction between G protein $\beta\gamma$-subunits and calcium channels; in contrast, ionotropic receptors affect release mainly by changing the presynaptic membrane potential. Accumulating evidence suggests that ionotropic receptors may also engage metabotropic cascades under some conditions. Presynaptic receptors can functionally reshape neural circuits by rapidly and reversibly changing the properties of synaptic transmission, and the specific expression of different receptors at different synapses allows each receptor subtype to have a distinct effect on neural processing.

Keywords Presynaptic receptors, transmitter release, ionotropic receptors, metabotropic receptors, neuromodulation.

Matthew Frerking
Neurological Sciences Institute, Oregon Health & Sciences University, Beaverton, OR, USA
e-mail: frerking@ohsu.edu

Up to this point, much of the focus of this book has been on mechanisms directly involved in the packaging, trafficking, and release of presynaptic vesicles containing neurotransmitters. This chapter changes focus somewhat and provides a broad overview of how neurochemical cues can modulate transmitter release, via activation of presynaptic receptors that regulate the release properties of the synapse. This chapter is unavoidably an incomplete exploration of this vast topic; we refer the interested reader to several topical reviews for additional information (1–11).

Presynaptic Receptors: Subtypes and Structure

Essentially all synapses express multiple distinct presynaptic receptors that can affect transmitter release; the substances to which these receptors bind range from classic neurotransmitters to neuropeptides, growth factors, lipids, and even recognition proteins on the postsynaptic cell. The receptors for these various ligands can be broadly divided into two major classes according to the mechanism by which they signal in response to ligand binding: metabotropic receptors, which couple to intracellular signaling cascades, and ionotropic receptors, which are ligand gated ion channels.

Metabotropic Receptors

The activation of metabotropic signaling cascades in the presynaptic terminal is perhaps the most common form of neuromodulation. G-protein–coupled receptors (GPCRs) are by far the most widespread and diverse class of presynaptic receptors. Other metabotropic receptors, most notably receptor-coupled kinases and phosphatases, have also been implicated in the acute regulation of neurotransmitter release. However, much less is known about these other metabotropic pathways with respect to presynaptic function.

The generic structure of GPCRs is defined by a canonical pattern of seven transmembrane α-helices. A range of pharmacologic, biochemical, and genetic approaches have identified several hundred GPCRs. This diversity is reflected in the extraordinary range of signals to which different GPCRs respond, including classical neurotransmitters, peptides, lipids, and ions (12). Ligand binding to the GPCR induces a conformational change in the receptor, which promotes the exchange of guanosine triphosphate (GTP) with guanosine diphosphate (GDP) that is bound to the α subunit of heterotrimeric G proteins. The binding of GTP enables dissociation of the α subunit from the β and γ subunits. Both the α-GTP and $\beta\gamma$ subunits are involved in the subsequent activation of a number of intracellular signaling cascades. GPCRs can also activate signaling cascades independent of G-protein activation, through mechanisms that remain poorly understood (13).

The superfamily of GPCRs can be divided into several classes, three of which are relevant to presynaptic neuromodulation (class A to C receptors) (14). Class

A receptors represent the overwhelming majority of GPCRs, including those that bind to most neuropeptides, lipid messengers, and neurotransmitters. Class B receptors are a small but structurally distinct group of receptors for selected peptides, such as calcitonin and corticotrophin-releasing factor (CRF). Class C receptors respond mainly to amino acids, with the most prominent members of the family being metabotropic glutamate receptors (mGluRs) and GABA$_B$ receptors (GABA$_B$Rs).

For many years, it was thought that GPCRs function as monomers, but this viewpoint has slowly been replaced by a more complex picture in which many GPCRs form oligomers—typically thought to be dimers—as a critical aspect of assembly and function (15). This finding was initially controversial, as many of the early reports on GPCR oligomerization were reported in heterologous systems. However, with the cloning of class C receptors, it was found that GABA$_B$Rs *must* form dimers (16,17). Subsequent studies reported several class A receptors that form dimers, including melatonin receptors, α- and β-adrenoceptors, and opioid receptors (18). At least some class B receptors also form obligatory multimers, although in this case the complex is a heterodimer in which the two components are unrelated. In these receptors, the ligand specificity is determined not only by a conventional GPCR subunit, but also by a family of accessory proteins known as receptor activity modifying proteins (RAMPs) (19). Thus, the same GPCR subunit contributes to signaling mediated by calcitonin, amylin, and calcitonin gene–related peptide (CGRP); the distinct receptors that distinguish between these ligands are defined by the incorporation of a particular RAMP into the receptor complex.

The dimerization of GPCRs has some interesting implications for GPCR function, one of which is that the individual subunits within the dimer need not be identical in their affinities for agonists, their specificity for G-protein coupling, or their association with accessory proteins that control subcellular localization, surface expression, or desensitization. This link between heteromeric composition and GPCR function is particularly pronounced for the interaction between class B receptors and RAMPs, as described above. Another way in which the heteromeric composition of GPCRs has proven to be important is in GPCR localization. Only two GABA$_B$R subunits (GABA$_B$R1 and GABA$_B$R2) have been described so far, and a functional GABA$_B$R must have both of them. However, the GABA$_B$R1 subunit has two splice variants (GABA$_B$R1a and GABA$_B$R1b), which determine specific subcellular localization of GABA$_B$Rs. Receptors containing the GABA$_B$R1a subunit are localized to the presynaptic terminal, while those containing the GABA$_B$R1b subunit are restricted to the somatodendritic region (20).

Thus, a particularly striking feature of GPCRs is their diversity, which comes not only from genetic distinctions between different receptor subtypes but also from the subtype-specific assembly of multimeric receptor complexes. However, the diversity in receptor types is not matched by a comparable diversity in the mechanisms by which GPCRs affect release, which occurs mainly through inhibition of presynaptic calcium channels, mediated by the βγ subunit of heterotrimeric G proteins (8). We will consider this surprising finding in greater detail below (see Presynaptic Inhibition).

Ionotropic Receptors

While it is clear that most presynaptic receptors are metabotropic, it is noteworthy that an ionotropic form of presynaptic inhibition, mediated by ionotropic $GABA_A$ receptors ($GABA_A$Rs), was the first identified form of presynaptic neuromodulation in the central nervous system (CNS) (6,21). It is generally difficult to study presynaptic ionotropic receptors directly because the presynaptic terminal is usually too small for electrophysiologic analyses, although there are a few exceptions (e.g., the calyx of Held, mossy fiber synapses of the hippocampus, and retinal bipolar cell terminals of the goldfish). Nevertheless, a large body of evidence implicates ionotropic receptors as modulators of transmitter release, both in the systems where presynaptic recordings can directly demonstrate this form of regulation and in the systems where the evidence is obtained indirectly by examining synaptic output.

Ligand-Gated Anion Channels

The inhibitory neurotransmitters GABA and glycine both activate chloride channels, and both GABARs and glycine receptors (GlyRs) have been found to act as presynaptic receptors in a number of systems, in addition to their more conventional postsynaptic contribution to inhibitory postsynaptic potentials (IPSPs). $GABA_A$R-mediated presynaptic currents have been observed in amacrine cells in culture (22) and mossy fiber boutons in situ, directly confirming their responsiveness to synaptically released GABA (23). Both immunohistologic and pharmacologic evidence suggests that presynaptic $GABA_A$Rs at mossy fiber synapses contain the $\alpha2$-subunit (23,24).

Presynaptic $GABA_A$Rs located on group I and II afferents inhibit glutamate release onto spinal motoneurons (6); they also inhibit transmitter release at the crayfish neuromuscular junction (25), neuropeptide release from pituitary terminals (26,27), and transmitter release from mossy fiber boutons (24). Presynaptic $GABA_C$Rs also tonically inhibit transmission from bipolar cells to ganglion or amacrine cells in the retina, via ambient GABA levels that are regulated by GABA uptake (28). However, not all actions of presynaptic GABARs are inhibitory. Early in development, $GABA_A$Rs enhance action potential-evoked release at the calyx of Held (29). Presynaptic $GABA_A$Rs also enhance the spontaneous quantal release of glycine in early postnatal rat dorsal horn neurons, although they inhibit release evoked by presynaptic spikes (30).

Although transmission at the calyx of Held is controlled by presynaptic $GABA_A$Rs early in development, the $GABA_A$Rs are replaced by GlyRs, which are also known to increase the frequency of spontaneous glutamate release (31). Presynaptic GlyRs also enhance GABA release in the ventral tegmental area of early postnatal rats, when GABAergic transmission onto dopamine (DA) cells is excitatory. When the intracellular chloride concentration shifts with development, the GABAergic response of DA neurons reverses polarity and becomes inhibitory; however, the polarity of flux through the presynaptic GlyRs also switches, and they switch from enhancing GABA release to inhibiting it. As a result, these GlyRs retain an excitatory effect on DA neurons over development (32).

Ligand-Gated Cation Channels

There are several ligand-gated cation channels that regulate transmitter release at various synapses in the CNS, including nicotinic acetylcholine receptors (nAChRs), purinergic P_{2X} receptors, 5-hydroxytryptamine-3 (5-HT$_3$) receptors, and ionotropic glutamate receptors (1). Here, we focus on nAChRs and ionotropic glutamate receptors, as these have been studied most extensively.

Nicotinic acetylcholine receptors (nAChRs) are found at presynaptic terminals throughout the CNS and peripheral nervous system (PNS), as demonstrated definitively using light and electron microscopy (25,33). Radiolabeled nAChR ligands and immunolabeling have shown localization of nAChRs along the length of the axon as well as anterograde transport of the receptors to the terminals. Physiologically, presynaptic nAChRs act as autoreceptors to enhance cholinergic transmission throughout the PNS and CNS. Many studies suggest the existence of multiple presynaptic receptors, with subunit compositions that are distinct from each other and from postsynaptic nAChRs (34). Presynaptic nAChRs are involved in heterosynaptic modulation of transmitter release as well, and enhance release of glutamate, dopamine, GABA, serotonin, and norepinephrine. These presynaptic nAChRs are located throughout several brain regions; notably, presynaptic nAChRs in the striatum enhance the release of dopamine, and may contribute to the addictive properties of nicotine.

The ionotropic glutamate receptors (iGluRs) can also regulate transmitter release, and distinct properties have been attributed to each of the iGluR subclasses: α-amino-3-hydroxy-5-methyl-4-isoxazole propionic acid (AMPA) receptors (AMPARs), N-methyl-D-aspartate (NMDA) receptors (NMDARs), and kainate receptors (KARs) (9). Presynaptic AMPARs inhibit glutamate release from the calyx of Held (35) and GABA release from stellate cells in the cerebellum (36); however, they have also been reported to facilitate transmitter release at reciprocal dendrodendritic synapses in the retina (37). There are several mechanisms by which the same ionotropic receptor might cause opposite effects at distinct synapses, and we will consider these in greater detail below (see Ionotropic Receptors).

Presynaptic NMDARs have also been found at several synapses. These receptors might be expected to directly induce transmitter release upon activation, because they act as a direct route of influx for presynaptic calcium; however, NMDAR channel opening requires a significant depolarization as well as glutamate, suggesting that these receptors will be active only under relatively specific circumstances. NMDAR subunit expression has been shown in mossy fiber terminals synapsing onto CA3 pyramidal cells and dorsal root ganglion (DRG) nerve terminals. Presynaptic NMDARs have also been shown to enhance release of dopamine in the striatum, norepinephrine in the cortex, and substance P in the spinal cord (9). An increasing body of evidence suggests that presynaptic NMDARs may play a role in long-term plasticity as well (38).

These studies implicate both AMPARs and NMDARs as presynaptic neuromodulators as well as direct mediators of the postsynaptic response; however, most experiments on presynaptic iGluRs have so far centered on KARs. Unlike the nearly ubiquitous involvement of AMPARs and NMDARs in postsynaptic reception, KARs contribute to excitatory postsynaptic currents (EPSCs) at only selected populations of glutamatergic synapses (5). However, KARs are expressed throughout the CNS, which raises the intriguing possibility that regulation of transmitter release might be their primary function. KARs were first found to inhibit glutamate release at Schaffer collateral synapses onto CA1 neurons (39), and subsequent studies have found a similar inhibition of release from a wide range of both excitatory and inhibitory synapses throughout the CNS (40). However, studies at mossy fiber synapses in the hippocampus have suggested a more complex effect, with low concentrations of KAR agonists facilitating release but higher concentrations depressing it (4). This bidirectional modulation has since been found at several synapses, and may be a consequence of presynaptic depolarization (see below).

Mechanisms of Regulating Transmitter Release

The preceding discussion provided an overview of the types of receptors that can modulate release; we now turn our attention to the mechanisms by which this modulation occurs.

Metabotropic Receptors

Given the great diversity of receptor subtypes and the coupling to many distinct effectors, one might expect a wide variety of mechanisms by which GPCRs regulate transmitter release. Surprisingly, the majority of GPCRs express their acute effects on synaptic transmission through a single general mechanism: the inhibition of presynaptic calcium channels by the heterotrimeric G-protein $\beta\gamma$ subunits following dissociation of the α-GTP subunit (41). We will consider some exceptions to this below (see Presynaptic Facilitation), but it should be kept in mind that GPCR-mediated facilitation is considerably less common than inhibition.

Presynaptic Inhibition

Early studies of transmitter release considered several possible mechanisms by which activation of presynaptic biochemical cascades might alter transmitter release; obvious possibilities include effects on presynaptic membrane potential, action potential waveform, calcium influx, or exocytotic mechanisms. The advent of calcium imaging, coupled with electrophysiologic recording, soon revealed that by far the most common mechanism for regulating transmitter release is the metabotropic downregulation of calcium influx. Calcium currents are subject to regulation by G-protein $\beta\gamma$ subunits, which slow the activation of calcium channels in response to depolarization

(8). This kinetic slowing of calcium currents is sufficient to substantially reduce calcium influx in response to the transient depolarization caused by action potentials. The $\beta\gamma$-dependence of this effect also provides an explanation for why several GPCRs cause mutually occlusive inhibition (42); the vast array of GPCRs converge onto a small number of $\beta\gamma$ subunits to mediate presynaptic inhibition.

A quantitative comparison of the inhibition of calcium currents and the inhibition of transmitter release indicates that most, and in some cases all, of the presynaptic inhibition mediated by GPCRs can be explained by effects on calcium channels (42). Three calcium channels contribute to transmitter release in most systems: $Ca_v2.1$, $Ca_v2.2$, and $Ca_v2.3$. Inhibition by the G-protein $\beta\gamma$ subunits is most pronounced for $Ca_v2.2$ (43,44), but $Ca_v2.1$ and $Ca_v2.3$ are also subject to G-protein–mediated inhibition and contribute to the GPCR-mediated presynaptic inhibition.

An alternative mechanism for presynaptic inhibition that had some early experimental support was the modulation of potassium channels by $\beta\gamma$ subunits. Consistent with this, GPCR-mediated postsynaptic inhibition occurs via the $\beta\gamma$-dependent activation of G-protein–activated inwardly rectifying potassium (GIRK) channels. However, genetic ablation of GIRK channels abolishes postsynaptic inhibition without affecting presynaptic inhibition. This argues strongly against a major role for GIRKs in presynaptic inhibition (45), but it remains possible that other potassium channels play a minor role in GPCR-mediated presynaptic inhibition.

Another alternative mechanism for presynaptic inhibition is a direct, biochemical modification of the exocytotic machinery as a result of GPCR-mediated signaling cascades. A key finding that supports this model is that many GPCRs inhibit the frequency of miniature postsynaptic responses that are produced by the spontaneous fusion of individual vesicles with the plasma membrane (46). These "minis" occur even when the pore of voltage-gated calcium channels is blocked; thus, a decrease in mini frequency is difficult to explain in terms of decreased calcium channel function.

An intriguing set of recent experiments suggests that this distinction between calcium channel function and spontaneous exocytosis may not be clear-cut, however. G-protein $\beta\gamma$ subunits bind not only to calcium channels but also to components of the exocytotic soluble N-ethylmaleimide–sensitive factor attachment receptor (SNARE) complex that primes synaptic vesicles for fusion with the plasma membrane, and the SNARE complex itself binds to calcium channels (47,48). Thus, these various components are bound together into a single large complex. The physical interaction of SNAREs with calcium channels affects the functional properties of both SNAREs and calcium channels (49,50), and it is possible that the effects on calcium influx and mini frequency are both generated by a single mechanism, with $\beta\gamma$ subunits affecting the interaction between SNAREs and calcium channels within the exocytotic complex.

Presynaptic Facilitation

Although it is generally the case that GPCR activation leads to an inhibition of transmitter release, there are some notably consistent exceptions to this general premise. A number of G_s-coupled GPCRs are known to facilitate exocytosis, in particular many of the class B GPCRs (3). The cyclic adenosine monophosphate (cAMP) signaling cascade facilitates transmitter release (51,52), and the cAMP effectors protein kinase A and Epac have been implicated in the effects of the G_s-coupled GPCRs. This suggests that facilitation requires activation of adenylate cyclase and production of cAMP, but the ultimate targets of this cAMP cascade have not yet been established conclusively (53).

Another set of presynaptic receptors that might be expected to facilitate transmitter release at first glance are those coupled to G_q. G_q-mediated activation of phospholipase C leads to the synthesis of inositol 1,4,5-*tris*-phosphate (IP_3) and diacylglycerol (DAG). IP_3 facilitates neurotransmitter release by releasing calcium from intracellular stores, while DAG does so through activation of PKC and direct interaction with Munc-18, a protein of the exocytotic machinery (54). Thus, it seems reasonable to predict that activation of G_q-coupled GPCRs would profoundly enhance release, and there are systems in which this is observed (55–57). However, the facilitatory effects of G_q-coupled GPCRs are surprisingly inconsistent, and G_q-coupled GPCRs as a general class are frequently observed to inhibit release as well (58–61).

The reasons for these surprising results remain obscure. One possible explanation is that G_q-coupled GPCRs might be excluded from the presynaptic terminal in most systems. In support of this idea, GPCR subfamilies such as the mGluRs have individual members that co-vary in their localization and coupling to specific $G\alpha$ subunits. mGluR1/5 are the only mGluRs that couple predominantly to G_q, and both of these mGluRs are restricted to the somatodendritic area in most cells that express them (62). In contrast, the other mGluRs, all of which couple to $G_{i/o}$, are located presynaptically in most cells.

An alternative explanation is that G_q may activate effectors that prevent the robust expression of presynaptic facilitatory effects. In support of this idea, PKC is well known to phosphorylate GPCRs, leading to uncoupling of the G protein from the receptor (63). Thus, G_q-linked GPCRs can elicit a rapid desensitization of GPCRs via PKC; we note with interest that this is well known to affect not only the G_q-coupled GPCR that initiates this cascade, but other GPCRs as well. One cautionary implication of this finding is that even where G_q-coupled GPCRs have been found to facilitate transmission, it may be due to heterologous desensitization of tonic presynaptic inhibition caused by another GPCR.

Ionotropic Receptors

At first glance, it might seem that ionotropic receptors have a simple and limited set of mechanisms by which they affect synaptic transmission: by either depolarizing or hyperpolarizing the presynaptic terminal. However, the effects of changing the voltage in the presynaptic terminal have been found to be surprisingly complex, and it is now clear that a purely ionotropic effect of these receptors can regulate transmitter release in a variety of ways. In addition to this, a few reports have provided evidence indicating that ionotropic receptors may also affect transmitter release in a surprising and unanticipated way: by activating heterotrimeric G proteins.

Voltage Changes

Changes in presynaptic voltage could, in principle, either increase or decrease synaptic transmission. Modest depolarization could enhance transmission by increasing axonal excitability to generate ectopic spiking, by slowing the action potential waveform to allow more calcium influx, or by leading to a modest tonic influx of calcium by weak activation of voltage-gated calcium channels. However, at high magnitudes, the depolarization could also lead to voltage-dependent inactivation of either sodium or calcium channels and thereby inhibit transmission (1,30). The overall effect will presumably depend on the identity of the permeant ions, the activation and inactivation ranges of different voltage-gated channels in the axon, and the resting membrane potential.

Thus, the relationship between presynaptic voltage and evoked transmitter release can be complex, and this is reflected in the effects of presynaptic ionotropic receptors at several synapses. At mossy fiber synapses onto CA3 pyramidal cells, low concentrations of kainate receptor agonists increase the amplitude of stimulus-evoked excitatory postsynaptic potentials (EPSPs) while higher concentrations of agonist decrease it. These changes in synaptic output are paralleled by changes in the size of the afferent fiber volley, an extracellular depolarization generated by the compound action potential in the stimulated presynaptic fibers (4).

The parallel effects on the EPSP and the fiber volley suggest that the change in EPSP size is downstream of effects on axonal excitability rather than a bona fide regulation of the synapse itself. Identical bidirectional changes in the fiber volley and EPSP are also observed when depolarizing the terminal with extracellular potassium, suggesting that depolarization is sufficient to explain these effects. A simple model that can explain both of these findings is that modest depolarization via presynaptic receptors increases fiber excitability, recruiting more afferent fibers to increase the number of activated synapses, while stronger depolarization leads to sodium channel inactivation or shunting that decreases fiber excitability (4). A similar bidirectional effect on transmitter release has been reported for both AMPARs and KARs at excitatory and inhibitory synapses in the dorsal horn (64), but the mechanisms involved have not yet been established in that system.

At some synapses, presynaptic ligand-gated cation channels can depolarize the axon sufficiently to induce ectopic spiking. Nicotine induces spontaneous GABA release from neurons in the interpeduncular nucleus even under conditions where the postsynaptic neuron and its presynaptic terminals are acutely isolated. Surprisingly, this effect of nicotine is blocked by tetrodotoxin (TTX). As is the case with effects on the fiber volley, this finding suggests a regulation of presynaptic excitability rather than a direct effect on transmitter release (25). A similar phenomenon takes place with KARs on hippocampal interneurons, where KAR agonists induce ectopic spiking in the axon that back-propagates to the soma (65).

In principle, ligand-gated chloride channels in the presynaptic terminal could either hyperpolarize or depolarize the presynaptic membrane, depending on the Cl⁻ reversal potential. Intracellular Cl⁻ levels are controlled by expression of chloride transporters, which are both developmentally and spatially regulated. Early in development, the chloride gradient leads to chloride efflux that depolarizes the cell, and presynaptic ligand-gated anion channels depolarize the synapse. Presynaptic GlyRs and GABA$_A$Rs enhance both spontaneous and evoked release at calyceal synapses by modestly depolarizing the terminal so that the resting calcium level in the terminal increases slightly, promoting asynchronous release and also engaging synaptic facilitation to raise the probability of spike-driven glutamate release (66,67). A similar enhancement in spontaneous release is caused by activation of presynaptic GABA$_A$Rs at synapses onto dorsal horn neurons, but in this case the receptors inhibit action potential–evoked release rather than facilitating it (68). It remains unclear whether this synapse-specific effect of GABA$_A$R activation on evoked release is due to differences in the ligand-induced depolarization or the expression of different voltage-gated channels that might respond to the same depolarization in different ways.

Shunting

An alternative mechanism by which presynaptic ionotropic receptors might affect release is through shunting of intracellular currents by the increase in "leakage" of currents from the cell through the open channels. The involvement of shunting in presynaptic regulation has been debated since the initial finding that GABA$_A$Rs are present in spinal cord primary afferents, and it should be noted that passive shunting and inactivation of active currents are not mutually exclusive as ionotropic mechanisms of presynaptic inhibition.

With that caveat in mind, the relative importance of voltage changes verses passive shunting as mechanisms by which GABA$_A$Rs mediate presynaptic inhibition has been carefully considered over the years, and evidence supporting both mechanisms has been reported (25). Recordings from pituitary secretory nerve endings (26) showed that depolarization alone, induced by injecting current through an electrode rather than by opening channels, was sufficient to cause the observed inhibition without shunting; detailed simulations also suggest that it would be difficult to achieve a sufficient change in conductance needed to elicit the observed level of inhibition by passive shunting (69).

However, other modeling studies show shunting without depolarization could play a major role in presynaptic inhibition (70,71). Furthermore, depolarization by current injection was unable to cause inhibition in crayfish sensory afferents (72), which indirectly supports a role for shunting. Thus, it seems that shunting may play a role in some systems but not others. In this context, it is noteworthy that the safety factor for axonal spike propagation depends on the axonal morphology (73,74). Reliable spike propagation also changes during high-frequency activity in at least some neuronal types (74,75). Thus, shunting may become more important under these circumstances.

Ligand-Gated Calcium Influx

Calcium entry through presynaptic ionotropic receptors plays a direct role in modulation of release at several synapses. This has been most extensively described for presynaptic nAChRs in area CA3 of the hippocampus, where acetylcholine increases the probability of release through a mechanism that is insensitive to blockade of both sodium and calcium channels (33; but see 76). This suggests that the calcium source for release is, at least in part, influx through the channel itself; it also suggests a close colocalization of these receptors with the release machinery. Calcium-induced calcium release from internal stores has also been reported to contribute to this facilitation (77).

Similar results have also been reported in other systems. AMPARs and KARs that lack posttranscriptional editing are also calcium permeable. Calcium entry is thought to be critical for the AMPAR-mediated regulation of transmitter release at dendrodendritic synapses in the retina (37), and for presynaptic KARs in the amygdala (78). Calcium flux through presynaptic NMDARs may also be important for the establishment of some forms of NMDAR-dependent long-term potentiation (LTP), but the mechanisms by which this takes place remain unclear (79).

Metabotropic Effects

Perhaps the most surprising mechanism by which presynaptic ionotropic receptors modulate transmission is through the activation of metabotropic signaling cascades, but evidence for this provocative new link between the two systems has now been found at several synapses with presynaptic KARs and AMPARs. To date, three lines of evidence suggest that these receptors have a direct metabotropic action. First, their effects are blocked by a variety of manipulations that interfere with signal transduction pathways, including kinase inhibitors and the highly specific $G_{i/o}$ inhibitor pertussis toxin (35,40). Second, the effects of these ionotropic receptors are both mimicked and occluded by heterologous activation of metabotropic pathways by GPCRs (80–82). Third, the metabotropic effects of these ionotropic receptors are not blocked by a wide assortment of approaches to prevent the indirect activation of GPCRs by kainate/AMPA receptor activation (reviewed in ref. 5).

Thus, evidence is mounting for the idea that ionotropic receptors can directly engage G-protein–mediated biochemical cascades, but this idea remains controversial and some degree of caution is warranted. In part, this is because of clear-cut cases where the metabotropic actions of ionotropic receptors are indirectly mediated by the depolarization-induced release of endogenous ligands for GPCRs (83,84). Another potential concern is that physiologic concentrations of intracellular Na^+, such as those expected during AMPAR or KAR activation, are known to promote G-protein heterotrimer dissociation and metabotropic actions (85,86), raising the possibility that G-protein activation might be a consequence of the channel's ionotropic activity.

As a result of these concerns, the assignment of AMPARs and KARs as "ionometabotropic" presynaptic receptors remains intriguing but has not yet been unequivocally established. Presuming that the metabotropic effects observed are, in fact, genuinely independent of ionotropic functions of these receptors, this implies that the proteins must interact physically in some way, either through direct binding or through an adaptor protein. The nature of this interaction and the proteins involved remain completely obscure, although various reports have implicated GluR1 for AMPARs (87) and GluR5 or KA2 for KARs (88,89).

Functional Roles of Presynaptic Receptors

We now discuss the function of neuromodulation mediated by presynaptic receptors, with our main emphasis on two ways in which presynaptic receptors can exert a profound influence over the processing of neural signals: by altering the synaptic response to patterns of activity that encode those signals, and by changing the neural pathways through which those signals are transmitted.

Activity-Dependent Signal Processing

All synapses described to date undergo multiple forms of activity-dependent synaptic plasticity. As a result, the output of the synapse is dynamic rather than static; the size of a postsynaptic potential (PSP) depends critically on forms of activity-dependent plasticity that are expressed at the synapse, and the history of activity preceding the PSP. On a time scale of seconds to minutes, activity-dependent short-term plasticity is the major determinant of synaptic dynamics, and most forms of this plasticity are due to presynaptic mechanisms. By interacting with these synaptic dynamics, presynaptic receptors can change the signal processing performed by the synapse.

One way in which this occurs is by the activity-dependent release of the receptor ligand. Neuropeptides, for example, are packaged into large dense-core vesicles that are located far from the calcium channels in the presynaptic terminal (90). As a result, dense-core vesicles are released with a higher threshold of activity than classic synaptic vesicles containing neurotransmitters. A similar dynamic can also be created by selective targeting of the receptor. For example, glutamatergic synapses in multiple parts of the brain express presynaptic mGluRs that are engaged during activity to enact a form of autoinhibition. At many of these synapses, this autoinhibition affects only high levels of activity because the presynaptic mGluRs are located outside the synaptic cleft, where they will only be activated by levels of glutamate release that are high enough to cause glutamate to spill out from the synapse (91,92).

A less obvious but more universal mechanism by which presynaptic receptors can affect activity-dependent signal processing is by changing the synaptic dynamics that are expressed. The pattern of synaptic responses in response to a high-frequency train of stimuli depends on the initial release probability of the synapse at the start of the train (2). Synapses with high release probabilities express a short-term depression in response to high-frequency trains, but as the release probability is reduced, this short-term depression is converted to a short-term facilitation. As a result, a presynaptic receptor that reduces the release probability will decrease the size of the postsynaptic responses at all frequencies of stimulation, but during high frequencies of stimulation this effect will be offset by an increase in short-term facilitation.

As a result, presynaptic inhibition selectively has the greatest inhibitory effect during low-frequency stimulation and spares synaptic transmission during high frequencies of presynaptic activity; in engineering terms, this is a form of high-pass filtering (93,94). Similarly, presynaptic neuromodulators that facilitate release would be expected to act as selective amplifiers of low-frequency activity. The filtering/amplification characteristics of presynaptic neuromodulators remain very poorly defined, but initial studies suggest that the filter imposed by $GABA_BR$-mediated presynaptic inhibition varies gradually over a range from 1 to 50 Hz (93). This frequency range overlaps with the neural responses to behaviorally relevant cues in many systems, and analytic studies suggest that the functional impact of this filter is to increase the contrast between synaptic responses to background levels of presynaptic activity, and responses to the presynaptic activity that occurs in response to behaviorally relevant cues (95).

Synapse-Dependent Signal Processing

Presynaptic receptors have direct effects on transmitter release only in the terminals that express them, and the expression of distinct receptor subtypes is subject to careful developmental and anatomic control. This is a mechanism by which the CNS can use a single ligand, released in a diffuse manner, to reversibly affect some synaptic connections while sparing others. Different presynaptic receptors are expressed on distinct subsets of synaptic connections; given the large heterogeneity in receptor subtypes, and the differential expression of individual receptor subtypes at different receptors, neural circuitry can be precisely and reversibly tuned by neurochemical control.

The hippocampus is a brain region in which several presynaptic receptors that exert control over distinct components of the neural circuit have been identified. Individual receptor subtypes in the hippocampus have been found to selectively control GABAergic (96) or glutamatergic (97) synapses. Similarly, distinct receptor subtypes control glutamate release from cortical projections onto hippocampal dentate granule cells (98); from granule cells onto pyramidal cells (99); and from pyramidal cells onto each other (76). The release of glutamate is also differentially regulated by presynaptic receptors according to whether the synapse is formed onto a pyramidal cell or an interneuron (100–102). Thus, distinct receptors control the transmission of neural signals through different regions of the hippocampus by regulating transmitter release based on the specific identities of the presynaptic and postsynaptic neurons.

Conclusion

Presynaptic receptors are found throughout the nervous system and regulate transmitter release in a wide range of systems. Presynaptic receptors fall into two distinct classes based on their effector mechanisms, with metabotropic receptors acting through biochemical cascades and ionotropic receptors acting through direct activation of ion fluxes across the plasma membrane; however, recent evidence suggests that ionotropic receptors may blur this distinction by directly engaging metabotropic functions. Presynaptic receptors affect release through a range of effects that include changes in membrane potential, direct interactions with the exocytotic machinery or calcium channels, and effects on axonal excitability. The diversity of presynaptic receptors is considerably larger than the diversity of mechanisms by which they affect release, suggesting that the functions of presynaptic receptors are related at least in part to the selective expression of different receptors in different locations or under different conditions. Thus, presynaptic receptors represent a broad class of molecules that can profoundly influence synaptic transmission, but do so with a high degree of synapse-specificity.

Acknowledgments The authors wish to acknowledge Robert Duvoisin for helpful discussions. M.F. is supported by a research grant from the National Institutes of Health/National Institute of Neurological Disorders and Stroke (NS045101).

References

1. Khakh BS, Henderson G. Modulation of fast synaptic transmission by presynaptic ligand-gated cation channels. J Auton Nerv Syst 2000;81(1–3):110–121.
2. Abbott LF, Regehr WG. Synaptic computation. Nature 2004;431(7010):796–803.
3. Harmar AJ. Family-B G-protein-coupled receptors. Genome Biol 2001;2(12):reviews 3013.
4. Schmitz D, Mellor J, Frerking M, Nicoll RA. Presynaptic kainate receptors at hippocampal mossy fiber synapses. Proc Natl Acad Sci U S A 2001;98(20):11003–11008.
5. Lerma J. Kainate receptor physiology. Curr Opin Pharmacol 2006;6(1):89–97.
6. Rudomin P, Schmidt RF. Presynaptic inhibition in the vertebrate spinal cord revisited. Exp Brain Res 1999;129(1):1–37.
7. Karnik SS, Gogonea C, Patil S, Saad Y, Takezako T. Activation of G-protein-coupled receptors: a common molecular mechanism. Trends Endocrinol Metab 2003;14(9):431–437.
8. Tedford HW, Zamponi GW. Direct G protein modulation of Cav2 calcium channels. Pharmacol Rev 2006;58(4):837–862.
9. Engelman HS, MacDermott AB. Presynaptic ionotropic receptors and control of transmitter release. Nat Rev Neurosci 2004;5(2):135–145.
10. Stevens CF. Presynaptic function. Curr Opin Neurobiol 2004;14(3):341–345.
11. Miller RJ. Presynaptic receptors. Annu Rev Pharmacol Toxicol 1998;38:201–227.
12. Jacoby E, Bouhelal R, Gerspacher M, Seuwen K. The 7 TM G-protein-coupled receptor target family. ChemMedChem 2006;1(8):761–782.
13. Heuss C, Gerber U. G-protein-independent signaling by G-protein-coupled receptors. Trends Neurosci 2000;23(10):469–475.
14. Kristiansen K. Molecular mechanisms of ligand binding, signaling, and regulation within the superfamily of G-protein-coupled receptors: molecular modeling and mutagenesis approaches to receptor structure and function. Pharmacol Ther 2004;103(1):21–80.
15. Pin JP, Neubig R, Bouvier M, et al. International Union of Basic and Clinical Pharmacology. LXVII. Recommendations for the recognition and nomenclature of G protein-coupled receptor heteromultimers. Pharmacol Rev 2007;59(1):5–13.
16. Kuner R, Kohr G, Grunewald S, Eisenhardt G, Bach A, Kornau HC. Role of heteromer formation in GABAB receptor function. Science 1999;283(5398):74–77.

17. White JH, Wise A, Main MJ, et al. Heterodimerization is required for the formation of a functional GABA(B) receptor. Nature 1998;396(6712):679–682.
18. Spedding M, Bonner TI, Watson SP. International Union of Pharmacology. XXXI. Recommendations for the nomenclature of multimeric G protein-coupled receptors. Pharmacol Rev 2002;54(2):231–232.
19. Parameswaran N, Spielman WS. RAMPs: The past, present and future. Trends Biochem Sci 2006;31(11):631–638.
20. Vigot R, Barbieri S, Brauner-Osborne H, et al. Differential compartmentalization and distinct functions of GABAB receptor variants. Neuron 2006;50(4):589–601.
21. Willis WD. John Eccles' studies of spinal cord presynaptic inhibition. Prog Neurobiol 2006;78(3–5):189–214.
22. Frerking M, Borges S, Wilson M. Variation in GABA mini amplitude is the consequence of variation in transmitter concentration. Neuron 1995;15(4):885–895.
23. Alle H, Geiger JR. GABAergic spill-over transmission onto hippocampal mossy fiber boutons. J Neurosci 2007;27(4):942–950.
24. Ruiz A, Fabian-Fine R, Scott R, Walker MC, Rusakov DA, Kullmann DM. GABAA receptors at hippocampal mossy fibers. Neuron 2003;39(6):961–973.
25. MacDermott AB, Role LW, Siegelbaum SA. Presynaptic ionotropic receptors and the control of transmitter release. Annu Rev Neurosci 1999;22:443–485.
26. Zhang SJ, Jackson MB. GABA-activated chloride channels in secretory nerve endings. Science 1993;259(5094):531–534.
27. Zhang SJ, Jackson MB. GABAA receptor activation and the excitability of nerve terminals in the rat posterior pituitary. J Physiol 1995;483(pt 3):583–595.
28. Hull C, Li GL, von Gersdorff H. GABA transporters regulate a standing GABAC receptor-mediated current at a retinal presynaptic terminal. J Neurosci 2006;26(26): 6979–6984.
29. Turecek R, Trussell LO. Reciprocal developmental regulation of presynaptic ionotropic receptors. Proc Natl Acad Sci U S A 2002;99(21):13884–13889.
30. Engelman HS, Anderson RL, Daniele C, Macdermott AB. Presynaptic alpha-amino-3–hydroxy-5–methyl-4–isoxazolepropionic acid (AMPA) receptors modulate release of inhibitory amino acids in rat spinal cord dorsal horn. Neuroscience 2006;139(2):539–553.
31. Turecek R, Trussell LO. Presynaptic glycine receptors enhance transmitter release at a mammalian central synapse. Nature 2001;411(6837):587–590.
32. Ye JH, Wang F, Krnjevic K, Wang W, Xiong ZG, Zhang J. Presynaptic glycine receptors on GABAergic terminals facilitate discharge of dopaminergic neurons in ventral tegmental area. J Neurosci 2004;24(41):8961–8974.
33. McGehee DS, Role LW. Presynaptic ionotropic receptors. Curr Opin Neurobiol 1996;6 (3):342–349.
34. Wonnacott S. Presynaptic nicotinic ACh receptors. Trends Neurosci 1997;20(2):92–98.
35. Takago H, Nakamura Y, Takahashi T. G protein-dependent presynaptic inhibition mediated by AMPA receptors at the calyx of Held. Proc Natl Acad Sci U S A 2005;102(20): 7368–7373.
36. Liu SJ. Biphasic modulation of GABA release from stellate cells by glutamatergic receptor sub-types. J Neurophysiol 2007;98:550–556.
37. Chavez AE, Singer JH, Diamond JS. Fast neurotransmitter release triggered by Ca influx through AMPA-type glutamate receptors. Nature 2006;443(7112):705–708.
38. Duguid I, Sjostrom PJ. Novel presynaptic mechanisms for coincidence detection in synaptic plasticity. Curr Opin Neurobiol 2006;16(3):312–322.
39. Chittajallu R, Vignes M, Dev KK, Barnes JM, Collingridge GL, Henley JM. Regulation of glutamate release by presynaptic kainate receptors in the hippocampus. Nature 1996;379(6560):78–81.
40. Huettner JE. Kainate receptors and synaptic transmission. Prog Neurobiol 2003;70(5):387–407.
41. Zamponi GW. Determinants of G protein inhibition of presynaptic calcium channels. Cell Biochem Biophys 2001;34(1):79–94.

42. Wu LG, Saggau P. Presynaptic inhibition of elicited neurotransmitter release. Trends Neurosci 1997;20(5):204–212.
43. Zhang C, Schmidt JT. Adenosine A1 and class II metabotropic glutamate receptors mediate shared presynaptic inhibition of retinotectal transmission. J Neurophysiol 1999;82(6):2947–2955.
44. Qian J, Saggau P. Presynaptic inhibition of synaptic transmission in the rat hippocampus by activation of muscarinic receptors: involvement of presynaptic calcium influx. Br J Pharmacol 1997;122(3):511–519.
45. Luscher C, Jan LY, Stoffel M, Malenka RC, Nicoll RA. G protein-coupled inwardly rectifying K+ channels (GIRKs) mediate postsynaptic but not presynaptic transmitter actions in hippocampal neurons. Neuron 1997;19(3):687–695.
46. Thompson SM, Capogna M, Scanziani M. Presynaptic inhibition in the hippocampus. Trends Neurosci 1993;16(6):222–227.
47. Gerachshenko T, Blackmer T, Yoon EJ, Bartleson C, Hamm HE, Alford S. Gbetagamma acts at the C terminus of SNAP-25 to mediate presynaptic inhibition. Nat Neurosci 2005;8(5):597–605.
48. Blackmer T, Larsen EC, Takahashi M, Martin TF, Alford S, Hamm HE. G protein betagamma subunit-mediated presynaptic inhibition: regulation of exocytotic fusion downstream of Ca2+ entry. Science 2001;292(5515):293–297.
49. Bezprozvanny I, Zhong P, Scheller RH, Tsien RW. Molecular determinants of the functional interaction between syntaxin and N-type Ca2+ channel gating. Proc Natl Acad Sci U S A 2000;97(25):13943–13948.
50. Jarvis SE, Zamponi GW. Masters or slaves? Vesicle release machinery and the regulation of presynaptic calcium channels. Cell Calcium 2005;37(5):483–488.
51. Weisskopf MG, Castillo PE, Zalutsky RA, Nicoll RA. Mediation of hippocampal mossy fiber long-term potentiation by cyclic AMP. Science 1994;265(5180):1878–1882.
52. Chavez-Noriega LE, Stevens CF. Increased transmitter release at excitatory synapses produced by direct activation of adenylate cyclase in rat hippocampal slices. J Neurosci 1994;14(1):310–317.
53. Seino S, Shibasaki T. PKA-dependent and PKA-independent pathways for cAMP-regulated exocytosis. Physiol Rev 2005;85(4):1303–1342.
54. Wierda KD, Toonen RF, de Wit H, Brussaard AB, Verhage M. Interdependence of PKC-dependent and PKC-independent pathways for presynaptic plasticity. Neuron 2007;54(2): 275–290.
55. Chen L, Yung KK, Yung WH. Neurotensin selectively facilitates glutamatergic transmission in globus pallidus. Neuroscience 2006;141(4):1871–1878.
56. Hasuo H, Matsuoka T, Akasu T. Activation of presynaptic 5–hydroxytryptamine 2A receptors facilitates excitatory synaptic transmission via protein kinase C in the dorsolateral septal nucleus. J Neurosci 2002;22(17):7509–7517.
57. Sikand P, Premkumar LS. Potentiation of glutamatergic synaptic transmission by protein kinase C-mediated sensitization of TRPV1 at the first sensory synapse. J Physiol 2007;581 (pt 2):631–647.
58. Buno W, Cabezas C, Fernandez de Sevilla D. Presynaptic muscarinic control of glutamatergic synaptic transmission. J Mol Neurosci 2006;30(1–2):161–164.
59. Lechner SG, Hussl S, Schicker KW, Drobny H, Boehm S. Presynaptic inhibition via a phospholipase C- and phosphatidylinositol bisphosphate-dependent regulation of neuronal Ca2+ channels. Mol Pharmacol 2005;68(5):1387–1396.
60. Kuang D, Yao Y, Maclean D, Wang M, Hampson DR, Chang BS. Ancestral reconstruction of the ligand-binding pocket of Family C G protein-coupled receptors. Proc Natl Acad Sci U S A 2006;103(38):14050–14055.
61. Edelbauer H, Lechner SG, Mayer M, Scholze T, Boehm S. Presynaptic inhibition of transmitter release from rat sympathetic neurons by bradykinin. J Neurochem 2005;93(5):1110–1121.
62. Hermans E, Challiss RA. Structural, signalling and regulatory properties of the group I metabotropic glutamate receptors: prototypic family C G-protein-coupled receptors. Biochem J 2001;359(pt 3):465–484.

63. Ferguson SS, Zhang J, Barak LS, Caron MG. Molecular mechanisms of G protein-coupled receptor desensitization and resensitization. Life Sci 1998;62(17–18):1561–1565.

64. Kerchner GA, Wang GD, Qiu CS, Huettner JE, Zhuo M. Direct presynaptic regulation of GABA/glycine release by kainate receptors in the dorsal horn: an ionotropic mechanism. Neuron 2001;32(3):477–488.

65. Semyanov A, Kullmann DM. Kainate receptor-dependent axonal depolarization and action potential initiation in interneurons. Nat Neurosci 2001;4(7):718–723.

66. Awatramani GB, Price GD, Trussell LO. Modulation of transmitter release by presynaptic resting potential and background calcium levels. Neuron 2005;48(1):109–121.

67. Awatramani GB, Turecek R, Trussell LO. Staggered development of GABAergic and glycinergic transmission in the MNTB. J Neurophysiol 2005;93(2):819–828.

68. Jang IS, Jeong HJ, Katsurabayashi S, Akaike N. Functional roles of presynaptic GABA(A) receptors on glycinergic nerve terminals in the rat spinal cord. J Physiol 2002;541(pt 2):423–434.

69. Graham B, Redman S. A simulation of action potentials in synaptic boutons during presynaptic inhibition. J Neurophysiol 1994;71(2):538–549.

70. Segev I. Computer study of presynaptic inhibition controlling the spread of action potentials into axonal terminals. J Neurophysiol 1990;63(5):987–998.

71. Cattaert D, El Manira A. Shunting versus inactivation: analysis of presynaptic inhibitory mechanisms in primary afferents of the crayfish. J Neurosci 1999;19(14):6079–6089.

72. Cattaert D, Libersat F, El Manira AA. Presynaptic inhibition and antidromic spikes in primary afferents of the crayfish: a computational and experimental analysis. J Neurosci 2001;21(3):1007–1021.

73. Luscher C, Streit J, Quadroni R, Luscher HR. Action potential propagation through embryonic dorsal root ganglion cells in culture. I. Influence of the cell morphology on propagation properties. J Neurophysiol 1994;72(2):622–633.

74. Mackenzie PJ, Murphy TH. High safety factor for action potential conduction along axons but not dendrites of cultured hippocampal and cortical neurons. J Neurophysiol 1998;80(4):2089–2101.

75. Luscher C, Streit J, Lipp P, Luscher HR. Action potential propagation through embryonic dorsal root ganglion cells in culture. II. Decrease of conduction reliability during repetitive stimulation. J Neurophysiol 1994;72(2):634–643.

76. Vogt KE, Regehr WG. Cholinergic modulation of excitatory synaptic transmission in the CA3 area of the hippocampus. J Neurosci 2001;21(1):75–83.

77. Le Magueresse C, Cherubini E. Presynaptic calcium stores contribute to nicotine-elicited potentiation of evoked synaptic transmission at CA3–CA1 connections in the neonatal rat hippocampus. Hippocampus 2007;17(4):316–325.

78. Braga MF, Aroniadou-Anderjaska V, Xie J, Li H. Bidirectional modulation of GABA release by presynaptic glutamate receptor 5 kainate receptors in the basolateral amygdala. J Neurosci 2003;23(2):442–452.

79. Sjostrom PJ, Turrigiano GG, Nelson SB. Neocortical LTD via coincident activation of presynaptic NMDA and cannabinoid receptors. Neuron 2003;39(4):641–654.

80. Satake S, Saitow F, Rusakov D, Konishi S. AMPA receptor-mediated presynaptic inhibition at cerebellar GABAergic synapses: a characterization of molecular mechanisms. Eur J Neurosci 2004;19(9):2464–2474.

81. Partovi D, Frerking M. Presynaptic inhibition by kainate receptors converges mechanistically with presynaptic inhibition by adenosine and GABAB receptors. Neuropharmacology 2006;51(6):1030–1037.

82. Negrete-Diaz JV, Sihra TS, Delgado-Garcia JM, Rodriguez-Moreno A. Kainate receptor-mediated presynaptic inhibition converges with presynaptic inhibition mediated by Group II mGluRs and long-term depression at the hippocampal mossy fiber-CA3 synapse. J Neural Transm 2007;114:1425–1431.

83. Schmitz D, Frerking M, Nicoll RA. Synaptic activation of presynaptic kainate receptors on hippocampal mossy fiber synapses. Neuron 2000;27(2):327–338.

84. Chergui K, Bouron A, Normand E, Mulle C. Functional GluR6 kainate receptors in the striatum: indirect downregulation of synaptic transmission. J Neurosci 2000;20(6):2175–2182.

85. Blumenstein Y, Maximyuk OP, Lozovaya N, et al. Intracellular Na+ inhibits voltage-dependent N-type Ca2+ channels by a G protein betagamma subunit-dependent mechanism. J Physiol 2004;556(pt 1):121–134.

86. Rishal I, Keren-Raifman T, Yakubovich D, et al. Na+ promotes the dissociation between Galpha GDP and Gbeta gamma, activating G protein-gated K+ channels. J Biol Chem 2003;278(6):3840–3845.

87. Wang Y, Small DL, Stanimirovic DB, Morley P, Durkin JP. AMPA receptor-mediated regulation of a Gi-protein in cortical neurons. Nature 1997;389(6650):502–504.

88. Rozas JL, Paternain AV, Lerma J. Noncanonical signaling by ionotropic kainate receptors. Neuron 2003;39(3):543–553.

89. Ruiz A, Sachidhanandam S, Utvik JK, Coussen F, Mulle C. Distinct subunits in heteromeric kainate receptors mediate ionotropic and metabotropic function at hippocampal mossy fiber synapses. J Neurosci 2005;25(50):11710–11718.

90. Scalettar BA. How neurosecretory vesicles release their cargo. Neuroscientist 2006; 12(2):164–176.

91. Scanziani M, Salin PA, Vogt KE, Malenka RC, Nicoll RA. Use-dependent increases in glutamate concentration activate presynaptic metabotropic glutamate receptors. Nature 1997;385(6617):630–634.

92. Piet R, Vargova L, Sykova E, Poulain DA, Oliet SH. Physiological contribution of the astrocytic environment of neurons to intersynaptic crosstalk. Proc Natl Acad Sci USA 2004;101(7):2151–2155.

93. Ohliger-Frerking P, Wiebe SP, Staubli U, Frerking M. GABA(B) receptor-mediated presynaptic inhibition has history-dependent effects on synaptic transmission during physiologically relevant spike trains. J Neurosci 2003;23(12):4809–4814.

94. Castro-Alamancos MA, Calcagnotto ME. High-pass filtering of corticothalamic activity by neuromodulators released in the thalamus during arousal: in vitro and in vivo. J Neurophysiol 2001;85(4):1489–1497.

95. Frerking M, Ohliger-Frerking P. Functional consequences of presynaptic inhibition during behaviorally relevant activity. J Neurophysiol 2006;96(4):2139–2143.

96. Vaughan CW, Ingram SL, Connor MA, Christie MJ. How opioids inhibit GABA-mediated neurotransmission. Nature 1997;390(6660):611–614.

97. Malva JO, Silva AP, Cunha RA. Presynaptic modulation controlling neuronal excitability and epileptogenesis: role of kainate, adenosine and neuropeptide Y receptors. Neurochem Res 2003;28(10):1501–1515.

98. Shigemoto R, Kinoshita A, Wada E, et al. Differential presynaptic localization of metabotropic glutamate receptor subtypes in the rat hippocampus. J Neurosci 1997;17 (19):7503–7522.

99. Yoshino M, Sawada S, Yamamoto C, Kamiya H. A metabotropic glutamate receptor agonist DCG-IV suppresses synaptic transmission at mossy fiber pathway of the guinea pig hippocampus. Neurosci Lett 1996;207(1):70–72.

100. Pelkey KA, Topolnik L, Lacaille JC, McBain CJ. Compartmentalized Ca(2+) channel regulation at divergent mossy-fiber release sites underlies target cell-dependent plasticity. Neuron 2006;52(3):497–510.

101. Sun HY, Dobrunz LE. Presynaptic kainate receptor activation is a novel mechanism for target cell-specific short-term facilitation at Schaffer collateral synapses. J Neurosci 2006;26(42):10796–10807.

102. Scanziani M, Gahwiler BH, Charpak S. Target cell-specific modulation of transmitter release at terminals from a single axon. Proc Natl Acad Sci U S A 1998;95(20):12004–12009.

Chapter 15
Transsynaptic Regulation of Presynaptic Release Machinery in Central Synapses by Cell Adhesion Molecules

Kensuke Futai and Yasunori Hayashi

Contents

Abstract Neuronal activity and resultant synaptic plasticity, such as long-term potentiation (LTP) and long-term depression (LTD), are accompanied by a dynamic regulation of the synaptic structure. At the same time, pre- and postsynaptic structures and functions are well coordinated at the individual synapse level. For example, large postsynaptic dendritic spines have a larger postsynaptic density with higher AMPA receptor number on their surface, while juxtaposing presynaptic terminals have a larger active zone and more docked vesicles. This indicates that structural modification seen in LTP and LTD must be coordinated at both pre- and postsynaptic structure, likely as a result of coordinated assembly of specific molecules on both sides of the synaptic cleft. Interestingly, there is evidence that the postsynaptic cell may be instructive to presynaptic functions. This review focuses on the postsynaptic mechanisms that retrogradely regulate presynaptic functionality and structure, emphasizing the role of neuronal adhesion molecules.

Yasunori Hayashi, MD PhD
RIKEN-MIT Neuroscience Research Center, The Picower Institute for Learning and Memory,
Department of Brain and Cognitive Sciences, Massachusetts Institute of Technology,
Cambridge, MA 02139, USA
e-mail: yhayashi@mit.edu

Z.-W. Wang (ed.) *Molecular Mechanisms of Neurotransmitter Release,*
© Humana Press 2008 a part of Springer Science+Business Media, LLC

Keywords Release probability, synaptic transmission, cell adhesion molecules, cadherin, catenin, neuroligin, neurexin, Eph receptor, ephrin, retrograde messenger.

The synapse is a highly specialized asymmetric structure that transmits information and stores it in the brain. The majority of synapses in the central nervous system are chemical synapses, which are physically separated into pre- and postsynaptic structures at the synaptic cleft. Although the two structures are physically separated, pre- and postsynaptic structures and functions are well coordinated at the individual synapse level. For example, in excitatory synapses on hippocampal pyramidal cells, large postsynaptic dendritic spines have a larger postsynaptic density with a greater number of α-amino-3-hydroxy-5-methyl-4-isoxazole propionic acid (AMPA) receptors on the surface. At the same time, juxtaposing presynaptic terminals have a larger active zone and more docked vesicles (1–4). Such coordination of postsynaptic and presynaptic structure and function ensures more efficient transmission. It has been reported that neuronal activity and resultant synaptic plasticity, such as long-term potentiation (LTP) and long-term depression (LTD), alter the efficiency of synaptic transmission in conjunction with postsynaptic structural changes (5), suggesting that synaptic plasticity can influence presynaptic structure and function. Therefore, it is extremely important to understand the mechanism of how presynaptic-postsynaptic coordination takes place in mature synapses. Most likely it is a result of the coordinated assembly of synaptic adhesion molecules on both sides of the synaptic cleft. Synaptically localized adhesion molecules have been reported as important mediators for organizing synaptic structure (6), and recent studies indicated that synaptic adhesion molecules modulate basal synaptic transmission and plasticity in matured synapses.

This chapter describes the history and possibilities of transsynaptic, especially retrograde, signaling on the expression mechanism of LTP, and discusses the molecules that support transsynaptic signaling, with an emphasis on cell adhesion molecules.

Historical Perspective on the Retrograde Regulation of Transmitter Release: Long-Term Potentiation Studies

Long-term potentiation (LTP) is a phenomenon in which a transient burst of synaptic input causes a long-lasting increase in subsequent synaptic transmission (7). It has been well established that LTP induction requires postsynaptic depolarization combined with the activation of N-methyl-D-aspartate (NMDA) receptors, and resultant influx of Ca^{2+}. This triggers a series of biochemical processes including the activation of calcium/calmodulin-dependent protein kinase II (CaMKII). Expression of LTP is achieved by increasing the number of AMPA receptors (AMPARs) at the synapse through the activity-dependent change of AMPAR trafficking pathway or by changing AMPAR channel properties via direct phosphorylation (8–10). Although this postsynaptic view is nowadays widely accepted, the presynaptic view was initially suggested by the observations of increased transmitter release and reduced failure rate after LTP induction, which are generally considered to reflect changes in release probability based on studies at the neuromuscular junction. Several diffusible molecules including nitric oxide (NO), arachidonic acids, carbon monoxide (CO), platelet-activating factor (PAF), and brain-derived neurotrophic factor (BDNF) have been suggested as possible retrograde messengers (11). However, these suggestions have often been questioned because either the reported results cannot be reproduced or the candidate molecules appear to lack sufficient specificities (12,13). Moreover, the studies from various knockout animals renounced the retrograde function of these molecules, at least in the context of LTP (14–16).

Although a decade of debate made the postsynaptic view of LTP current prevailing, it does not positively rule out the presynaptic view, and further new evidence is accumulating (16–19). In view of structural changes occurring at the synapse, as early as 1977, only four years after LTP was reported (7), a pioneering electron microscopic study by Fifková's group (20) reported that the induction of LTP in the dentate gyrus increases the size of dendritic spines, which is followed by an increase in the dimension of the presynaptic terminus after a transient disparity. In fact, the presynaptic structures (length of active zone and number of synaptic vesicles) and postsynaptic structures (length of postsynaptic density and the dimension of postsynaptic density) in naive tissue appear well coordinated (1–4). At some point after LTP induction, pre- and postsynaptic structures must necessarily be coordinated to maintain the proportion observed *in vivo*.

The presence of retrograde modulation of presynaptic function and structure is also suggested by observations outside of LTP studies. For example, analyses of connections made between a Schaffer collateral axon from a CA3 pyramidal neuron targeting CA1 pyramidal neurons or inhibitory interneurons indicate that the type of the postsynaptic target neuron can dictate the presynaptic properties (21). A similar observation was made between synapses formed between a single presynaptic pyramidal cell and two different types of postsynaptic cells (22). The presynaptic termini in a single cell can have different protein components depending on postsynaptic cell type, and this ability appears to be involved in target cell-specific presynaptic function (23). Furthermore, the alteration in the activity level of a specific postsynaptic neuron can change presynaptic properties. For example, in hippocampal dissociated culture, increasing postsynaptic CaMKII activity by transfecting its active forms results in the remodeling of presynaptic input by increasing the number of synaptic contacts between pairs of neuron, while decreasing the total number of connected cells (24). Similar retrograde action of CaMKII activity has also been reported in *Drosophila* (25,26). Postsynaptically localized synaptotagmin 4 (Syt 4), a calcium sensor for membrane fusion, is a candidate molecule for the release of retrograde messengers in *Drosophila* (27). Yoshihara *et al.* reported that Syt 4 triggered the release of retrograde messengers that enhanced presynaptic function through the activation of the presynaptic cyclic adenosine monophosphate (cAMP)-dependent kinase pathway. These observations exemplify the ability of a postsynaptic neuron to retrogradely influence functional properties of the presynaptic terminal. Thus, postsynaptic neurons must be equipped with mechanisms to retrogradely regulate the presynaptic release probability, though these mechanisms may not take place in relatively early phase of LTP (<30 min after induction).

Transsynaptic Adhesion Molecules

Cadherin-Catenin–Mediated Transsynaptic Signaling

The cadherin superfamily consists of more than 100 members in vertebrates. They are classified into subfamilies that are called classical cadherins, desmosomal cadherins, protocadherins, Flamingo/CELSRs (*c*adherin, *e*pidermal growth factor [EGF]-like, *l*aminin A globular-like [LAG], and *s*even-pass *r*eceptors), and Fat cadherin (28). Cadherins make homophilic adhesion between cells expressing the same class of cadherin through their extracellular domain containing the repetitive cadherin repeats, including the calcium-binding domain. Classical cadherins have been most extensively studied, and their cytoplasmic domain binds to β-catenin and p120 catenins (29,30). β-catenin associates with α-catenin, which is known as an actin-binding protein. These protein–protein interactions likely underlie the mechanism of cadherin-mediated synapse formation and spine stability.

Postsynaptic overexpression of the dominant-negative form of N-cadherin, which has a deletion in the extracellular domain, reduced the number of presynaptic puncta and changed spine morphology concomitant with the reduction of frequency of miniature excitatory postsynaptic currents (mEPSCs) (31). A neuronal culture differentiated from mouse embryonic stem (ES) cells lacking N-cadherin showed that the absence of N-cadherin enhanced synaptic depression in response to paired-pulse or high-frequency stimulation, although evoked postsynaptic currents (EPSCs) in response to a single stimulus and the mean amplitude of mEPSCs were indistinguishable between neurons with and those without N-cadherin (32). Synaptic structures were also not altered in neurons lacking N-cadherin, consistent with the analysis of a conditional knockout of N-cadherin in hippocampal neurons (33). These observations suggest that N-cadherin controls short-term synaptic plasticity transsynaptically. Interestingly, the same synaptic phenotypes were observed when the deficiency of N-cadherin was restricted to postsynaptic neurons in experiments of coculturing wild-type neurons and the ES cell-derived neurons, suggesting that postsynaptic N-cadherin retrogradely controls presynaptic release (32). These studies suggested that N-cadherin is involved in vesicle recruitment from the readily releasable pool to the active zone and in vesicle recycling pathways (31,32). The entire process likely involves N-cadherin binding proteins. A conditional knockout of β-catenin reduced the number of releasable vesicles and exacerbated synaptic depression during high-frequency stimulation (34). Conversely, postsynaptic overexpression of β-catenin resulted in an increase in mEPSC frequency, suggesting a retrograde regulation by postsynaptic β-catenin/cadherin interaction, although there is the alternative possibility that β-catenin overexpression increased the number of functional synapses in this case (35).

It has also been reported that spine stability and spine density are altered in knockout mice of α-N-cadherin and p120 catenin, respectively, but precise electrophysiological analyses of these animals have not been performed (36–38). Interestingly, δ-catenin knockout mice showed reduced paired-pulse facilitation (PPF) in hippocampal neurons consistent with the ES cell study for N-cadherin (39). Like N-cadherin, other classical cadherins are also important for the formation of synapses and synaptic function. Knockout of cadherin 11 enhanced LTP in the hippocampal CA1 region without changes in paired-pulse facilitation (PPF), indicating that the absence of cadherin 11 may increase the flexibility of the synaptic structure, allowing it to receive more AMPA receptors (40). Knockout of cadherin 8, which is specifically expressed in the spinal cord, led to loss of menthol-induced enhancement of AMPAR-mediated mEPSC frequency (41). RNA interference (RNAi) based knockdown of cadherin 11 and 13 indicates the importance of these molecules on the formation and function of the glutamatergic synapse (42).

Recently two studies showed that N-cadherin formed a protein complex with AMPA receptors *in vivo* (43), and the extracellular N-terminal domain of GluR2, a key subunit of AMPA receptors, can interact directly with N-cadherin (44). It is unclear whether this interaction is mediated by *cis*- or *trans*-synaptic manner. Nevertheless, this heterophilic interaction could be an important mechanism for AMPA receptor trafficking, retrograde regulation of synaptic transmission, and coordination between pre- and postsynaptic function.

Neuroligin-Neurexin-Mediated Transsynaptic Signaling

Neurexins (Nrxns) were isolated as a family of brain membrane surface proteins that bind α-latrotoxin, which is a neurotoxin from black widow spiders and functions as a potent trigger of neurotransmitter release (45,46). Nrxns are encoded by three genes *(Nrxn1–3),* each consisting of two isoforms (α- and β-) with different product lengths. Both α- and β-Nrxns have a single transmembrane domain and bind to CASK (mLin-2) intracellularly through a PSD-95/Dlg/ZO-1 homology (PDZ) domain binding consensus sequence (47). CASK further interacts with Mint, syntenin, and synaptotagmin. Through these three interacting proteins, CASK is eventually linked to other proteins of the presynaptic vesicle release machinery. Extracellularly, both α- and β-Nrxns bind to neuroligin (NL) through their LNS (laminin, nectin, sex-hormone binding globulin) domains (48,49). The NLs are encoded by five different genes in humans, and they have in common one transmembrane region and an extracellular domain that is homologous to acetylcholinesterase but is catalytically inactive (46,50). Intracellularly, NLs have PDZ domain binding consensus sequences that bind to PSD-95, SAP102, Shank, S-SCAM, PICK1, SPAR, and GOPC, which are major components of the postsynaptic structure (51–54). Through these interactions, Nrxns and NLs bridge the presynaptic release machinery and the postsynaptic receptor complex.

In vitro experiments suggest that Nrxns and NLs regulate synapse formation bidirectionally. Nrxns expressed in nonneuronal cells or coated on beads induced

dendritic clustering of proteins involved in excitatory and inhibitory synaptic transmission in contacting dendrites (55). The NLs, in contrast, induced presynaptic
differentiation to recruit presynaptic proteins (56–58). Knockout mouse of α-Nrxns
or NLs showed serious functional but no apparent structural deficits. Triple knockout of NL1–3 reduced the frequencies of both miniature excitatory and inhibitory
postsynaptic currents (mEPSCs and mIPSCs). Since spine densities and mean
amplitudes of the miniature postsynaptic currents were normal in the triple knockout compared with wild-type mice, the decreased frequencies of mEPSCs and
mIPSCs reflect reduced presynaptic release probability (59).

Recently it has been reported that postsynaptic NL1 is implicated in the modulation of presynaptic release probability by cooperating with postsynaptic PSD-95 and
presynaptic Nrxn. Futai *et al* (60) showed that manipulating postsynaptic expression
levels of PSD-95 and NL1 altered presynaptic release probability in organotypic hippocampal slice culture, suggesting that PSD-95-NL1 interaction retrogradely regulates presynaptic release probability. Paired pre- and postsynaptic recordings of two
CA3 pyramidal neurons indicate that presynaptic overexpression of a dominant-negative form of β-Nrxn reduced the release probability. Therefore, the effect is most
likely through the interaction between presynaptic β-Nrxn and postsynaptic NL.
However, presynaptic overexpression of β-Nrxn did not mimic the effect of postsynaptic overexpression of PSD-95 or NLG, suggesting that β-Nrxn exists in redundancy
and postsynaptic PSD-95–NLG complex has an instructive role for this transsynaptic
mechanism. Since α-Nrxn modulates presynaptic calcium channel, it might be possible that α-Nrxn is involved in some way. However, NLG1 used in this study does not
bind to α-Nrxn (61), but still fully exerts its effects. Therefore, the effects of NLG1
observed in our assays do not require direct interaction with presynaptic α-Nrxn,
though we do not rule out indirect involvement.

Ephrin Receptor-Ephrin Ligand Mediated Transsynaptic Signaling

Both Eph receptors, which are tyrosine kinase receptors, and their ligands are
divided into to subclasses: A and B. The ephrinA ligands are tethered to the membrane through glycosylphosphatidylinositol (GPI)-linkage anchors, and specifically
bind to EphA receptors, while the ephrinB ligands associate with the plasma membrane through a transmembrane domain, and preferentially bind to EphB receptors.
The intracellular carboxy-terminal tail of Eph receptors contains the tyrosine kinase
domain, a SAM protein interaction domain, and a consensus motif for binding to
PDZ domain-containing proteins. Interestingly, several Eph receptors bind synaptic
PDZ domain proteins such as the glutamate receptor interacting protein GRIP1, the
protein kinase C–interacting protein PICK1, the syndecan-binding protein syntenin,
and the Ras-binding protein AF-6 (62,63). The ephrinB ligands also have PDZ
domain-binding motifs in the carboxy terminal region, which can mediate association with syntenin, PICK1, GRIP1, and GRIP2 (63–65). Thus, the Eph receptors

and the ephrinB ligands may be linked to the synaptic scaffold through PDZ-mediated protein interactions. Both EphA and EphB receptors have been detected mainly in postsynaptic sites (62,66,67), but some of the Eph receptors are also expressed in presynaptic terminals (68). In contrast, there is little evidence for the synaptic localization of ephrin ligands, and the pattern of expression is different among different subtypes. In the adult hippocampus, for example, ephrin-B2 is expressed mainly in CA1 pyramidal cells, and is more abundant at the postsynaptic side (69–71), whereas ephrin-B3 is expressed in dentate gyrus granule cells and is targeted to mossy fiber axons and terminals (69,71,72). It has been reported that transsynaptic retrograde signaling from postsynaptic EphB receptors to presynaptic ephrinB ligands contributes to the induction of an NMDA receptor (NMDAR)-independent LTP between hippocampal mossy fibers and CA3 pyramidal neurons. Interfering with EphB/ephrinB transsynaptic signaling by the intracellular application of the carboxyl-terminal peptide of EphB2 receptor blocked mossy fiber LTP, while expression of a dominant-negative form of ephrinB3 ligand reduced LTP (72,73). On the other hand, extracellular application of soluble EphB2 receptor and ephrinB1 ligand to activate EphB/ephrinB transsynaptic signaling occluded LTP. Interestingly, ephrinB3 knockout mice exhibited normal mossy fiber LTP (72). This lack of effect may be due to redundant functions of other ephrinBs.

Transsynaptic Signaling Mediated by Other Candidate Molecules

Neuronal specific immunoglobulin superfamily protein, SynCAM, works as a homophilic cell adhesion molecule at the synapse. The intracellular domain of SynCAM binds to PDZ-domain proteins such as CASK (74). Expression of SynCAM in HEK293 cells that were cocultured with hippocampal neurons induced synaptogenesis in these nonneuronal cells, while postsynaptic overexpression of SynCAM in hippocampal neurons increased the frequency of mEPSCs without changing the number of synapse, indicative of presynaptic site of modification (75). Also postsynaptic overexpression of SAP97 and Shank1 increased staining intensity of presynaptic sites with an amphipathic fluorescent (FM) dyes and increased the frequency of mEPSC (76,77), suggesting a retrograde regulation of the release machinery by these molecules. These proteins are localized intracellularly, however, and the actual mechanism that transmits signaling is unknown.

How Do Cell-Adhesion Molecules Change the Presynaptic Functionality?

Recent findings show that dendritic spines expand rapidly and persistently after LTP induction, which is accompanied by synaptic translocation of other molecules such as AMPA receptor, CaMKIIα, β-catenin, and actin (10,35,78,79).

These observations suggest that LTP might be accompanied by an increase in synaptic components in general. Therefore, it is likely that the cell adhesion molecules are translocated to the synapse as part of a process of rebuilding larger postsynaptic structures. The increased number of postsynaptic cell adhesion molecules will then recruit more presynaptic counterparts, which may stabilize synaptic structure by further recruiting synaptic components. This may lead to an increased number of synaptic vesicles as well as active zone components, thereby increasing the number of synaptic vesicles released per action potential. The presynaptic binding partner of postsynaptic neuroligin, β-Nrxn, binds to the PDZ domain of CASK through its intracellular carboxyl terminus. N-cadherin also binds to CASK indirectly through the interaction with β-catenin and LIN-7/Veli/Mals, which makes a complex with CASK (80). CASK then links β-Nrxn and N-cadherin to synaptic vesicle trafficking via binding with Mint1 (X11), which directly interacts with Munc18, a functional regulator of neurotransmitter release. Mutations in CAMGUK, the *Drosophila* CASK homologue, caused a serious presynaptic functional deficit (81). Knockout mice of CASK showed a change in the frequency of spontaneous release events with no structural abnormalities (82).

In the hippocampal CA1 synapse, a multivesicular release has been recently proposed, as opposed to the monovesicular release, which was originally proposed for this synapse (83,84). Therefore, it is reasonable to assume that the presynaptic terminus has the capacity to regulate the number of released vesicles by changing the number of active zones rather than by increasing the probability of release per vesicle without changing the total number of vesicles. An increased number of vesicles released per action potential can explain the observed increase in cleft glutamate concentration (60). Because AMPA receptors at the synapse are not saturated with glutamate (85), the change in glutamate concentration can change postsynaptic response properties. In this way, a qualitative change in the synaptic vesicles can change the temporal pattern of synaptic transmission, which has been measured as presynaptic release probability. Unlike originally proposed retrograde messengers, which are presumed to activate signaling cascades, changing the number of synaptic cell adhesion molecules can provide a way to change the efficacy of synaptic transmission. The effect will persist as long as a constant number of molecules exist, and does not require a mechanism to persistently alter biochemical signaling.

In the future, it is highly desired to elucidate the constructive process of synapse modification after LTP induction, from changes in synaptic cell adhesion molecules to rearrangements of presynaptic structures and vesicular release machineries. With such information in hand, we would then be able to truly understand pre- and postsynaptic roles in LTP.

Acknowledgments We thank Ms. Honor Hsin and Mr. John C. Howard for their comments on the manuscript. Y.H. was supported by grants from RIKEN, the National Institutes of Health (R01DA17310), and the Ellison Medical Foundation. K.F. is a recipient of a Special Postdoctoral Researchers Fellowship from RIKEN.

References

1. Conti R, Lisman J. The high variance of AMPA receptor- and NMDA receptor-mediated responses at single hippocampal synapses: evidence for multiquantal release. Proc Natl Acad Sci U S A 2003;100:4885–4890.
2. Matsuzaki M, Ellis-Davies GC, Nemoto T, Miyashita Y, Iino M, Kasai H. Dendritic spine geometry is critical for AMPA receptor expression in hippocampal CA1 pyramidal neurons. Nat Neurosci 2001;4:1086–1092.
3. Shepherd GM, Harris KM. Three-dimensional structure and composition of CA3–>CA1 axons in rat hippocampal slices: implications for presynaptic connectivity and compartmentalization. J Neurosci 1998;18:8300–8310.
4. Schikorski T, Stevens CF. Quantitative ultrastructural analysis of hippocampal excitatory synapses. J Neurosci 1997;17:5858–5867.
5. Matsuzaki M. Factors critical for the plasticity of dendritic spines and memory storage. Neurosci Res 2007;57:1–9.
6. Yamagata M, Sanes JR, Weiner JA. Synaptic adhesion molecules. Curr Opin Cell Biol 2003;15:621–632.
7. Bliss TV, Lømo T. Long-lasting potentiation of synaptic transmission in the dentate area of the anaesthetized rabbit following stimulation of the perforant path. J Physiol (Lond) 1973;232:331–356.
8. Malinow R, Malenka RC. AMPA receptor trafficking and synaptic plasticity. Annu Rev Neurosci 2002;25:103–126.
9. Malenka RC, Bear MF. LTP and LTD: an embarrassment of riches. Neuron 2004;44:5–21.
10. Futai K, Hayashi Y. Dynamism of postsynaptic proteins as the mechanism of synaptic plasticity. In: Hensch T, Fagiolini M, eds. Excitatory-inhibitory balance. New York: Kluwer Academic/Plenum Publishers, 2004:45–58.
11. Fitzsimonds RM, Poo MM. Retrograde signaling in the development and modification of synapses. Physiol Rev 1998;78:143–170.
12. Gribkoff VK, Lum-Ragan JT. Evidence for nitric oxide synthase inhibitor-sensitive and insensitive hippocampal synaptic potentiation. J Neurophysiol 1992;68:639–642.
13. Selig DK, Segal MR, Liao D, et al. Examination of the role of cGMP in long-term potentiation in the CA1 region of the hippocampus. Learn Mem 1996;3:42–48.
14. Kobayashi K, Ishii S, Kume K, Takahashi T, Shimizu T, Manabe T. Platelet-activating factor receptor is not required for long-term potentiation in the hippocampal CA1 region [In Process Citation]. Eur J Neurosci 1999;11:1313–1316.
15. Poss KD, Thomas MJ, Ebraldize AK, O'Dell TJ, Tonegawa S. Hippocampal long-term potentiation is normal in heme oxygenase-2 mutant mice. Neuron 1995;15:867–873.
16. Zakharenko SS, Patterson SL, Dragatsis I, et al. Presynaptic BDNF required for a presynaptic but not postsynaptic component of LTP at hippocampal CA1–CA3 synapses. Neuron 2003;39:975–990.
17. Choi S, Klingauf J, Tsien RW. Postfusional regulation of cleft glutamate concentration during LTP at "silent synapses." Nat Neurosci 2000;3:330–336.
18. Emptage NJ, Reid CA, Fine A, Bliss TV. Optical quantal analysis reveals a presynaptic component of LTP at hippocampal Schaffer-associational synapses. Neuron 2003;38:797–804.
19. Lauri SE, Palmer M, Segerstrale M, Vesikansa A, Taira T, Collingridge GL. Presynaptic mechanisms involved in the expression of STP and LTP at CA1 synapses in the hippocampus. Neuropharmacology 2007;52:1–11.
20. Wilson CJ, Groves PM, Fifková E. Monoaminergic synapses, including dendro-dendritic synapses in the rat substantia nigra. Exp Brain Res 1977;30:161–174.
21. Sun HY, Lyons SA, Dobrunz LE. Mechanisms of target-cell specific short-term plasticity at Schaffer collateral synapses onto interneurones versus pyramidal cells in juvenile rats. J Physiol 2005;568:815–840.

22. Reyes A, Lujan R, Rozov A, Burnashev N, Somogyi P, Sakmann B. Target-cell-specific facilitation and depression in neocortical circuits. Nat Neurosci 1998;1:279–285.

23. Shigemoto R, Kulik A, Roberts JD, et al. Target-cell-specific concentration of a metabotropic glutamate receptor in the presynaptic active zone. Nature 1996;381:523–525.

24. Pratt KG, Watt AJ, Griffith LC, Nelson SB, Turrigiano GG. Activity-dependent remodeling of presynaptic inputs by postsynaptic expression of activated CaMKII. Neuron 2003;39:269–281.

25. Kazama H, Morimoto-Tanifuji T, Nose A. Postsynaptic activation of calcium/calmodulin-dependent protein kinase II promotes coordinated pre- and postsynaptic maturation of Drosophila neuromuscular junctions. Neuroscience 2003;117:615–625.

26. Haghighi AP, McCabe BD, Fetter RD, Palmer JE, Hom S, Goodman CS. Retrograde control of synaptic transmission by postsynaptic CaMKII at the Drosophila neuromuscular junction. Neuron 2003;39:255–267.

27. Yoshihara M, Adolfsen B, Galle KT, Littleton JT. Retrograde signaling by Syt 4 induces presynaptic release and synapse-specific growth. Science 2005;310:858–863.

28. Takeichi M. The cadherin superfamily in neuronal connections and interactions. Nat Rev Neurosci 2007;8:11–20.

29. Wheelock MJ, Johnson KR. Cadherins as modulators of cellular phenotype. Annu Rev Cell Dev Biol 2003;19:207–235.

30. Takeichi M, Abe K. Synaptic contact dynamics controlled by cadherin and catenins. Trends Cell Biol 2005;15:216–221.

31. Bozdagi O, Valcin M, Poskanzer K, Tanaka H, Benson DL. Temporally distinct demands for classic cadherins in synapse formation and maturation. Mol Cell Neurosci 2004;27:509–521.

32. Jungling K, Eulenburg V, Moore R, Kemler R, Lessmann V, Gottmann K. N-cadherin transsynaptically regulates short-term plasticity at glutamatergic synapses in embryonic stem cell-derived neurons. J Neurosci 2006;26:6968–6978.

33. Kadowaki M, Nakamura S, Machon O, Krauss S, Radice GL, Takeichi M. N-cadherin mediates cortical organization in the mouse brain. Dev Biol 2007;304:22–33.

34. Bamji SX, Shimazu K, Kimes N, et al. Role of beta-catenin in synaptic vesicle localization and presynaptic assembly. Neuron 2003;40:719–731.

35. Murase S, Mosser E, Schuman EM. Depolarization drives beta-Catenin into neuronal spines promoting changes in synaptic structure and function. Neuron 2002;35:91–105.

36. Togashi H, Abe K, Mizoguchi A, Takaoka K, Chisaka O, Takeichi M. Cadherin regulates dendritic spine morphogenesis. Neuron 2002;35:77–89.

37. Abe K, Chisaka O, Van Roy F, Takeichi M. Stability of dendritic spines and synaptic contacts is controlled by alpha N-catenin. Nat Neurosci 2004;7:357–363.

38. Elia LP, Yamamoto M, Zang K, Reichardt LF. p120 catenin regulates dendritic spine and synapse development through Rho-family GTPases and cadherins. Neuron 2006;51:43–56.

39. Israely I, Costa RM, Xie CW, Silva AJ, Kosik KS, Liu X. Deletion of the neuron-specific protein delta-catenin leads to severe cognitive and synaptic dysfunction. Curr Biol 2004;14:1657–1663.

40. Manabe T, Togashi H, Uchida N, et al. Loss of cadherin-11 adhesion receptor enhances plastic changes in hippocampal synapses and modifies behavioral responses. Mol Cell Neurosci 2000;15:534–546.

41. Suzuki SC, Furue H, Koga K, et al. Cadherin-8 is required for the first relay synapses to receive functional inputs from primary sensory afferents for cold sensation. J Neurosci 2007;27:3466–3476.

42. Paradis S, Harrar DB, Lin Y, et al. An RNAi-based approach identifies molecules required for glutamatergic and GABAergic synapse development. Neuron 2007;53:217–232.

43. Nuriya M, Huganir RL. Regulation of AMPA receptor trafficking by N-cadherin. J Neurochem 2006;97:652–661.

44. Saglietti L, Dequidt C, Kamieniarz K, et al. Extracellular interactions between GluR2 and N-cadherin in spine regulation. Neuron 2007;54:461–477.

45. Ushkaryov YA, Petrenko AG, Geppert M, Südhof TC. Neurexins: synaptic cell surface proteins related to the alpha-latrotoxin receptor and laminin. Science 1992;257:50–56.

46. Craig AM, Kang Y. Neurexin-neuroligin signaling in synapse development. Curr Opin Neurobiol 2007;17:43–52.
47. Lise MF, El-Husseini A. The neuroligin and neurexin families: from structure to function at the synapse. Cell Mol Life Sci 2006;63:1833–1849.
48. Ichtchenko K, Hata Y, Nguyen T, et al. Neuroligin 1: a splice site-specific ligand for beta-neurexins. Cell 1995;81:435–443.
49. Boucard AA, Chubykin AA, Comoletti D, Taylor P, Südhof TC. A splice code for trans-synaptic cell adhesion mediated by binding of neuroligin 1 to alpha- and beta-neurexins. Neuron 2005;48:229–236.
50. Dean C, Dresbach T. Neuroligins and neurexins: linking cell adhesion, synapse formation and cognitive function. Trends Neurosci 2006;29:21–29.
51. Hirao K, Hata Y, Ide N, et al. A novel multiple PDZ domain-containing molecule interacting with N-methyl-D-aspartate receptors and neuronal cell adhesion proteins. J Biol Chem 1998;273:21105–21110.
52. Iida J, Hirabayashi S, Sato Y, Hata Y. Synaptic scaffolding molecule is involved in the synaptic clustering of neuroligin. Mol Cell Neurosci 2004;27:497–508.
53. Irie M, Hata Y, Takeuchi M, et al. Binding of neuroligins to PSD-95. Science 1997;277:1511–1515.
54. Meyer G, Varoqueaux F, Neeb A, Oschlies M, Brose N. The complexity of PDZ domain-mediated interactions at glutamatergic synapses: a case study on neuroligin. Neuropharmacology 2004;47:724–733.
55. Graf ER, Zhang X, Jin SX, Linhoff MW, Craig AM. Neurexins induce differentiation of GABA and glutamate postsynaptic specializations via neuroligins. Cell 2004;119:1013–1026.
56. Dean C, Scholl FG, Choih J, et al. Neurexin mediates the assembly of presynaptic terminals. Nat Neurosci 2003;6:708–716.
57. Levinson JN, Chery N, Huang K, et al. Neuroligins mediate excitatory and inhibitory synapse formation: involvement of PSD-95 and neurexin-1beta in neuroligin-induced synaptic specificity. J Biol Chem 2005;280:17312–17319.
58. Scheiffele P, Fan J, Choih J, Fetter R, Serafini T. Neuroligin expressed in nonneuronal cells triggers presynaptic development in contacting axons. Cell 2000;101:657–669.
59. Varoqueaux F, Aramuni G, Rawson RL, et al. Neuroligins determine synapse maturation and function. Neuron 2006;51:741–754.
60. Futai K, Kim MJ, Hashikawa T, Scheiffele P, Sheng M, Hayashi Y. Retrograde modulation of presynaptic release probability through signaling mediated by PSD-95–neuroligin. Nat Neurosci 2007;10:186–195.
61. Boucard AA, Chubykin AA, Comoletti D, Taylor P, Sudhof TC. A splice code for trans-synaptic cell adhesion mediated by binding of neuroligin 1 to alpha- and beta-neurexins. Neuron 2005;48:229–236.
62. Buchert M, Schneider S, Meskenaite V, et al. The junction-associated protein AF-6 interacts and clusters with specific Eph receptor tyrosine kinases at specialized sites of cell-cell contact in the brain. J Cell Biol 1999;144:361–371.
63. Torres R, Firestein BL, Dong H, et al. PDZ proteins bind, cluster, and synaptically colocalize with Eph receptors and their ephrin ligands. Neuron 1998;21:1453–1463.
64. Lin D, Gish GD, Songyang Z, Pawson T. The carboxyl terminus of B class ephrins constitutes a PDZ domain binding motif. J Biol Chem 1999;274:3726–3733.
65. Bruckner K, Pablo Labrador J, Scheiffele P, Herb A, Seeburg PH, Klein R. EphrinB ligands recruit GRIP family PDZ adaptor proteins into raft membrane microdomains. Neuron 1999;22:511–524.
66. Murai KK, Nguyen LN, Irie F, Yamaguchi Y, Pasquale EB. Control of hippocampal dendritic spine morphology through ephrin-A3/EphA4 signaling. Nat Neurosci 2003;6:153–160.
67. Martone ME, Holash JA, Bayardo A, Pasquale EB, Ellisman MH. Immunolocalization of the receptor tyrosine kinase EphA4 in the adult rat central nervous system. Brain Res 1997;771:238–250.
68. Henderson JT, Georgiou J, Jia Z, et al. The receptor tyrosine kinase EphB2 regulates NMDA-dependent synaptic function. Neuron 2001;32:1041–1056.

69. Grunwald IC, Korte M, Wolfer D, et al. Kinase-independent requirement of EphB2 receptors in hippocampal synaptic plasticity. Neuron 2001;32:1027–1040.

70. Grunwald IC, Korte M, Adelmann G, et al. Hippocampal plasticity requires postsynaptic ephrinBs. Nat Neurosci 2004;7:33–40.

71. Liebl DJ, Morris CJ, Henkemeyer M, Parada LF. mRNA expression of ephrins and Eph receptor tyrosine kinases in the neonatal and adult mouse central nervous system. J Neurosci Res 2003;71:7–22.

72. Armstrong JN, Saganich MJ, Xu NJ, Henkemeyer M, Heinemann SF, Contractor A. B-ephrin reverse signaling is required for NMDA-independent long-term potentiation of mossy fibers in the hippocampus. J Neurosci 2006;26:3474–3481.

73. Contractor A, Rogers C, Maron C, Henkemeyer M, Swanson GT, Heinemann SF. Trans-synaptic Eph receptor-ephrin signaling in hippocampal mossy fiber LTP. Science 2002; 296: 1864–1869.

74. Biederer T, Sara Y, Mozhayeva M, et al. SynCAM, a synaptic adhesion molecule that drives synapse assembly. Science 2002;297:1525–1531.

75. Sara Y, Biederer T, Atasoy D, et al. Selective capability of SynCAM and neuroligin for functional synapse assembly. J Neurosci 2005;25:260–270.

76. Regalado MP, Terry-Lorenzo RT, Waites CL, Garner CC, Malenka RC. Transsynaptic signaling by postsynaptic synapse-associated protein 97. J Neurosci 2006;26:2343–2357.

77. Sala C, Piech V, Wilson NR, Passafaro M, Liu G, Sheng M. Regulation of dendritic spine morphology and synaptic function by Shank and Homer. Neuron 2001;31:115–130.

78. Otmakhov N, Tao-Cheng JH, Carpenter S, et al. Persistent accumulation of calcium/calmodulin-dependent protein kinase II in dendritic spines after induction of NMDA receptor-dependent chemical long-term potentiation. J Neurosci 2004;24:9324–9331.

79. Okamoto K, Nagai T, Miyawaki A, Hayashi Y. Rapid and persistent modulation of actin dynamics regulates postsynaptic reorganization underlying bidirectional plasticity. Nat Neurosci 2004;7:1104–1112.

80. Olsen O, Moore KA, Nicoll RA, Bredt DS. Synaptic transmission regulated by a presynaptic MALS/Liprin-alpha protein complex. Curr Opin Cell Biol 2006;18:223–227.

81. Zordan MA, Massironi M, Ducato MG, et al. Drosophila CAKI/CMG protein, a homolog of human CASK, is essential for regulation of neurotransmitter vesicle release. J Neurophysiol 2005;94:1074–1083.

82. Atasoy D, Schoch S, Ho A, et al. Deletion of CASK in mice is lethal and impairs synaptic function. Proc Natl Acad Sci U S A 2007;104:2525–2530.

83. Christie JM, Jahr CE. Multivesicular release at Schaffer collateral-CA1 hippocampal synapses. J Neurosci 2006;26:210–216.

84. Tong G, Jahr CE. Multivesicular release from excitatory synapses of cultured hippocampal neurons. Neuron 1994;12:51–59.

85. Liu G, Choi S, Tsien RW. Variability of neurotransmitter concentration and nonsaturation of postsynaptic AMPA receptors at synapses in hippocampal cultures and slices. Neuron 1999; 22:395–409.

Chapter 16
Differential Regulation of Small Clear Vesicles and Large Dense-Core Vesicles

Tao Xu and Pingyong Xu

Contents

Abstract The many differences in the properties of small clear vesicles (SCVs) and large dense-core vesicles (LDCVs) suggest that these two classes of secretory organelles employ different sets of molecules in exocytosis. Relatively little is known, however, about the factors that differentially participate in SCV and LDCV release. This chapter briefly reviews the differences between SCV and LDCV exocytosis, and discusses key molecules that are possibly involved in the differential regulation of the trafficking, docking, priming, and fusion of SCVs and LDCVs.

Keywords Small clear vesicle (SCV), large dense-core vesicle (LDCV), exocytosis, endocytosis, docking, priming, tethering, fusion, vesicle biogenesis, vesicle translocation.

Tao Xu
National Laboratory of Biomacromolecules, Institute of Biophysics, Chinese Academy of Sciences, Beijing 100101, China
e-mail: xutao@sun5.ibp.ac.cn

Pingyong Xu
National Laboratory of Biomacromolecules, Institute of Biophysics, Chinese Academy of Sciences, Beijing 100101, China
e-mail: pyxu19742@yahoo.com

Z.-W. Wang (ed.) *Molecular Mechanisms of Neurotransmitter Release,*
© Humana Press 2008 a part of Springer Science+Business Media, LLC

Neurons communicate with one another through the release of molecules from synaptic small clear vesicles (SCVs) and large dense-core vesicles (LDCVs, also called dense-core granules). Classic neurotransmitters are packaged in SCVs and undergo fast phasic release at active zones of the nerve terminal. In contrast, secretory proteins, specifically neuropeptides, are synthesized in the cell body and condensed in LDCVs. LDCVs can be released in the soma as well as in the nerve terminals away from active zones. Initial formation of immature LDCVs occurs at the *trans*-Golgi network (TGN). Once formed, immature LDCVs must be processed and remodeled to form mature LDCVs, which will then be transported to underneath the plasma membrane waiting to be released. SCVs, however, can be locally supplied in the synaptic terminal via endocytic pathways and be reloaded by vesicular transporters. Furthermore, SCVs and LDCVs differ in speeds and latencies for exocytosis upon Ca^{2+} stimulation.

Apparently, SCVs and LDCVs are distinct organelles responsible for different types of neurosecretion. Surprisingly, despite the differences, the exocytosis of SCVs and LDCVs share conserved features. For example, both SCVs and LDCVs are triggered to release by Ca^{2+}, and synaptotagmin I has been shown to be required for the Ca^{2+} sensing of both types of release (1). Likewise, the same set of soluble *N*-ethylmaleimide–sensitive factor attachment receptor (SNARE) protein is used by both SCVs and LDCVs (2,3). Furthermore, Munc18 proteins, which are involved in the docking as well as priming of vesicles, are dispensable for both SCV and LDCV exocytosis (4). Finally, both SCV and LDCV exocytosis are sensitive to various regulations, such as Ca^{2+}-dependent priming (5,6), protein kinase C (PKC)- and PKA-dependent facilitation (7–10), etc.

Despite the ever-increasing list of factors that are involved in the transportation, docking, priming, and fusion of regulated exocytosis, relatively little is known about the factors that differentially participate in SCV and LDCV exocytosis. This chapter is not intended to discuss the conserved molecular mechanisms that are shared by SCVs and LDCVs in their exocytotic pathway. Readers interested in this aspect may refer to other chapters in this book for more details. We limit our discussion here to our current understanding of factors that are differentially used by SCVs and LDCVs.

The Exocytotic Pathway

Biogenesis

The biogenesis of SCVs and LDCVs is a complex orchestration of events culminating in a vesicle population responsible for the uptake, storage, and regulated secretion of neurotransmitters and neuropeptides. Due to space limitations, we only briefly discuss the major differences in the biogenesis of LDCVs and SCVs here. Readers are referred to several reviews (11–13) for in-depth information.

In order for efficient storage of large amounts of peptides and other cargoes in an osmotically inert form, the secretory peptides are highly condensed, which gives rise to the dense-core appearance visualized under electron microscopy. The LDCVs in most cell types represent a distinct class of organelle in the biosynthetic pathway. However, in various hemopoietic cells and certain other cell types, LDCVs share several features with lysosomes and possess lysosomal markers (14), and hence are also called secretory lysosomes. This suggests that a convergence of biosynthetic and endocytic lysosomal biogenesis is required for LDCV formation in such cells. The mechanistic basis of LDCV biogenesis has not been demonstrated. Initial formation of immature LDCVs occurs at the *trans*-Golgi network (TGN). It is less clear whether LDCV formation from TGN requires a coat-driven budding process. It is hypothesized that membrane deformation may result from the aggregation of secretory proteins in the TGN. The granin family, a unique group of acidic, soluble secretory proteins including chromogranins and secretogranins, is thought to be essential for this process. Granins tend to bind Ca^{2+} with low affinity but high capacity and then aggregate *in vitro* at low pH in the presence of Ca^{2+}. The aggregation of granins may allow wrapping of the TGN membrane around the forming aggregate. It has been shown that downregulation of chromogranin A in PC12 cells reduces LDCV number and expression of chromogranin A in fibroblasts induces the formation of dense-core vesicles of around 100 nm in diameter (15). Budding granules must subsequently be pinched off from TGN to form immature LDCVs. Depletion of cholesterol appears to arrest LDCV biogenesis at a late stage with dense-core buds observed at the TGN (16). It has been shown that dynamin II may control the LDCV formation in the final scission process at the TGN (17). Once formed, immature LDCVs must be further processed to form mature LDCVs by fusing with other immature LDCVs and removing missorted material via budding. For example, syntaxin 6 is required for immature LDCV fusion (18), and is removed from mature LDCVs by budding of adaptor protein AP-1/clathrin-coated vesicles (19). Interestingly, synaptotagmin IV present on immature LDCVs is thought to inhibit the exocytotic Ca^{2+} sensor synaptotagmin I (20), with its removal during maturation enabling normal Ca^{2+}-dependent release (21).

In contrast to LDCVs, which are de novo synthesized at the TGN, SCVs can be supplied locally in the synaptic terminal, that is, independent of the endoplasmic reticulum (ER) and Golgi complex machineries, in order to sustain prolonged synaptic activity at high frequency. New vesicles need to be endowed with all the molecular components, which make them capable of efficient coupling between stimulus and neurotransmission. The molecular components of SCVs, however, are thought to be synthesized in the cell body and transported to the nerve terminal. It has been shown that synaptophysin, a major membrane protein of SCVs, is transported down the axon from the TGN to the nerve terminal via membrane carriers larger than SCVs (22). It has been revealed that motor proteins of the kinesin superfamily mediate anterograde axonal transport. Following its first cell surface appearance, newly synthesized synaptophysin undergoes multiple cycles of endocytosis-exocytosis until it eventually becomes segregated into SCVs. It remains to be investigated whether other newly synthesized SCV membrane proteins, such as SV2, synaptobrevin, and vesicular transporter, take the same routing pathway and to what extent this model can be applied to SCV biogenesis in general.

Current models of synaptic vesicle biogenesis suggest that at least two pathways exist for the formation of SCVs: either indirectly via an intermediate endosomal compartment or directly from the plasma membrane. Several lines of evidence point to the involvement of an intracellular compartment, most likely an endosomal intermediate, in the formation of SCVs (23,24). It has been shown that SCV proteins are first colocalized with transferrin receptors after endocytosis from the plasma membrane, subsequently sorted away from non-SCV proteins at early endosomes, and become selectively enriched in tubular extensions that function as donor compartments for the budding of new SCVs. The budding of SCVs has been shown to require adenosine diphosphate (ADP) ribosylation factor-1 (ARF1) and adaptor protein complex AP3, but not clathrin (25–27). Another member of the ARF guanosine triphosphatase (GTPase) family, ARF6, has also been implicated in SCV biogenesis (28). An alternative pathway of SCV biogenesis has been proposed to derive directly from a special compartment distinct from the transferrin receptor-containing endosome and to be connected to the plasma membrane via narrow continuity (29). Unlike the biogenesis of SCVs from endosomes, the formation of plasma membrane–derived SCVs uses the adaptor protein AP2 instead of AP3 and requires clathrin and dynamin but not guanosine triphosphate (GTP) hydrolysis by ARF1 (27,30). The severe phenotype observed at synapses of *Drosophila* α-adaptin (a subunit of AP2) mutants compared to the relatively mild neuronal phenotype of AP3 null mice seems to imply that the AP2 pathway is more relevant for SV formation than the AP3 pathway in certain neurons (31,32).

The SCVs that go through the endocytic recycling step are those that release their entire content through full collapse into the presynaptic membrane during exocytosis. However, SCVs may also release neurotransmitters by forming a transient fusion pore with the plasma membrane without losing its identity and rapidly returning to the readily releasable pool (RRP) for reuse. This mode of exo-endocytotic cycle is termed "kiss-and-run" (33). As an alternative to the kiss-and-run mode, an even faster recycling mechanism is thought to occur in which SCVs stay at the release sites after transient open of the fusion pore without undocking from the active zone, hence named "kiss-and-stay" (34). Kiss-and-run and its variation kiss-and-stay are thought to allow rapid and repeated reuse and to preserve the ability of terminals to maintain synaptic transmission during high frequency firings. However, the significance of the kiss-and-run endocytosis by SCVs is still debated (35–38). Currently the molecular mechanism underlying the choice between full fusion and kiss-and-run is unknown. Overexpression of different domains of synaptotagmin I and IV has been shown to control the choice between full fusion and kiss-and-run. After full fusion, the membrane components of LDCVs are thought to be transported en route back to the TGN where LDCVs are generated, possibly passing through an endosomal sorting compartment (39). However, recent experiments also suggest a kiss-and-stay (also called "cavicapture") mode of fusion for LDCVs (40), implying that the membrane components of LDCVs can be retreated intact after fusion. It is unclear how LDCVs could be restrained in the open configuration without collapsing into the plasma membrane and what triggers the closure of the fusion pore.

Translocation

Once SCVs and LDCVs are formed, they have to undergo sequential steps before they finally fuse with the plasma membrane. These functionally distinct sequential steps involve physical translocation of vesicles to the subplasmalemmal region of the cell, tethering and then docking at release sites on the plasma membrane, conversion to a fusion competent state after priming, and finally triggered membrane fusion.

Rab proteins comprise the largest family within the Ras superfamily of small GTPase. Rab proteins increase from 11 members in yeast to 63 members in human, closely correlating the evolution with increasing endomembrane complexity. Individual Rab proteins are localized to distinct, characteristic organelles, suggesting that each regulates a particular trafficking step of a particular vesicle type. A wide variety of biologic activities arises from the combinatorial interactions of a given Rab with a wide array of downstream effectors and their respective binding partners. Rab effectors have been shown to be involved in the initial tethering of vesicles to target membrane, in the movement along microtubule via motor proteins, and in actin-based mobility through interactions with class V myosins (41). Hence, SCVs and LDCVs are likely to use different Rab proteins to coordinate translocation along different tracks.

Recent work has established an important role for Rab27 in secretory lysosome and LDCV exocytosis in melanocytes, cytotoxic T lymphocytes, and neuroendocrine cells. In melanocytes, Rab27a is localized to the pigment-containing melanosome granules, which is a type of secretory lysosome, and is essential for their transportation to the cell periphery. The Rab27a effector melanophilin links Rab27a-positive granules to the actin motor myosin-Va. Without myosin-Va-dependent capture of these organelles on actin filaments, melanosomes cannot be transferred to the cell periphery. In addition, mice and patients with mutations in Rab27a also lack the ability to secrete from the lytic granules of cytotoxic T lymphocytes (42,43). Rab27 has also been implicated in regulation of LDCV exocytosis in various endocrine and neuroendocrine cells (44,45).

The SCVs contain members of at least three families of Rab proteins: Rab3 (Rab3A, 3B, 3C, and 3D), Rab5, and Rab11 (46). Of these, Rab3 proteins are the most abundant. Rab3A alone accounts for ~25% of the total Rab GTP binding in brain. Rab3A has been shown to regulate neurotransmission by recruiting SCVs into the RRP during repetitive stimulation (47). In a genetic analysis of Rab3 proteins, it was shown that Rab3 is required for survival in mice and that the four Rab3 proteins are functionally redundant in this role. Furthermore, Rab3 proteins are not in themselves essential for SCV exocytosis but function to modulate the basic release machinery. Unlike the role of Rab27 in the translocation of LDCVs, it is unclear at present whether Rab3 participates in the translocation of SCVs to underneath the terminal membrane. Rab3 mutants in *Caenorhabditis elegans* are viable but demonstrate less SCVs close to the active zone, suggesting a role for Rab3 in SCV translocation or tethering (48).

Tethering/Docking

Probably the best-characterized Rab effectors are involved in the initial tethering of vesicles to target membranes. These include the exocyst complex (Sec4 effector in yeast exocytosis) (49,50), the HOPS protein complex (Ypt7 effector in transport to the vacuole) (51,52), p115 (Rab1 effector in Golgi transport) (53), and EEA1 (Rab5 effector in endocytosis) (54,55). It is thus perceptible that Rab27 and Rab3, together with their specific effectors, could function in the tethering/docking of LDCVs and SCVs to the plasma membrane. Analysis of ashen mice, which are characterized by a single point mutation that prevents the proper splicing of Rab27a, has revealed involvement of Rab27a in the membrane tethering/docking step of the LDCVs in pancreatic β cells (56) and of secretory lysosomes in cytotoxic T-lymphocytes (42,43). The synaptotagmin-like protein (Slp) family, which includes Slp1/JFC1, Slp2-a, Slp3-a, Slp4/granuphilin, Slp5, and rabphilin, has been identified as one group of Rab27 effectors. The members in Slp family contain an N-terminal Rab27-binding Slp homology domain (SHD) and C-terminal tandem C2 domains. Although the SHD of Slp4-a interacts with three distinct Rab species (Rab3, Rab8, and Rab27) *in vitro*, Slp4-a functions as a Rab27A effector during dense-core vesicle (DCV) exocytosis under physiologic conditions (57). In Slp4/granuphilin knockout mice, a decrease in the number of plasma membrane-docked insulin-containing vesicles has been observed. Despite a decrease in docking, however, Slp4/granuphilin-deficiency enhances insulin secretion. Biochemical analysis has shown that Slp4 interacts with Munc18-1 or Munc18-1 and Syntaxin-1 complex. Thus it has been proposed that Slp4 negatively regulates LDCV exocytosis by forcing the vesicle into a nonfunctional docked state. Unlike Slp4, the other four Slps, including Slp1, 2, 3, and 5, have been reported to specifically interact with Rab27 and do not interact with other Rabs, including Rab3. Slp2 is most abundantly expressed in the gastric surface mucous cells. Analysis of Slp2-a mutant mice has revealed a reduced number of mucus granules at the apical plasma membrane in the mucous cells, probably due to reduced docking. Thus, it has been hypothesized that Rab27 and its effector Slp proteins may participate in putative docking machineries in different types of cells where they are endogenously expressed (58). However, it is not clear whether all members of the Slp family participate in the docking, or whether Slp proteins participate only in a nonproductive docking as suggested by the phenotype of Slp4-deficiency. Rabphilin had long been recognized as the effector of Rab3 as well as Rab27. Deletion of rabphilin produced no detectable effect in mice (59) and only a mild phenotype in *C. elegans* (60). A recent study suggests that the binding of rabphilin to synaptosome-associated protein of 25 kDa (SNAP-25) accelerates the exocytosis of SVs only after the RRP has been exhausted (61). Apparently, the exact functions of Slp proteins and how Rab27/Rab3 mediates the docking of vesicles to the plasma membrane remain to be further explored.

Priming

After docking at the plasma membrane, vesicles undergo a priming step to prepare them for fusion in response to Ca^{2+} signal. The priming of vesicles into a fusion-competent state is thought to involve, at least in part, the assembly of *trans*-SNARE complexes (62,63). The precise mechanism by which priming is catalyzed remains to be identified. Studies of knockout mutants of worms, flies, and mice have demonstrated an essential role of Munc13 proteins in SCV priming. The requirement of Munc13 proteins for LDCV exocytosis, however, is less clear. Although exogenously expressed Munc13-1 strongly stimulates LDCV secretion in chromaffin cells, LDCV secretion remains relatively normal in chromaffin cells isolated from Munc13-1 knockouts. Our recent study in pancreatic β cells suggests that Munc13-1 is required in accelerated priming of LDCVs. However, the basal maintenance of fusion competent RRP does not seem to require Munc13-1. The involvement of Munc13 proteins in neuropeptide release from dense-core vesicles has also been confirmed in *unc-13* mutants of *C. elegans* (64).

Besides rabphilin, RIM has been identified as another effector of Rab3 (65). RIM-deficient mouse and *C. elegans* (*unc-10* mutant) exhibit reduced synaptic transmission, defects in synaptic plasticity but normal SCV docking (66,67), suggesting a postdocking role for RIM in SCV exocytosis. RIM forms a tripartite complex with Munc13-1 and Rab3 (68). Given the RIM-Munc13 interaction, it is plausible that RIM may function in SCV priming. Ca^{2+}-dependent activator protein for secretion (CAPS) was identified as an essential protein required for LDCV exocytosis (69). CAPS is highly conserved in evolution: a single CAPS isoform (UNC-31) is found in *C. elegans*, whereas two closely related isoforms are expressed in vertebrates: CAPS1 and CAPS2. CAPS contains a conserved MH domain, which is also found in members of the Munc13 family. CAPS appears to be required for LDCV but not SCV exocytosis (70,71). A recent study, however, demonstrated that CAPS1 is probably involved in the uptake or storage of monoamines into LDCVs, but not in the Ca^{2+}-triggered LDCV exocytosis per se. This study, however, has not addressed the redundancy of CAPS2, which is expressed at eightfold higher levels than CAPS1 in adrenal glands. By contrast, recent experiments using *unc-31* mutant of *C. elegans* (64,72) and our recent paper (73) clearly demonstrated a requirement of CAPS for LDCV exocytosis. Understanding the mechanism of action of CAPS should provide insight into key differences between SCV and LDCV exocytosis.

Fusion

It is well documented that the latencies to fusion and fusion rates for Ca^{2+}-triggered SCV and LDCV exocytosis are quite different. Estimate of the latencies to fusion, which is the time difference between instantaneous elevation of Ca^{2+} and the detection of fusion, provides an indication of the binding rate of Ca^{2+} to the Ca^{2+} sensor and the execution time for fusion events. The latencies to fusion are estimated to be ~10 times shorter for SCV exocytosis (0.06 to 1.5 ms) (74–76) than those for LDCV exocytosis (3 to 50 ms) (77–80). The exocytotic fusion rates of RRP vesicles, measured by the exponential fits for the pool depletion, are also notably shorter for SCV exocytosis than those for LDCV exocytosis. Furthermore, the dependence of exocytosis on Ca^{2+} also differs between SCV and LDCV exocytosis. It is suggested that a fourth- or higher order relationship between Ca^{2+} and SCV exocytosis is necessary for synchronizing neurotransmitter release with presynaptic Ca^{2+} influx, whereas hormone and peptide release may require a shallower Ca^{2+}-dependence (74, 76, 80–82). These differences suggest that, even after vesicles are docked and primed, the Ca^{2+}-triggered fusion machineries may differ between SCVs and LDCVs.

Current evidence indicates that synaptotagmin proteins are the key molecular components that confer Ca^{2+} sensing of membrane fusion (83, 84). At least 16 isoforms of synaptotagmins have been identified in mammalians. It is speculated that differential localization of synaptotagmins to different types of vesicles may form fusion mechanisms with various Ca^{2+}-sensitivities. Synaptotagmin I is best characterized as an abundant synaptic vesicle-associated protein essential for rapid synchronous synaptic vesicle exocytosis. Synaptotagmin I also exists on LDCVs in neuroendocrine and endocrine cells, and has been shown to be involved in Ca^{2+}-dependent LDCV exocytosis. Synaptotagmin IX has been postulated to function as a major Ca^{2+} sensor for LDCV exocytosis in neuroendocrine cells. Synaptotagmin IX represents a close homologue to synaptotagmin I on sequence alignments. Nevertheless, the unique binding properties of synaptotagmin IX with Ca^{2+}, phospholipid, and SNARE complex suggest a substantially different biologic role from that of synaptotagmin I. Because the presence of multiple synaptotagmin genes (85) and the existence of multiple synaptotagmin isoforms on single vesicles (86), it remains a challenge to demonstrate whether and how synaptotagmin compositions confer the different Ca^{2+}-sensing properties of SCV and LDCV fusion.

Membrane fusion upon exocytosis requires the formation of a fusion pore, which connects the vesicle lumen and the extracellular fluid. The fusion pore represents a pivotal intermediate that might control the amount of release and that can be subjected to physiologic regulation. Although our understanding of the composition of fusion pores and dynamics of fusion pore dilation are quite limited, it is possible that the mechanisms for fusion pore formation differ between SCVs and LDCVs. It has been estimated that the conductance of SCV fusion pores is 11 times smaller than that of LDCV fusion pores (87). It is also noted that the so-called prespike "foot" is absent in amperometric recording for SCV exocytosis, which is present in many LDCV exocytotic events (88). These differences suggest that the fusion pores formed by SCVs and LDCVs also has a different molecular composition. It should be mentioned that synaptotagmins not only serve as the Ca^{2+} sensors for exocytosis, but also are postulated to function in the formation, dilation, and closure of fusion pore.

Regulation

Both SCV and LDCV exocytosis are subjected to regulation by second messenger pathways. A large number of studies on many different cell types have implicated protein phosphorylation in the control of regulated exocytosis. PKA and PKC have been shown to enhance triggered exocytosis in essentially all cell types examined including neurons, neuroendocrine cells, endocrine cells, platelets, and so on. An array of exocytotic proteins has been identified as the substrates for PKA and PKC *in vitro*, and to a lesser extent *in vivo*. Because of the apparent co-localization of SCVs and LDCVs in the same neuron, it is unclear whether the specificity of regulation is achieved by activation of different isoforms of protein kinases or by spatial-restricted activation of the same protein kinase. A recent study in *C. elegans* has shed light on how the specificity of regulation is achieved. The PKC-1 protein of *C. elegans*, which is an orthologue of vertebrate PKCε and PKCη isoforms, has been shown to regulate exocytosis of neuropeptide-containing DCVs in *C. elegans* motor neurons. By contrast, SCV release occurred normally in *pkc-1* mutants. Similar neuropeptide secretion defects of the *pkc-1* mutants were found in mutants lacking *unc-31* (encoding the protein CAPS) or *unc-13* (encoding Munc13). This finding suggests that it is likely that different isoforms of PKC may differentially regulate SCV and LDCV exocytosis, which adds another layer of regulation of these two types of secretory organelles to fulfill their distinct physiologic functions.

Conclusion

The last decade has seen a remarkable explosion in our knowledge of the many proteins that are required for the regulated exocytosis and that regulate the process. It is now acknowledged that LDCV exocytosis occurs through mechanisms with many aspects in common with SCV exocytosis and most likely uses the same basic protein components. Further studies are expected to reveal the factors that contribute to the differences in the biogenesis, trafficking pathway, docking/priming, Ca^{2+}-triggered fusion, as well as regulation by second messengers, of SCVs and LDCVs.

References

1. Voets T, Moser T, Lund PE, et al. Intracellular calcium dependence of large dense-core vesicle exocytosis in the absence of synaptotagmin I. Proc Natl Acad Sci USA 2001;98(20): 11680–11685.
2. Jena BP. Cell secretion and membrane fusion. Domest Anim Endocrinol 2005;29(1):145–165.
3. Sorensen JB. SNARE complexes prepare for membrane fusion. Trends Neurosci 2005; 28(9):453–455.

4. Toonen RF. Role of Munc18–1 in synaptic vesicle and large dense-core vesicle secretion. Biochem Soc Trans 2003;31(pt 4):848–850.

5. Schneggenburger R, Neher E. Presynaptic calcium and control of vesicle fusion. Curr Opin Neurobiol 2005;15(3):266–274.

6. von Ruden L, Neher E. A Ca-dependent early step in the release of catecholamines from adrenal chromaffin cells. Science 1993;262(5136):1061–1065.

7. Chen C, Regehr WG. The mechanism of cAMP-mediated enhancement at a cerebellar synapse. J Neurosci 1997;17(22):8687–8694.

8. Gillis KD, Mossner R, Neher E. Protein kinase C enhances exocytosis from chromaffin cells by increasing the size of the readily releasable pool of secretory granules. Neuron 1996;16(6):1209–1220.

9. Stevens CF, Sullivan JM. Regulation of the readily releasable vesicle pool by protein kinase C. Neuron 1998;21(4):885–893.

10. Waters J, Smith SJ. Phorbol esters potentiate evoked and spontaneous release by different presynaptic mechanisms. J Neurosci 2000;20(21):7863–7870.

11. Bonanomi D, Benfenati F, Valtorta F. Protein sorting in the synaptic vesicle life cycle. Prog Neurobiol 2006;80(4):177–217.

12. Burgoyne RD, Morgan A. Secretory granule exocytosis. Physiol Rev 2003;83(2):581–632.

13. Hannah MJ, Schmidt AA, Huttner WB. Synaptic vesicle biogenesis. Annu Rev Cell Dev Biol 1999;15:733–798.

14. Blott EJ, Griffiths GM. Secretory lysosomes. Nat Rev Mol Cell Biol 2002;3(2):122–131.

15. Kim T, Tao-Cheng JH, Eiden LE, Loh YP. Chromogranin A, an "on/off" switch controlling dense-core secretory granule biogenesis. Cell 2001;106(4):499–509.

16. Wang Y, Thiele C, Huttner WB. Cholesterol is required for the formation of regulated and constitutive secretory vesicles from the trans-Golgi network. Traffic 2000;1(12):952–962.

17. Yang Z, Li H, Chai Z, et al. Dynamin II regulates hormone secretion in neuroendocrine cells. J Biol Chem 2001;276(6):4251–4260.

18. Wendler F, Page L, Urbe S, Tooze SA. Homotypic fusion of immature secretory granules during maturation requires syntaxin 6. Mol Biol Cell 2001;12(6):1699–1709.

19. Klumperman J, Kuliawat R, Griffith JM, Geuze HJ, Arvan P. Mannose 6-phosphate receptors are sorted from immature secretory granules via adaptor protein AP-1, clathrin, and syntaxin 6–positive vesicles. J Cell Biol 1998;141(2):359–371.

20. Littleton JT, Serano TL, Rubin GM, Ganetzky B, Chapman ER. Synaptic function modulated by changes in the ratio of synaptotagmin I and IV. Nature 1999;400(6746):757–760.

21. Eaton BA, Haugwitz M, Lau D, Moore HP. Biogenesis of regulated exocytotic carriers in neuroendocrine cells. J Neurosci 2000;20(19):7334–7344.

22. Regnier-Vigouroux A, Tooze SA, Huttner WB. Newly synthesized synaptophysin is transported to synaptic-like microvesicles via constitutive secretory vesicles and the plasma membrane. EMBO J 1991;10(12):3589–3601.

23. Clift-O'Grady L, Linstedt AD, Lowe AW, Grote E, Kelly RB. Biogenesis of synaptic vesicle-like structures in a pheochromocytoma cell line PC-12. J Cell Biol 1990;110(5):1693–1703.

24. Bauerfeind R, Huttner WB. Biogenesis of constitutive secretory vesicles, secretory granules and synaptic vesicles. Curr Opin Cell Biol 1993;5(4):628–635.

25. Salem N, Faundez V, Horng JT, Kelly RB. A v-SNARE participates in synaptic vesicle formation mediated by the AP3 adaptor complex. Nat Neurosci 1998;1(7):551–556.

26. Faundez V, Horng JT, Kelly RB. ADP ribosylation factor 1 is required for synaptic vesicle budding in PC12 cells. J Cell Biol 1997;138(3):505–515.

27. Shi G, Faundez V, Roos J, Dell'Angelica EC, Kelly RB. Neuroendocrine synaptic vesicles are formed in vitro by both clathrin-dependent and clathrin-independent pathways. J Cell Biol 1998;143(4):947–955.

28. Powelka AM, Buckley KM. Expression of ARF6 mutants in neuroendocrine cells suggests a role for ARF6 in synaptic vesicle biogenesis. FEBS Lett 2001;501(1):47–50.

29. Schmidt A, Hannah MJ, Huttner WB. Synaptic-like microvesicles of neuroendocrine cells originate from a novel compartment that is continuous with the plasma membrane and devoid of transferrin receptor. J Cell Biol 1997;137(2):445–458.
30. Shupliakov O, Ottersen OP, Storm-Mathisen J, Brodin L. Glial and neuronal glutamine pools at glutamatergic synapses with distinct properties. Neuroscience 1997;77(4):1201–1212.
31. Gonzalez-Gaitan M, Jackle H. Role of Drosophila alpha-adaptin in presynaptic vesicle recycling. Cell 1997;88(6):767–776.
32. Kantheti P, Qiao X, Diaz ME, et al. Mutation in AP-3 delta in the mocha mouse links endosomal transport to storage deficiency in platelets, melanosomes, and synaptic vesicles. Neuron 1998;21(1):111–122.
33. Fesce R, Grohovaz F, Valtorta F, Meldolesi J. Neurotransmitter release: fusion or 'kiss-and-run'? Trends Cell Biol 1994;4(1):1–4.
34. Sudhof TC. The synaptic vesicle cycle. Annu Rev Neurosci 2004;27:509–547.
35. Li Z, Burrone J, Tyler WJ, Hartman KN, Albeanu DF, Murthy VN. Synaptic vesicle recycling studied in transgenic mice expressing synaptopHluorin. Proc Natl Acad Sci USA 2005;102 (17):6131–6136.
36. Dickman DK, Horne JA, Meinertzhagen IA, Schwarz TL. A slowed classical pathway rather than kiss-and-run mediates endocytosis at synapses lacking synaptojanin and endophilin. Cell 2005;123(3):521–533.
37. Wienisch M, Klingauf J. Vesicular proteins exocytosed and subsequently retrieved by compensatory endocytosis are nonidentical. Nat Neurosci 2006;9(8):1019–1027.
38. He L, Wu XS, Mohan R, Wu LG. Two modes of fusion pore opening revealed by cell-attached recordings at a synapse. Nature 2006;444(7115):102–105.
39. Tooze SA, Stinchcombe JC. Biogenesis of secretory granules. Semin Cell Biol 1992;3 (5):357–366.
40. Taraska JW, Perrais D, Ohara-Imaizumi M, Nagamatsu S, Almers W. Secretory granules are recaptured largely intact after stimulated exocytosis in cultured endocrine cells. Proc Natl Acad Sci USA 2003;100(4):2070–2075.
41. Grosshans BL, Ortiz D, Novick P. Rabs and their effectors: achieving specificity in membrane traffic. Proc Natl Acad Sci USA 2006;103(32):11821–11827.
42. Stinchcombe JC, Barral DC, Mules EH, et al. Rab27a is required for regulated secretion in cytotoxic T lymphocytes. J Cell Biol 2001;152(4):825–834.
43. Haddad EK, Wu X, Hammer JA 3rd, Henkart PA. Defective granule exocytosis in Rab27a-deficient lymphocytes from Ashen mice. J Cell Biol 2001;152(4):835–842.
44. Tsuboi T, Fukuda M. Rab3A and Rab27A cooperatively regulate the docking step of dense-core vesicle exocytosis in PC12 cells. J Cell Sci 2006;119(pt 11):2196–2203.
45. Tolmachova T, Anders R, Stinchcombe J, et al. A general role for Rab27a in secretory cells. Mol Biol Cell 2004;15(1):332–344.
46. Fischer von Mollard G, Stahl B, Li C, Sudhof TC, Jahn R. Rab proteins in regulated exocytosis. Trends Biochem Sci 1994;19(4):164–168.
47. Geppert M, Bolshakov VY, Siegelbaum SA, et al. The role of Rab3A in neurotransmitter release. Nature 1994;369(6480):493–497.
48. Nonet ML, Staunton JE, Kilgard MP, et al. Caenorhabditis elegans rab-3 mutant synapses exhibit impaired function and are partially depleted of vesicles. J Neurosci 1997;17(21):8061–8073.
49. Itzen A, Rak A, Goody RS. Sec2 is a highly efficient exchange factor for the Rab protein Sec4. J Mol Biol 2007;365(5):1359–1367.
50. Novick P, Brennwald P, Walworth NC, et al. The cycle of SEC4 function in vesicular transport. Ciba Found Symp 1993;176:218–228; discussion 229–232.
51. Stroupe C, Collins KM, Fratti RA, Wickner W. Purification of active HOPS complex reveals its affinities for phosphoinositides and the SNARE Vam7p. EMBO J 2006;25(8):1579–1589.
52. Bugnicourt A, Froissard M, Sereti K, Ulrich HD, Haguenauer-Tsapis R, Galan JM. Antagonistic roles of ESCRT and Vps class C/HOPS complexes in the recycling of yeast membrane proteins. Mol Biol Cell 2004;15(9):4203–4214.

53. Allan BB, Moyer BD, Balch WE. Rab1 recruitment of p115 into a cis-SNARE complex: programming budding COPII vesicles for fusion. Science 2000;289(5478):444–448.
54. Christoforidis S, McBride HM, Burgoyne RD, Zerial M. The Rab5 effector EEA1 is a core component of endosome docking. Nature 1999;397(6720):621–625.
55. Simonsen A, Lippe R, Christoforidis S, et al. EEA1 links PI(3)K function to Rab5 regulation of endosome fusion. Nature 1998;394(6692):494–498.
56. Kasai K, Ohara-Imaizumi M, Takahashi N, et al. Rab27a mediates the tight docking of insulin granules onto the plasma membrane during glucose stimulation. J Clin Invest 2005;115 (2):388–396.
57. Fukuda M, Kanno E. Analysis of the role of Rab27 effector Slp4-a/granuphilin-a in dense-core vesicle exocytosis. Methods Enzymol 2005;403:445–457.
58. Fukuda M. Rab27 and its effectors in secretory granule exocytosis: a novel docking machinery composed of a Rab27.effector complex. Biochem Soc Trans 2006;34(pt 5):691–695.
59. Schluter OM, Schnell E, Verhage M, et al. Rabphilin knock-out mice reveal that rabphilin is not required for rab3 function in regulating neurotransmitter release. J Neurosci 1999;19(14): 5834–5846.
60. Staunton J, Ganetzky B, Nonet ML. Rabphilin potentiates soluble N-ethylmaleimide sensitive factor attachment protein receptor function independently of rab3. J Neurosci 2001;21(23):9255–9264.
61. Deak F, Shin OH, Tang J, et al. Rabphilin regulates SNARE-dependent re-priming of synaptic vesicles for fusion. EMBO J 2006;25(12):2856–2866.
62. Xu T, Binz T, Niemann H, Neher E. Multiple kinetic components of exocytosis distinguished by neurotoxin sensitivity. Nat Neurosci 1998;1(3):192–200.
63. Xu T, Rammner B, Margittai M, Artalejo AR, Neher E, Jahn R. Inhibition of SNARE complex assembly differentially affects kinetic components of exocytosis. Cell 1999;99(7): 713–722.
64. Sieburth D, Madison JM, Kaplan JM. PKC-1 regulates secretion of neuropeptides. Nat Neurosci 2007;10(1):49–57.
65. Wang Y, Okamoto M, Schmitz F, Hofmann K, Sudhof TC. Rim is a putative Rab3 effector in regulating synaptic-vesicle fusion. Nature 1997;388(6642):593–598.
66. Schoch S, Castillo PE, Jo T, et al. RIM1alpha forms a protein scaffold for regulating neurotransmitter release at the active zone. Nature 2002;415(6869):321–326.
67. Koushika SP, Richmond JE, Hadwiger G, Weimer RM, Jorgensen EM, Nonet ML. A post-docking role for active zone protein Rim. Nat Neurosci 2001;4(10):997–1005.
68. Dulubova I, Lou X, Lu J, et al. A Munc13/RIM/Rab3 tripartite complex: from priming to plasticity? EMBO J 2005;24(16):2839–2850.
69. Walent JH, Porter BW, Martin TF. A novel 145 kd brain cytosolic protein reconstitutes Ca(2+)-regulated secretion in permeable neuroendocrine cells. Cell 1992;70(5):765–775.
70. Berwin B, Floor E, Martin TF. CAPS (mammalian UNC-31) protein localizes to membranes involved in dense-core vesicle exocytosis. Neuron 1998;21(1):137–145.
71. Cai T, Fukushige T, Notkins AL, Krause M. Insulinoma-associated protein IA-2, a vesicle transmembrane protein, genetically interacts with UNC-31/CAPS and affects neurosecretion in Caenorhabditis elegans. J Neurosci 2004;24(12):3115–3124.
72. Speese S, Petrie M, Schuske K, et al. UNC-31 (CAPS) is required for dense-core vesicle but not synaptic vesicle exocytosis in Caenorhabditis elegans. J Neurosci 2007;27(23):6150–6162.
73. Zhou KM, Dong YM, Ge Q, Zhu D, et al. PKA activation bypasses the requirement for UNC-31 in the docking of dense core vesicles from C. elegans neurons. Neuron 2007;56(4):657–669.
74. Schneggenburger R, Neher E. Intracellular calcium dependence of transmitter release rates at a fast central synapse. Nature 2000;406(6798):889–893.
75. Sabatini BL, Regehr WG. Timing of neurotransmission at fast synapses in the mammalian brain. Nature 1996;384(6605):170–172.
76. Heidelberger R, Heinemann C, Neher E, Matthews G. Calcium dependence of the rate of exocytosis in a synaptic terminal. Nature 1994;371(6497):513–515.
77. Hsu SF, Jackson MB. Rapid exocytosis and endocytosis in nerve terminals of the rat posterior pituitary. J Physiol 1996;494 (pt 2):539–553.

78. Thomas P, Wong JG, Lee AK, Almers W. A low affinity Ca2+ receptor controls the final steps in peptide secretion from pituitary melanotrophs. Neuron 1993;11(1):93–104.

79. Chow RH, von Ruden L, Neher E. Delay in vesicle fusion revealed by electrochemical monitoring of single secretory events in adrenal chromaffin cells. Nature 1992;356(6364):60–63.

80. Voets T. Dissection of three Ca2+-dependent steps leading to secretion in chromaffin cells from mouse adrenal slices. Neuron 2000;28(2):537–545.

81. Beutner D, Voets T, Neher E, Moser T. Calcium dependence of exocytosis and endocytosis at the cochlear inner hair cell afferent synapse. Neuron 2001;29(3):681–690.

82. Yang H, Zhang C, Zheng H, et al. A simulation study on the Ca2+-independent but voltage-dependent exocytosis and endocytosis in dorsal root ganglion neurons. Eur Biophys J 2005;34(8):1007–1016.

83. Shin OH, Rizo J, Sudhof TC. Synaptotagmin function in dense core vesicle exocytosis studied in cracked PC12 cells. Nat Neurosci 2002;5(7):649–656.

84. Chapman ER. Synaptotagmin: a Ca(2+) sensor that triggers exocytosis? Nat Rev Mol Cell Biol 2002;3(7):498–508.

85. Sugita S, Shin OH, Han W, Lao Y, Sudhof TC. Synaptotagmins form a hierarchy of exocytotic Ca(2+) sensors with distinct Ca(2+) affinities. EMBO J 2002;21(3):270–280.

86. Lynch KL, Martin TF. Synaptotagmins I and IX function redundantly in regulated exocytosis but not endocytosis in PC12 cells. J Cell Sci 2007;120(pt 4):617–627.

87. Klyachko VA, Jackson MB. Capacitance steps and fusion pores of small and large-dense-core vesicles in nerve terminals. Nature 2002;418(6893):89–92.

88. Bruns D, Jahn R. Real-time measurement of transmitter release from single synaptic vesicles. Nature 1995;377(6544):62–65.

Index